ATLAS OF 3D ECHOCARDIOGRAPHY

ATLAS OF 3D ECHOCARDIOGRAPHY

Edward A. Gill MD, FAHA, FASE, FACP, FACC, FNLA

*Professor of Medicine, Department of Medicine, Division of Cardiology;
Adjunct Professor of Radiology, Director of Echocardiography,
Harborview Medical Center, University of Washington
Clinical Professor of Diagnostic Ultrasound, Seattle University,
Seattle, Washington*

ELSEVIER
SAUNDERS

1600 John F. Kennedy Blvd.
Ste 1800
Philadelphia, PA 19103-2899

ATLAS OF 3D ECHOCARDIOGRAPHY   ISBN: 978-1-4377-2699-2

Library of Congress Cataloging-in-Publication Data

Atlas of 3D Echocardiography / [edited by] Edward A. Gill.
    p. ; cm.
   3D echocardiography
   Includes bibliographical references and index.
   ISBN 978-1-4377-2699-2 (hardcover : alk. paper)
   I. Gill, Edward A.   II. Title: 3D echocardiography.
   [DNLM: 1. Echocardiography, Three-Dimensional—methods—Atlases.   2. Cardiovascular Diseases—ultrasonography—Atlases.   WG 17]
   616.1'207543—dc23

                   2012016293

Executive Content Strategist: Dolores Meloni
Content Development Specialist: Taylor Ball
Publishing Services Manager: Patricia Tannian
Project Manager: Carrie Stetz
Design Direction: Louis Forgione

Printed in China

Last digit is the print number: 9 8 7 6 5 4 3 2 1

DEDICATION

To my late friend James E. Weiel, PhD, who died suddenly and unexpectedly of cardiac causes during Thanksgiving week 2011, and whose unrelenting dedication to his two passions of science and photography was unequaled.

Preface

Three-dimensional (3D) echocardiography has arguably been the most significant development for echocardiography in the past two decades and has been very important for the development of cardiology in general. When I was a medical resident in the late 1980s, echocardiography inspired me to pursue a fellowship in cardiology. The reason was clear: no technology at that time allowed such complete evaluation of cardiac structure and function and displayed it in such an exquisite fashion. Fast forward to today, and this opinion hasn't changed; echocardiography never fails to advance its technology and organize it in such an eye-pleasing fashion. 3D echocardiography is the flagship example. When the first versions of 3D echocardiography began to enter the clinical cardiology market in the early 1990s, it was clear to me that I wanted this technology for our echocardiography laboratory. Since the early gated transthoracic 3D transesophageal echocardiography acquisition in 1995 and on to real-time transthoracic 3D in 2002 and real-time transesophageal 3D in 2007, I have been particularly privileged to help with the development and feedback of this technology and ultimately to institute it in everyday clinical use. *Atlas of 3D Echocardiography* is the culmination of years of work applying 3D technology to thousands of interesting clinical cases. I believe this atlas will enable readers to greatly enhance their understanding and appreciation of 3D echocardiography.

Edward A. Gill

Acknowledgments

I acknowledge the tireless efforts of the contributing authors who, by sharing their expertise and experience, have made this project complete. I also thank Carla Griswold, my administrative assistant, for her expertise and dedication with the preparation of all manuscripts, figures, references, and additional material. I thank all of the Harborview Medical Center cardiac sonographers for helping capture images for this book: Elenese Berther, Alicia Bourne, Rachel Karl, Denise McRee, Eric Sisk, and Terese Tognazzi-Evans. Special thanks to all the administrators at Harborview Medical Center who supported the development of three-dimensional echocardiography at our institution. Finally, but most importantly, I thank my parents, without whose support medical school would have been only a dream, let alone writing this book. Thanks also to my immediate family—my wife, Kathy, and our two sons, Matt and Marcus—for their unending love, support, and most of all, patience with this project.

Foreword

On October 29, 1953, Inge Edler, inspired by the use of radar technology in World War II, recorded the first "ultrasound cardiogram" and published his group's findings 1 year later. Since then, the technology of echocardiography has never failed to progress and excite. Just when echocardiography is deemed mature, a noteworthy breakthrough emerges. To say that real-time three-dimensional echocardiography (RT3DE) was such a breakthrough is, realistically, a major understatement. RT3DE, as it emerged in the transthoracic version in 2002, followed by the transesophageal version in 2007, is arguably the most important technologic breakthrough for cardiology to date in the twenty-first century. From a cultural standpoint, it is so timely that its development and introduction coincide with the beginning of Generation AO, the "always on" generation.

It was exceedingly important for echocardiography to develop a clinically useful 3D technique because other cardiac imaging modalities, notably cardiac magnetic resonance imaging and, to a greater extent, computed tomography, also have the ability to display information in three dimensions. However, the two unique aspects of RT3DE are the ability to display in real time and the clear superiority of valvular visualization, particularly mitral valve visualization by RT3D transesophageal echocardiography (TEE).

RT3DE is now a technology that is appreciated for its benefits worldwide. It has been interesting to see RT3DE flourish to a somewhat greater extent in Europe and Asia than in the United States, at least partly due to economic barriers for the institution of new imaging technology in the latter.

In this atlas, Dr. Gill and his coauthors have brought 3DE to life in a comprehensive publication that will serve as an indispensable learning tool for the novice as well as the expert in 3DE. Dr. Gill has covered everything from the technology and history of 3DE to the basic examination and its advanced uses, including the use of RT3DTEE in interventional procedures. Indeed, 3DE has evolved dramatically. It has gone from a novelty that produced intriguing and awe-inspiring pictures to a technology that is absolutely essential for some advanced interventional procedures, notably procedures that involve manipulation of the mitral valve—such as placing mitral clips and positioning vascular plugs to occlude periprosthetic regurgitation.

Bernhard Mumm
Roberto M. Lang, MD
September 2012

Contributors

Tara Bharucha, MB Bchir, MA (Cantab)
Congenital Cardiac Centre, University Hospital Southampton NHS Foundation Trust, Southampton, United Kingdom

Nicole M. Bhave, MD
Cardiovascular Imaging Fellow, Section of Cardiology, Noninvasive Cardiac Imaging Laboratories, University of Chicago Medical Center, Chicago, Illinois

Alicia A. Bourne, BS, RDCS
Harborview Medical Center Echocardiography Laboratory, University of Washington, Seattle, Washington

Jennifer L. Dorosz, MD
Assistant Professor of Medicine, Division of Cardiology, University of Colorado Denver, Aurora, Colorado

Renata G. Ferreira, MD
Assistant Professor of Anesthesiology, University of Washington Medical School, Staff Anesthesiologist, Department of Anesthesiology and Pain Medicine, University of Washington Medical Center, Seattle, Washington

Edward A. Gill, MD
Professor of Medicine, Department of Medicine, Division of Cardiology; Adjunct Professor of Radiology, Director of Echocardiography, Harborview Medical Center, University of Washington; Clinical Professor of Diagnostic Ultrasound, Seattle University, Seattle, Washington

Judy Hung, MD
Associate Director of Echocardiography, Department of Medicine, Division of Cardiology, Massachusetts General Hospital, Boston, Massachusetts

Carly Jenkins, PhD
Senior Research Fellow, Cardiac Imaging Group, University of Queensland, Queensland, Australia

Rachel Karl, RDCS
Harborview Medical Center Echocardiography Laboratory, University of Washington, Seattle, Washington

Cliona Kenny, MB
Cardiology SpR & Echocardiography Fellow, King's College Hospital, London, United Kingdom

Berthold Klas, BS
TomTec Corporation, Chicago, Ilinois

Roberto M. Lang, MD
Professor of Medicine, Past President, American Society of Echocardiography, Director, Noninvasive Cardiac Imaging Laboratories, University of Chicago Medical Center, Chicago, Illinois

G. Burkhard Mackensen, MD
Chief, Division of Cardiothoracic Anesthesiology, UW Medicine Research & Education Endowed Professor in Anesthesiology, Adjunct Professor of Medicine, Department of Anesthesiology & Pain Medicine, UW Medicine Regional Heart Center, University of Washington, Seattle, Washington

Gary S. Mak, MD
Echocardiography Fellow, Cardiac Ultrasound Laboratory, Massachusetts General Hospital, Harvard Medical School, Boston, Massachusetts

Denise McRee, RDCS
Harborview Medical Center Echocardiography Laboratory, University of Washington, Seattle, Washington

Luc Mertens, MD, PhD
Division of Cardiology, The Hospital for Sick Children, Toronto, Ontario, Canada

Mark J. Monaghan, PhD
Professor of Echocardiography, Director of Non-Invasive Cardiology, King's College Hospital, London, United Kingdom

Ernesto E. Salcedo, MD
Professor of Medicine, Division of Cardiology, University of Colorado Denver; Director of Echocardiography, University of Colorado Hospital, Aurora, Colorado

Ivan S. Salgo, MD
Chief, Cardiovascular Investigations, Research & Development, Ultrasound, Philips Healthcare, Andover, MA

Florence H. Sheehan, MD
Research Professor, Department of Medicine, Division of Cardiology, University of Washington, Seattle, Washington

Eric J. Sisk, BA, RDCS
Harborview Medical Center Echocardiography Laboratory, University of Washington, Seattle, Washington

Lissa Sugeng, MD, MPH
Associate Professor of Medicine, Section of Cardiovascular Medicine, Yale School of Medicine, New Haven, Connecticut

Terese Tognazzi-Evans, RDCS
Harborview Medical Center Echocardiography Laboratory, University of Washington, Seattle, Washington

Mary-Pierre Waiss, BS, RDCS
Vice President for Clinical Development, Ventripoint, Inc., Seattle, Washington

Lynn Weinert, BS, RDCS
Research Technician, University of Chicago Hospitals, Chicago, Illinois

Elisa Zaragosa-Macias, MD
Cardiovascular Disease Fellow, University of Washington, Seattle, Washington

Contents

To view corresponding videos, visit the *Atlas of 3D Echocardiography* collection online at expertconsult.com.

Historical Perspective on Three-Dimensional Echocardiography

Edward A. Gill and Berthold Klas

INTRODUCTION

Three-dimensional echocardiography (3DE) has been in existence since the 1970s, albeit with images that barely resembled a heart at that time. Throughout the 1970s and 1980s, 3DE was limited by computing power, both at the workstation and at the ultrasound level. In the 1990s, as both two-dimensional echocardiography (2DE) image quality and computing power dramatically improved, 3DE began to make strides as a possible clinical entity. During these early attempts at 3DE, it was never real time and was approached from the perspective of capturing multiple 2D images of the heart and either tracing a wire frame of the heart or melding the 2D images together using interpolation methods to create a 3D image. The first attempts at real-time 3DE were undertaken by von Ramm et al at Duke University in the 1990s. The major transition from research to clinical tool for 3DE happened in 2002 when the first reasonably user-friendly version of real-time 3DE (RT3DE) was introduced. This was also the first version of RT3DE to have diagnostic-quality 3DE images performed by an ultrasound system that was capable of both 2DE and 3DE.

EARLIEST APPROACHES

3DE had its beginnings in the 1970s with primitive equipment and equally primitive images. By the mid-1980s, there was early 3DE performed with standard B-mode ultrasound and tracking devices designed to locate the transducer in space. The initial approach to 3D echo was to obtain multiple 2D images and reconstruct them into a 3D image. This was accomplished by registering the 2D images such that it could be discerned how the individual images fit together to form the 3D image. Such registration of the images was achieved by tracking the transducer in space via mechanical, acoustic, electromagnetic, or optical detection apparatus. In the mechanical approach, the transducer had an actual mechanical arm attached to it and therefore dictated movement in space (**Figure 1-1**). Dekker and colleagues[1] are credited with this first iteration of 3DE using the mechanical arm approach in 1974. Next came an acoustic attempt at location, the "spark gap" technique by Moritz and Shreve[2] in 1976. In this technique, the transducer was located by sending pulsed acoustic signals from a device holding the transducer, called a spark gap to a Cartesian locator grid (**Figure 1-2**). This approach, in theory, allowed free-hand scanning—meaning that the transducer did not have to follow a predetermined pathway and, indeed, was the precursor to free-hand scanning using an electromagnetic locator. Both electrocardiography and respiratory gating were often used, or images were acquired with breath holding. Initially, only end-diastolic and end-systolic images of the left ventricle (LV) were obtained. Over time, complete cardiac cycles could be obtained.[3,4] Several groups published articles during this period using a variety of primitive transducer tracking systems and the resultant less than pleasing 3D imaging.[5-10]

In 1977, Raab and colleagues[11] developed the magnetic locator, which ultimately led to the most advanced type of free-hand scanning, but this method for transducer location never

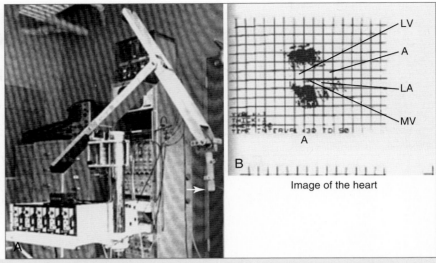

Figure 1-1 A, The mechanical arm used by Dekker and colleagues[1] for tracking the ultrasound transducer in space. Note the *arrow* depicting the actual ultrasound transducer. As might be imagined, this apparatus was not well received by sonographers because moving the transducer around was physically taxing, given the weight and awkwardness of the mechanical arm. **B,** Image of the heart. Note that the image shows only mild resemblance to the actual heart and heart chambers. A, aorta; LA, left atrium; LV, left ventricle; MV, mitral valve.

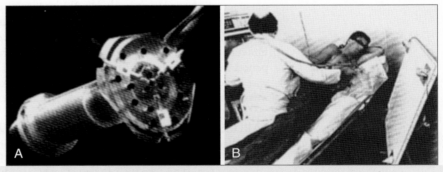

Figure 1-2   An acoustic "spark gap" apparatus used by Moritz and Shreve[2] for locating the transducer for three-dimensional echocardiography. **A,** Actual device housing the transducer, with the audio signal sent from the trifurcating mechanism. **B,** The device in practice, with the coordinates shown on the board to the right of the user.

caught on until the mid-1990s. This method is still used today by some labs, predominantly for research purposes (**Figure 1-3;** see also Figures 1-13, 1-14).

In between the spark gap and the free-hand magnetic approaches were myriad tactics that used the technique of transducer movement in a preprogrammed, stepwise fashion while attempting to keep the patient and the sonographer as stationary as possible. The mechanical devices then moved the transducer in a linear, fanlike, or rotational direction. An example of a fanlike acquisition is shown in **Figure 1-4.**

Fanlike Scanning

Fanlike scanning was, in theory, advantageous for evaluating the right ventricle (RV) compared with rotational or linear scanning, since the RV is not easily accessed from the apex and often is best imaged from the RV inflow tract using a more rightward direction of scanning from the standard parasternal view.[12]

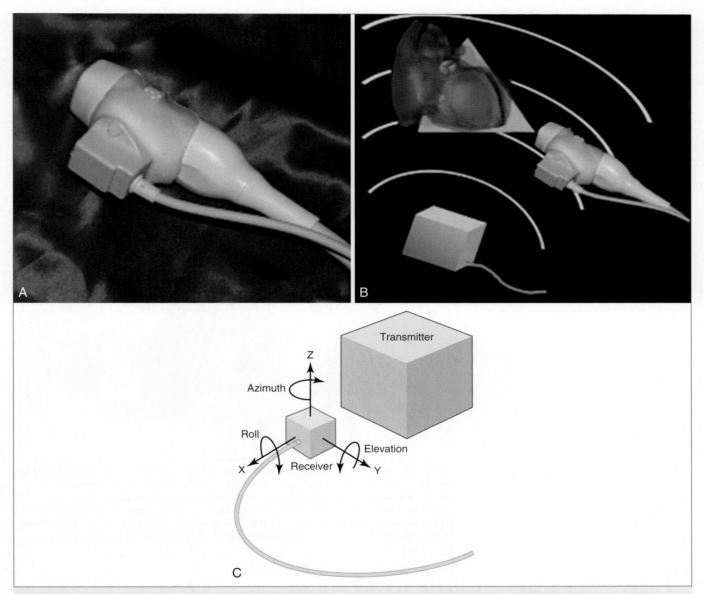

Figure 1-3   A, Electromagnetic locator device. The sensor is shown attached to a holder for the transducer. **B,** Summary of the electromagnetic sensor system. The magnet is located in the box, which serves as the transmitter. The magnet is connected to the sensor and indirectly to the ultrasound system. **C,** The location of the transducer is tracked by the electromagnetic sensor.

Rotational Scanning

The rotational approach used a cylinder-like mechanical apparatus that those in the industry at that time referred to as the "bazooka" (**Figure 1-5**). This device had a mechanical stepper motor that moved the transducer sequentially through a semicircular or 180-degree scan with stops every two to three degrees to acquire a 2D image. The acquisition of roughly 60 images was followed by computer software processing, initially using a polar coordinate approach to meld the images into a 3D image. The computer software used significant interpolation between images. The result was frequent "stitch" artifact caused by deficiencies in image line-up from patient movement, transducer movement outside the prespecified position, respiratory or cardiac gating artifact, or all of these factors. Although innovative and potentially very powerful for this era, clear limitations remained. Hence, clinical applicability was very limited.[13]

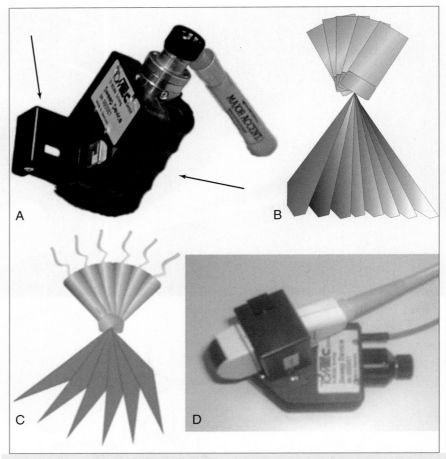

Figure 1-4 A, A fanlike device for three-dimensional acquisition. This device, made by TomTec, Inc., stepped the transducer through a fanlike motion. The transducer was held by the square apparatus (*arrows*), and the user held the device in a manner similar to a pistol grip. **B,** The stepwise approach to fanlike scanning. **C,** Ultrasound transducer being held by the fanlike mechanical device in the direction of acquisition. **D,** Mechanical fan device and transducer within. (**B,** Courtesy TomTec, Inc., Munich, Germany.)

Linear or Parallel Scanning

In linear scanning, the transducer was sequentially stepped along a line and obtained images every few millimeters, as opposed to degrees with the rotational and fanlike scans (**Figures 1-6** to **1-9**). Examples of linear scanning using an intravascular ultrasound, predominantly for coronary imaging, as well as a transthoracic echocardiography (TTE) device are shown in the figures. A device, known as "lobster tail," for linear pullback using transesophageal echocardiography (TEE) was available as well. In similar fashion as the previously described linear devices, the lobster tail operated by stepwise pullback of the TEE probe in the esophagus, with imaging at each stop. This TEE probe, developed by TomTec, Inc. (Munich, Germany), included both the TEE probe and the "stepper," that is, the device that moved the probe sequentially (see Figures 1-8 and 1-9). There were several iterations of this technique, including one that involved placing the TEE probe in a water bath within the esophagus to serve as a "standoff" to improve acoustic effects and sharpen the images (see Figure 1-8). The rotational method of scanning with the lobster tail is summarized in Figure 1-9. Further summaries regarding the various types of scanning, early fetal ultrasound, and early computer hardware are shown in **Figures 1-10** to **1-12**.

Text continued on page 11

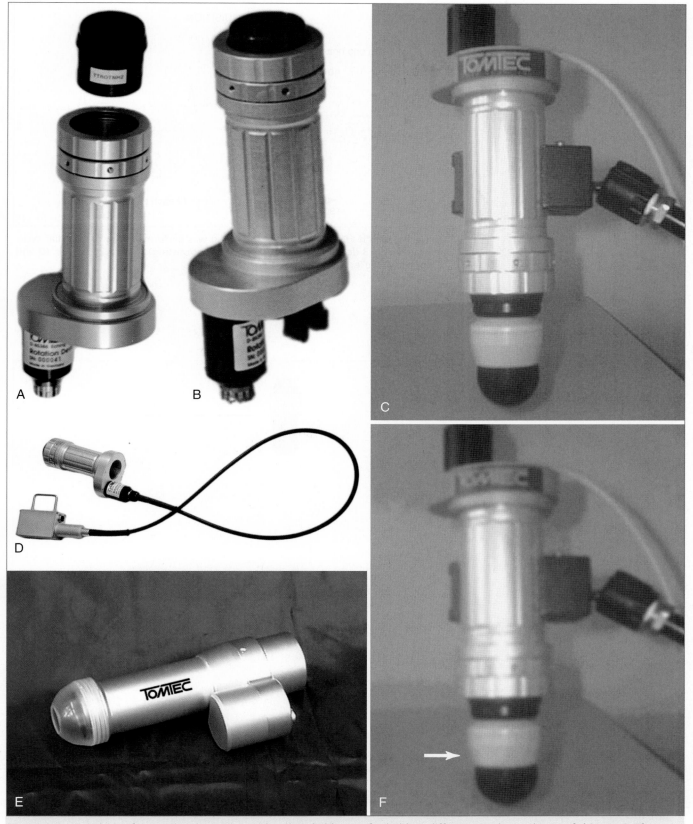

Figure 1-5 A, A device for rotational scanning with a detachable part for holding different-sized transducers of this era. **B,** The detachable transducer holder is back in place. **C,** A transducer (an older mechanical transducer) is shown held in place. **D,** The rotational device with the attached hardware for connecting to the computer that operated the motor on the rotation stepper. **E,** Another version of the rotation device produced by TomTec, Inc. **F,** Rotational scanner shown in close-up. The *arrow* shows the transducer.

Continued

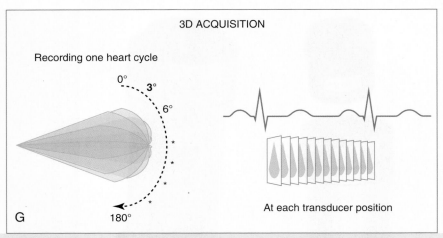

Figure 1-5, cont'd G, How rotational scanning was performed with one cardiac cycle obtained every 3 degrees and each cardiac cycle consisting of 15 to 20 frames. (**D** and **G,** Courtesy TomTec, Inc., Munich, Germany.)

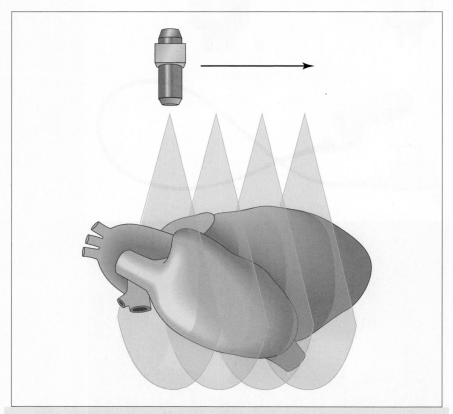

Figure 1-6 Parallel, or linear, scanning. In this schematic, the transducer is sequentially "stepped" through the heart following a linear motion.

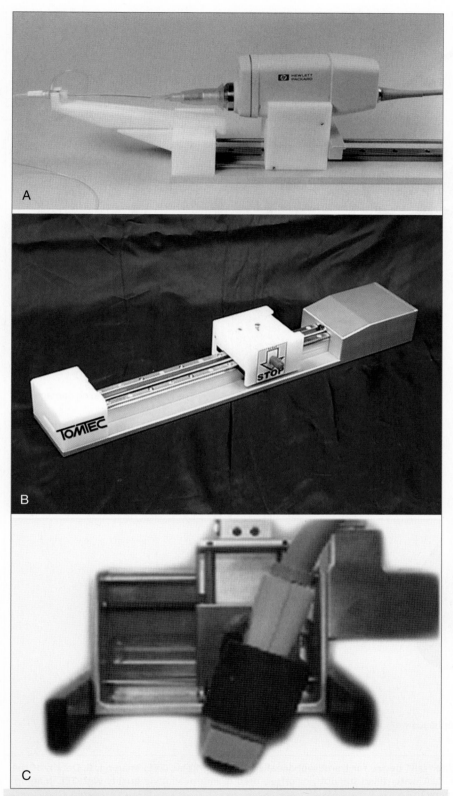

Figure 1-7   Parallel, or linear, scanning. In these iterations of three-dimensional scanning, the transducer was moved in a linear, stepwise fashion. **A** and **B,** The linear stepper device for use with an intravascular ultrasound device. **C,** A linear stepper for a transthoracic transducer. (Courtesy TomTec, Inc., Munich, Germany.)

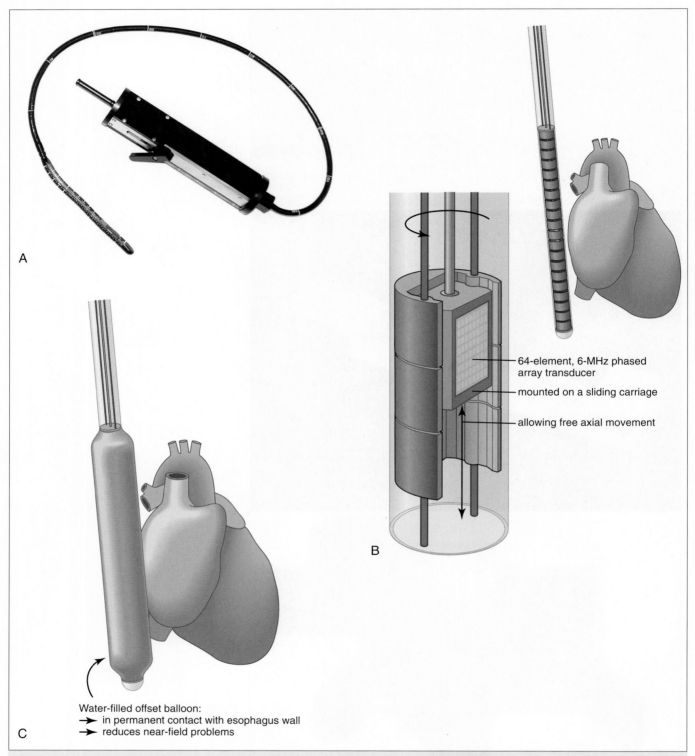

64-element, 6-MHz phased array transducer

mounted on a sliding carriage

allowing free axial movement

Water-filled offset balloon:
→ in permanent contact with esophagus wall
→ reduces near-field problems

Figure 1-8 **A,** Linear scanning using the "lobster tail" device for transesophageal echocardiographic (TEE) imaging. **B,** Details of the TEE probe and how it slides within a carriage. **C,** A water-filled standoff, or offset, used to improve image quality with TEE imaging. (**B** and **C,** Courtesy TomTec, Inc., Munich, Germany.)

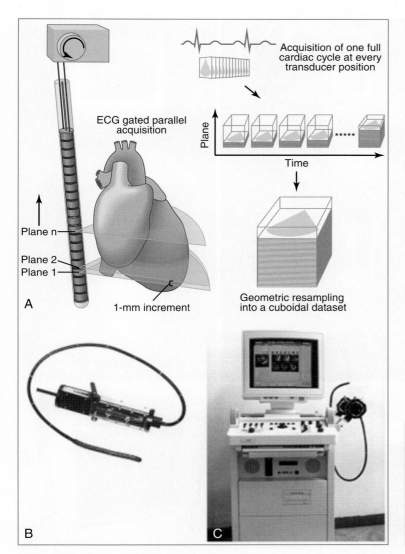

Figure 1-9 Summary of acquisition and processing of three-dimensional data using the linear approach with the "lobster tail" transesophageal echocardiography system. **A,** Acquisition hardware acquires one full cardiac cycle (14 to 20 frames) at every transducer position and then processes the information into a cube, or volume, of data. **B** and **C,** The hardware. (Courtesy TomTec, Inc., Munich, Germany.) ECG, electrocardiographic.

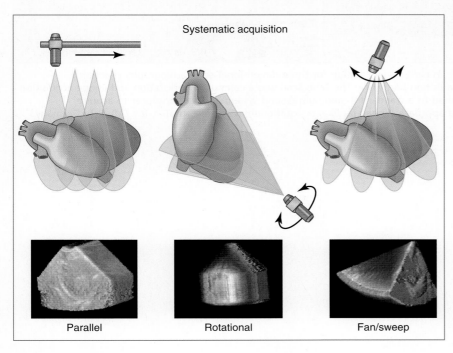

Figure 1-10 Summary of linear (parallel), rotational, and fanlike scanning. (Courtesy TomTec, Inc., Munich, Germany.)

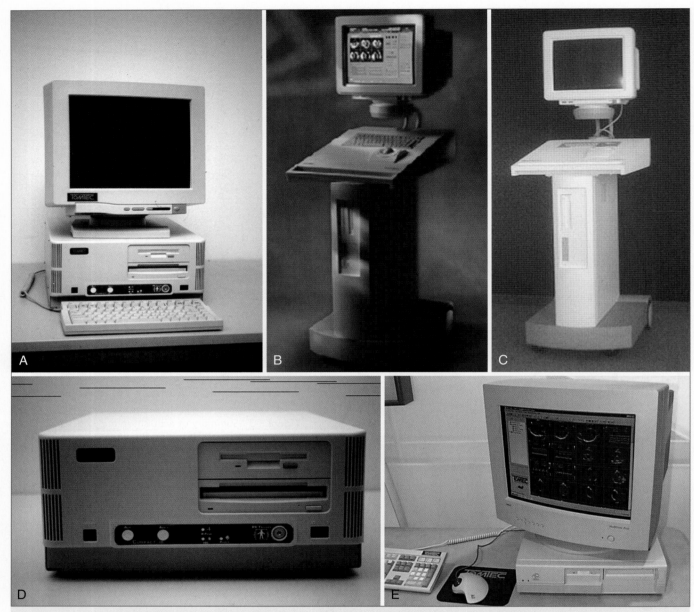

Figure 1-11 A and **D,** The Compact 3D Review, an early review station for three-dimensional echocardiography processing. **B, C,** and **E,** Early review stations and image acquisition hardware. The Echo-Scan was a computer workstation and image acquisition device combined. The Echo-Scan could be attached to a standard B-mode ultrasound system and its transducer to acquire two-dimensional images in the preprogrammed approach (linear, fanlike, or rotational). (Courtesy TomTec, Inc., Munich, Germany.)

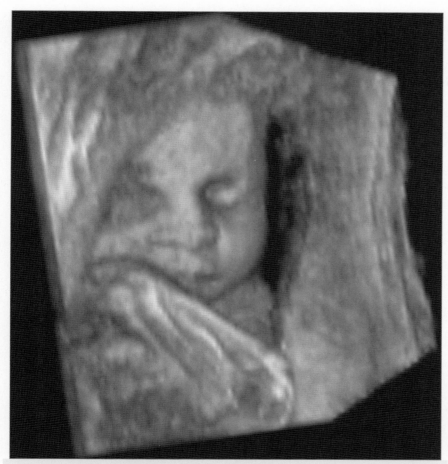

Figure 1-12   Early fetal images performed using standard B-mode ultrasound and the TomTec Echo-Scan system. (Courtesy TomTec, Inc., Munich, Germany.)

MORE ADVANCED FREE-HAND SCANNING

Later, using the technology developed by Raab, free-hand scanning became commercially available from TomTec and from 3D Echo Tech (Boulder, CO; later acquired by GE Medical systems). Both systems used an enhanced version of the electromagnetic detector described by Raab in 1977 (**Figures 1-13** and **1-14**; see also Figure 1-3). A magnet was enclosed in a plastic housing and placed close to the patient. The electromagnetic locator was electrically wired to a sensor that was placed on the ultrasound transducer and connected to a microcomputer and the commercially available ultrasound system. This enhanced version of the electromagnetic detector is still commercially available today through Ascension Technologies (Milton, VT). Before using this device for free-hand scanning, a calibration must be performed, typically using a phantom that had multiple wires passing through a water bath (see Figure 1-14). This process is tedious and time consuming and is a major reason for the lack of clinical acceptance. Currently, companies that use the electromagnetic sensor for free-hand scanning often hire out the calibration process so the user does not need to become involved in the process. An example of quantitative left ventricular imaging using the method the electromagnetic locator is provided by Legget et al.[14] As computing power improved in the late 1980s and early 1990s, the data processing algorithms for 2D images became advanced and allowed direct conversion of basic images from a polar coordinate system to the cartesian coordinate system. With the evolution of interpolation, gaps between images could be filled, and with the addition of

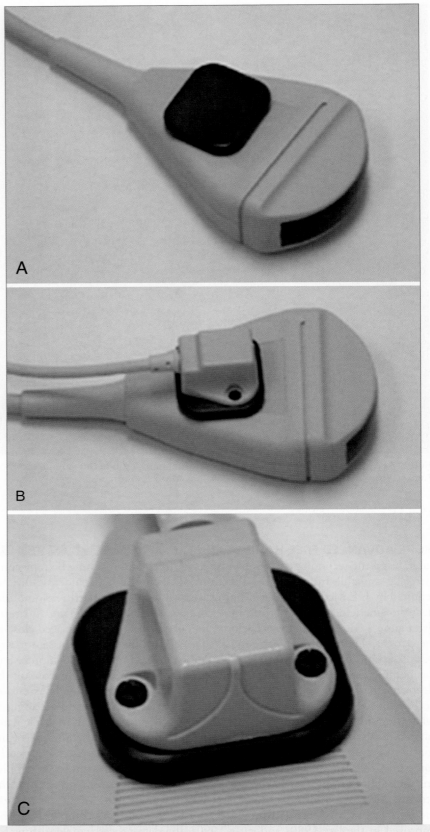

Figure 1-13 **A** to **C,** Electromagnetic sensor placed on a general ultrasound transducer. (Courtesy TomTec, Inc., Munich, Germany.)

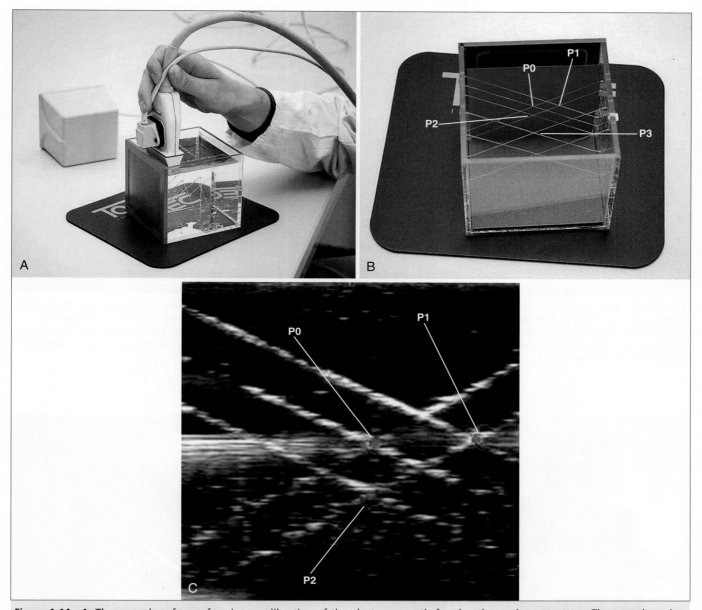

Figure 1-14   A, The procedure for performing a calibration of the electromagnetic free-hand scanning apparatus. The transducer is scanning in a water bath; the wires in the bath are set at a known distance and are used as calibration points. **B,** More details of the wires used for calibration. **C,** How the wires appear in ultrasound imaging. (**A** and **C,** Courtesy TomTec, Inc., Munich, Germany.)

smoothing algorithms, the images could be more systematically reconstructed to resemble an entire heart—or at least individual ventricles.

ON-BOARD ROTATIONAL 3D TRANSESOPHAGEAL AND TRANSTRACHEAL ECHOCARDIOGRPHY

In 1993, TomTec partnered with Hewlett-Packard (HP, Palo Alto, CA) to develop a rotation motor for the existing HP TEE multiple probe (Omniplane I) (**Figure 1-15**). This allowed rotational scanning using an already available TEE probe. In 1995, the partnership between TomTec and HP progressed even further and led to the development of software that was embedded in the HP 5500 Ultrasound system (**Figure 1-16**). The technique for this system is summarized in **Figure 1-17**. Examples of some of the images obtained with the rotational TEE approach are shown in **Figures 1-18** to **1-23**. In addition, HP developed a transthoracic

Text continued on page 18

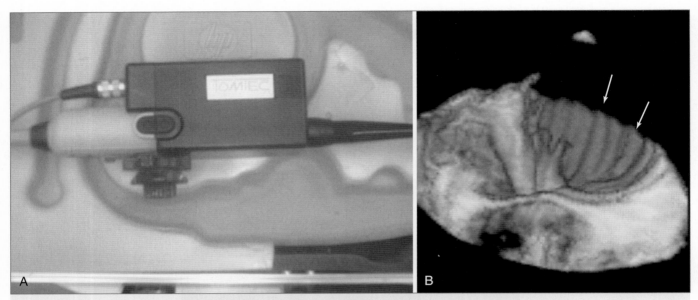

Figure 1-15 **A,** A standard transesophageal echocardiography (TEE) probe (Omniplane I, Hewlett-Packard, Palo Alto, CA) fitted with a stepper motor made by TomTec used to drive the Omniplane TEE through a rotation, with preprogrammed stops at every few angle advancements (typically 3 degrees). **B,** A grayscale image of a three-dimensional image acquired with the Omniplane TEE and the rotational stepper motor. Note the rotational artifacts (*arrows*) caused by interpolation of the two-dimensional images between angle stops. (Courtesy TomTec, Inc., Munich, Germany.)

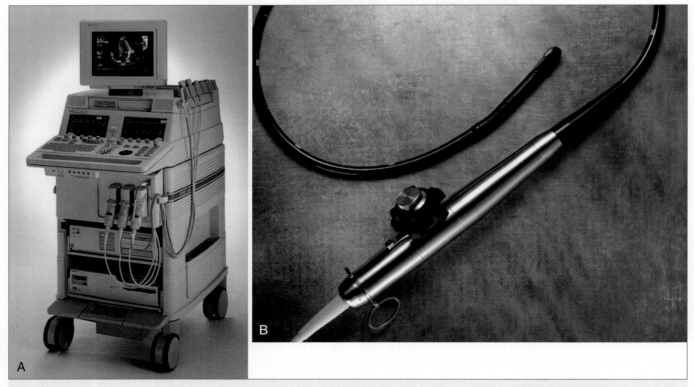

Figure 1-16 Later, Hewlett-Packard and TomTec, Inc. partnered to use a standard ultrasound system (the HP 5500, **A**) and standard transesophageal echocardiography (TEE) probe (the Omni II, **B**) and an onboard software program that achieved the same result as shown in Figure 1-15 without needing external hardware to drive the TEE probe. (Courtesy TomTec, Inc., Munich, Germany.)

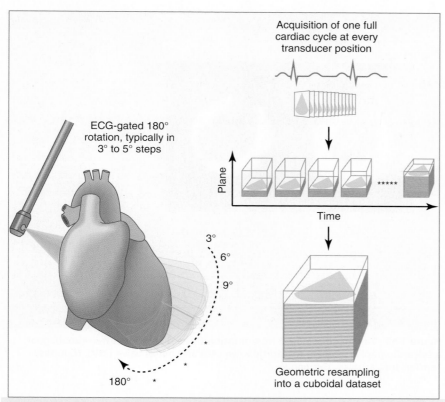

Figure 1-17 A summary of how rotational three-dimensional (3D) transesophageal echocardiography was performed. An electrocardiography (*ECG*)-gated 180-degree rotation was performed with stops every 3 degrees to acquire a two-dimensional (2D) image. The 2D images were collected and, using computer interpolation, contained into a volume of data that could then be rendered into 3D images and cut in multiple planes. (Courtesy TomTec, Inc., Munich, Germany.)

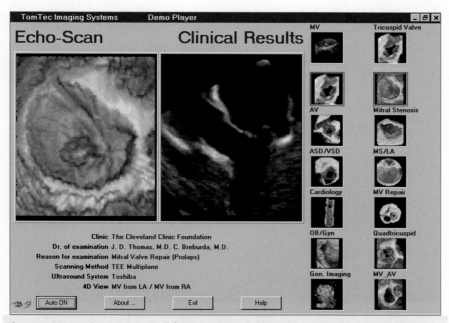

Figure 1-18 An image acquired from rotational three-dimensional transesophageal echocardiography showing mitral valve prolapse. (Courtesy TomTec, Inc., Munich, Germany.)

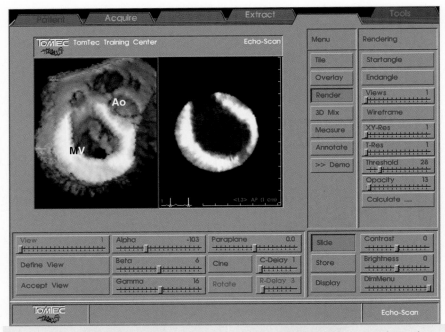

Figure 1-19 An image acquired from rotation three-dimensional transesophageal echocardiography showing the aortic valve (*Ao*) and mitral valve (*MV*). (Courtesy TomTec, Inc., Munich, Germany.)

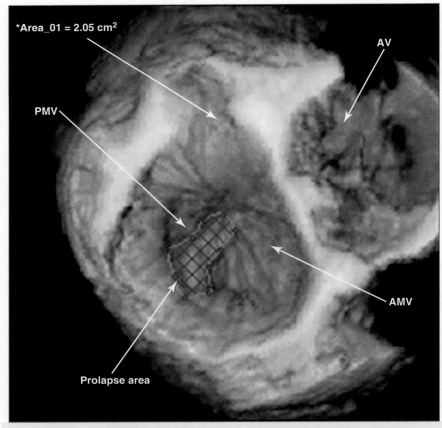

Figure 1-20 An image of mitral valve prolapse obtained using rotational three-dimensional transesophageal echocardiography imaging. AMV, anterior mitral valve; AV, aortic valve; PMV, posterior mitral valve. (Courtesy TomTec, Inc., Munich, Germany.)

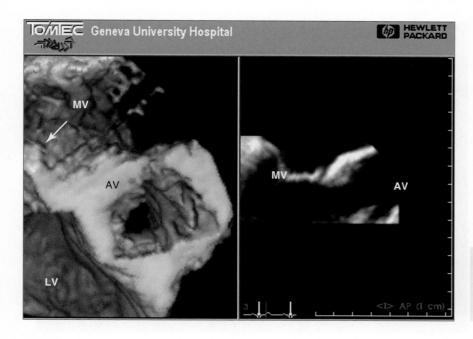

Figure 1-21 Rotational three-dimensional transesophageal echocardiography imaging showing the aortic valve (*AV*), left ventricle (*LV*), and mitral valve (*MV*). (Courtesy TomTec, Inc., Munich, Germany.)

VENTRICULAR MV/LVOT

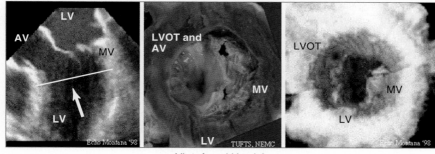

View from LV to LA

Figure 1-22 Mitral valve (*MV*) prolapse shown from the left ventricular side. The left image shows two-dimensional posterior MV prolapse. The center image shows MV prolapse in a pathologic specimen viewed from the left ventricular side. The right image shows the three-dimensional image of MV prolapse from the ventricular side as well as the left ventricular outflow tract (*LVOT*). AV, aortic valve; LV, left ventricle. (Courtesy TomTec, Inc., Munich, Germany.)

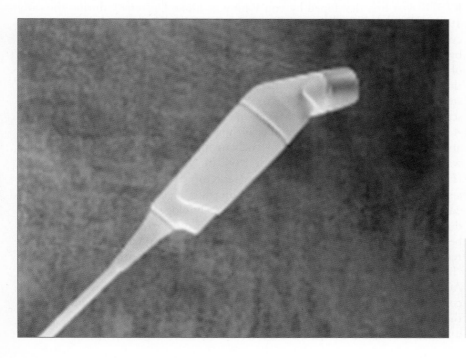

Figure 1-23 Rotational transthoracic transducer. A transducer developed by Hewlett Packard used software on board a standard ultrasound system (HP 5500) developed by TomTec, Inc., to rotate the transducer. (Courtesy Hewlett-Packard, Palo Alto, CA.)

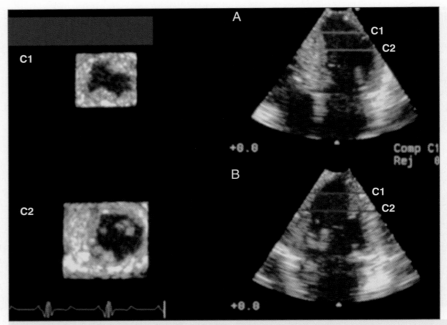

Figure 1-24 Images obtained using the Volumetrics three-dimensional system. The system was originally developed by Duke University and then commercialized by Volumetrics (Chapel Hill, NC). (Courtesy David Adams, Duke University, Durham, NC.)

transducer during the same period (see Figure 1-23). Although a transducer with the rotational mechanism contained within the ultrasound probe was much less cumbersome than holding a conventional probe within the rotational device (shown in Figure 1-5), the image quality was not found to be superior and this transducer was short lived. For the next 7 years or so, 3DE would mostly be performed with the rotational TEE approach. This approach occasionally was quite impressive in the evaluation of the mitral valve but did not offer much for evaluating LV function and size, particularly for quantification.[15,16]

REAL-TIME THREE-DIMENSIONAL METHODS

RT3DE was first developed by von Ramm at Duke University during the early 1990s.[17,18] With RT3DE, an entire cardiac volume was obtained in one cardiac cycle. Since only one cardiac cycle was used, there was no "stitch" artifact caused by interpolation between multiple 2D images. The good news was that a volume of data had been acquired. The bad news, however, was that the output was in the form of multiple cross-sectional views of the LV that had the look of parasternal short-axis views. This gave rise to the term *C scan* (**Figure 1-24**). Each C scan was a cross-sectional cut through the 3D dataset. Note that in Figure 1-24, *A* and *B*, the four- and two-chamber orthogonal views are shown, as well as C1 and C2, the sequential short-axis or axial cuts through the heart. This technology was made commercially available in 1997 by Volumetrics (Chapel Hill, NC) (**Figure 1-25**). However, the ultrasound system was very large and did not have a separate transducer for performing 2D imaging. Hence, only what was supposedly 3D imaging could be performed. This technology used a sparse-array transducer, as shown in **Figure 1-26**, with not all of the area of the transducer head being connected to individual elements. In addition, to derive true 3D volume rendering, an offline workstation had to be used. Hence, there were no truly "live" 3D echo images. Volumetrics did show RT3DE rendering at the 2000 American Heart Association meetings, but within months after this showing, the company ceased operations. Undoubtedly, this was a business decision based on the knowledge that a similar, yet much more advanced product was already well into the development stage at HP. The development stage for RT3DE began at

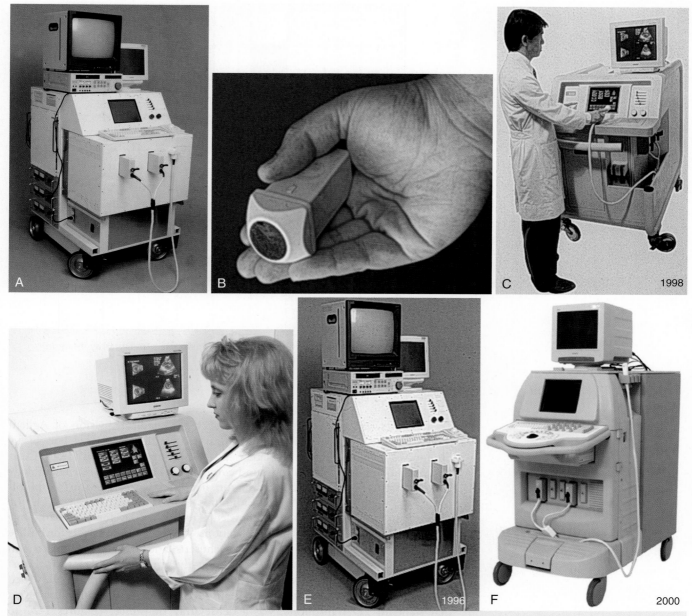

Figure 1-25 **A,** The Volumetrics (Chapel Hill, NC) prototype three-dimensional (3D) imaging system. This prototype developed by Duke University was very large and made exclusively for 3D imaging. It did not have transducers exclusive for two-dimensional imaging. As a result, it was largely purchased by organizations that wanted to perform research studies rather than for clinical use. **C,** This Model 1 instrument was the first production model by Volumetrics, Inc., circa 1998. **B** and **D-F,** The progression of Volumetrics 3D imaging from 1996 to 2000. The company folded shortly after the introduction of the model shown in **F.** (Courtesy David Adams, Duke University, Durham, NC.)

HP around 1996. As mentioned earlier, HP had already been a force in the industry when the company co-developed rotational 3D TEE scanning with TomTec and released that product to the general market in 1995. By late 1998, HP had a working prototype for transthoracic RT3DE; it was undoubtedly being tested at specialized 3D centers such as those at the thorax center in Rotterdam, The Netherlands; by Dr. Andreas Francke in Hannover, Germany; and at the University of Chicago echocardiography lab in the United States. HP began showing the prototypes to luminary customers by 1999. A major development in the history of RT3DE came in 1999 when HP spun off its medical division and other computer technology divisions into an entity called Agilent

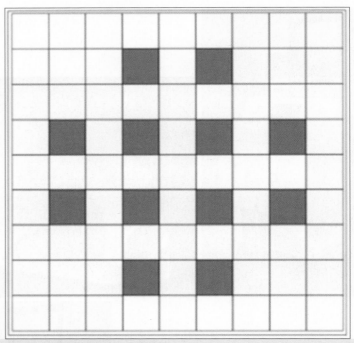

Figure 1-26 The Volumetrics (Chapel Hill, NC) system used sparse-array imaging, which limited image resolution.

Technologies (Andover, MA). The next year, the medical division of Agilent (excluding the measurement and chemical testing divisions) was bought by Philips Medical Systems of The Netherlands, now known as Philips Health Care. Philips had bought another ultrasound company in 1998, Advanced Technology Laboratories (ATL) of Bothell, Washington, in 1998. Hence, after the HP spinoff to Agilent, the purchase of Agilent by Philips and the already existing ATL, the plan was to merge the ultrasound knowledge to further develop 3D technology as well as other echocardiography applications. The U.S. headquarters for Philips Health was established in Andover, Massachusetts, and the sales headquarters in Bothell, Washington. Thereafter, in 2002, at the time of the American Heart Association meetings, Philips released the first generation of its RT3DE, which used a transthoracic transducer. This transducer, which was significantly larger that standard 2D transducers, was a dense-array transducer (**Figures 1-27** to **1-29**) and had more than 3000 elements, as opposed to the 256 in the sparse-array unit.

Two years later, at the 2004 American Heart Association meetings, General Electric Health Care (Chalfont St. Giles, United Kingdom) would follow suit with its versions of RT3DE. Similarly, Toshiba introduced RT3DE at the 2007 American College of Cardiology Annual Scientific Sessions in New Orleans, Louisiana. Siemens (Erlangen, Germany) and the U.S. ultrasound group in Issaquah, Washington, would introduce their transthoracic RT3DE system in late 2008. All these RT3DE systems use a transthoracic transducer as well as a matrix-type, dense-array transducer. Because of this approach, the transducer in these products is considerably larger than that used in 2D imaging.

In 2004 and in 2006, Philips Medical Systems released significant upgrades to the 3D systems with the introduction of the ie33 imaging system; General Electric also made major upgrades in 2008 and in 2010, with the introduction of the i9 imaging system.

The greatest impact on patient care with regard to 3D and RT3DE happened when Philips introduced the RT3DTEE probe in 2007 at the American Heart

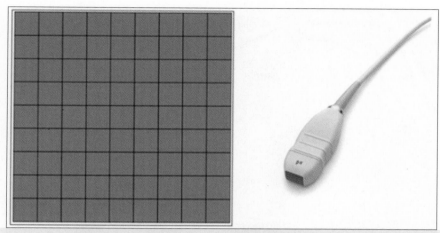

Figure 1-27   Dense-array imaging. Real-time three-dimensional imaging, first introduced in 2002 by Philips Medical Systems (now Philips Health Care, Andover, MA) used dense-array imaging.

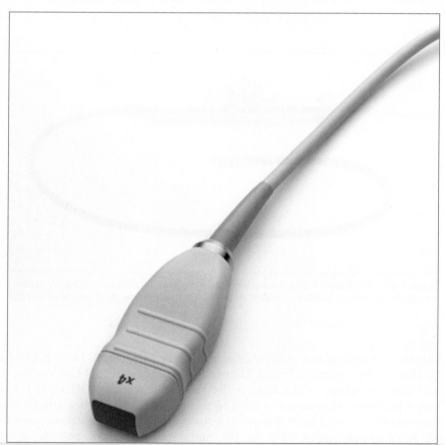

Figure 1-28   The matrix transducer used for dense-array imaging by Philips Medical Systems (now Philips Health Care, Andover, MA).

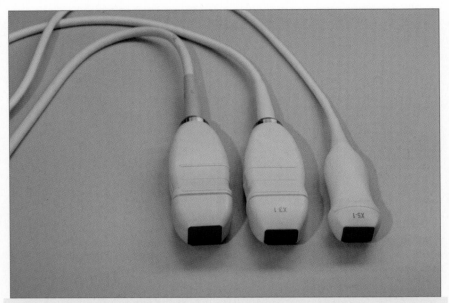

Figure 1-29   The first-generation Matrix (Philips Health Care, Andover, MA) transducer (*left*), second-generation Matrix transducer (*middle*), and third-generation Matrix transducer, with the latter similar to the standard two-dimensional transducer.

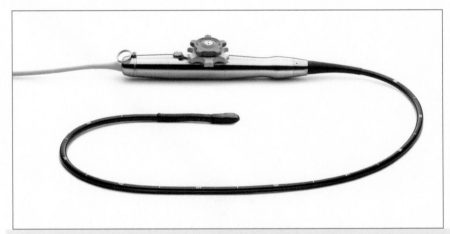

Figure 1-30   The Matrix three-dimensional transesophageal echocardiography probe introduced by Philips Medical Systems (now Philips Health Care, Andover, MA) in 2007.

Association meetings and earlier that year in Europe (**Figures 1-30** to **1-34**). At the time of this writing, General Electric is releasing an RT3DTEE system, 5 years after the release of the first one by Philips Health Care. RT3DTEE has been a particular advance with regard to patient treatment, particularly for the treatment of structural heart disease in the interventional lab. Treatments involving percutaneous intervention on the mitral valve are now possible using RT3DTEE guidance. The use of RT3DTEE in the interventional lab is outlined in Chapter 15.

Finally, in 2010, Philips Health Care introduced a TTE transducer for both RT2D and RT3DE imaging (**Figure 1-35**). The X5 transducer is the world's first miniaturized matrix-type transducer that allows the user to perform both 2D and 3D echocardiographic imaging without switching transducers, with comparable 2D and 3D image quality.

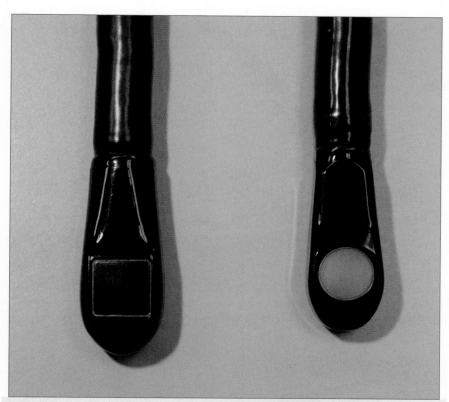

Figure 1-31   The Matrix transesophageal echocardiography (TEE) probe (*left*) and the standard Omni III two-dimensional (2D) TEE probe (*right*) (both Philips Health Care, Andover, MA). Note that control of the Matrix TEE probe is entirely electronic, as opposed to mechanical in the previous 2D echocardiography probe.

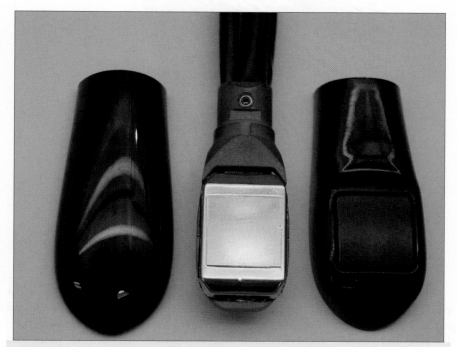

Figure 1-32   The Matrix transesophageal echocardiography transducer shown with the external covering front and back (at *left* and *right*) and the internal electronic mechanics (*center*).

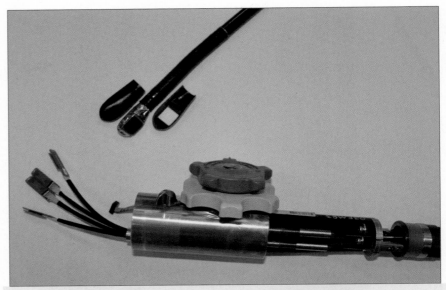

Figure 1-33 Steering mechanism for the Matrix three-dimensional transesophageal echocardiography probe (Philips Health Care, Andover, MA).

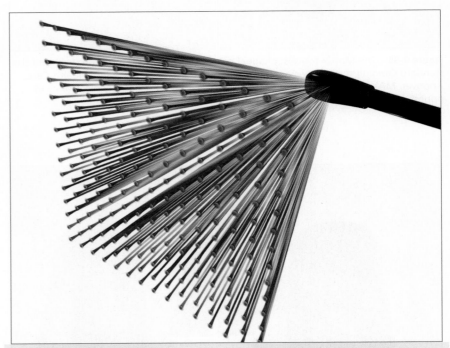

Figure 1-34 Schematic of how the Matrix three-dimensional transesophageal echocardiography probe (Philips Health Care, Andover, MA) sends out parallel scan lines on the lateral and elevation plane, creating a volume or, more properly, a frustum, of imaging data.

The development of RT3DE in 2002 by Philips Health Care was a step that made the greatest impact toward 3DE being used on a regular basis by clinical cardiologists and not merely in the research arena. With its 2002 introduction, RT3DE has become more commonplace throughout the United States and worldwide. In fact, 3D technology has proliferated more widely and quickly into Europe and Asia than in United States. Further proliferation continues on a near exponential curve as the technology continues to improve, becomes more

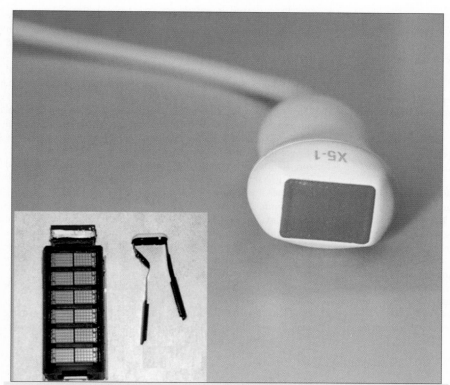

Figure 1-35   The X5 transducer, the third-generation and latest Matrix transthoracic three-dimensional transducer for transthoracic imaging (Philips Health Care, Andover, MA). It is similar in size and shape to the same-level two-dimensional transducer, the S5.

miniaturized, and develops more user-friendly interfaces with clearer integration into clinical practice without affecting the general workflow. This fact is discussed in more detail in Chapter 3.

In January 2006, two new 3D ultrasound billing codes were introduced: (1) RT3DE acquisition and analysis, and (2) offline analysis using a separate workstation. How this coding evolves over time will also have an impact on the clinical practice of echocardiography in the years to come.

Since the initial release of RT3DE by Philips in 2002, the volume of data generated from research in the field is enormous, with more than 3000 articles on 3DE cited on Medline during this period. A position paper and summary paper were published by the American Society of Echocardiography in 2007 to guide clinicians in the use of 3DE.[19,20] The European Society of Cardiology has provided a website called 3D Echo Box to guide clinicians through all the articles that describe the use of 3D echocardiography (http://www.escardio.org/communities/EAE/3d-echo-box/Pages/welcome.aspx). The most recent guidelines were published in the January 2012 issue of the *Journal of the American Society of Echocardiography*.[21]

References

1. Dekker DL, Piziali RL, Dong B Jr: A system for ultrasonically imaging the human heart in three dimensions. *Compt Biomed Res* 7:544–553, 1974.
2. Mortiz WE, Shreve PL: A microprocessor-based spatial locating system for use with diagnostic ultrasound IEEE. *Trans Biomed Eng* 64:966–974, 1976.
3. King DL, King DL Jr, Shao MYC: Three-dimensional spatial registration and interactive display of position and orientation of real-time ultrasound images. *J Ultrasound Med* 9:525–532, 1990.
4. Gopal AS, King DL, Katz J, et al: Three-dimensional echocardiographic volume computation by polyhedral surface reconstruction: In vitro validation and comparison to magnetic resonance imaging. *J Am Soc Echocardiogr* 5:115–124, 1992.
5. Geiser EA, Lypkiewics SM, Christi LG, et al: A framework for three-dimensional time varying reconstruction of the human left ventricle: Sources of error and estimation of their magnitude. *Compt Biomed Res* 13:225–241, 1980.
6. Matsumoto M, Matsuo H, Kitabatake A, et al: Three-dimensional echocardiograms and two-dimensional echocardiographic images at

desired planes by a computerized system. *Ultrasound Med Biol* 3:163–178, 1977.

7. Pearlman AS, Mortiz WE, Medema DK, et al: Three-dimensional reconstruction of the formalin-fixed ventricle using nonparallel two-dimensional ultrasonic scans. *Circulation* 64(Suppl IV):65, 1981.

8. Ghosh A, Nanda NC, Maurer G: Three-dimensional reconstruction of echocardiographic images using the rotation method. *Ultrasound Med Biol* 8:655–661, 1982.

9. Maurer G, Nanda NC: Two dimensional echocardiographic evaluation of exercise-induced left and right ventricular asynergy: Correlation with thallium scanning. *Am J Cardiol* 48:720–727, 1981.

10. Linker DT, Mortiz WE, Pearlman AS: A new three-dimensional echocardiographic method of right ventricular volume measurement: In vitro validation. *J Am Coll Cardiol* 8:101–106, 1986.

11. Raab FH, Blood EB, Steiner TO, et al: Magnetic position and orientation tracking system. *IEEE Trans Aerosp Electron Syst* AES-15:709–718, 1979.

12. Delabays A, Pandian NG, Cao QL, et al: Transthoracic real-time three-dimensional echocardiography using a fan-like scanning approach for data acquisition: Methods, strengths, problems, and initial clinical experience. *Echocardiography* 12:49–59, 1995.

13. Salustri A, Roelandt JR: Ultrasonic three-dimensional reconstruction of the heart. *Ultrasound Med Biol* 21:281–293, 1995.

14. Legget ME, Leotta DF, Bolson EL, et al: System for quantitative three-dimensional echocardiography of the left ventricle based on a magnetic-field position and orientation sensing system. *IEEE Trans Biomed Engineer* 45:494–504, 1998.

15. Nanda N, Pinheiro L, Sanyal R, et al: Multiplane transesophageal echocardiographic imaging and three-dimensional reconstruction. *Echocardiography* 9:667–676, 1992.

16. Chen Q, Nosir YF, Vletter WB, et al: Accurate assessment of mitral valve area in patients with mitral stenosis by three-dimensional echocardiography. *J Am Soc Echocardiogr (Official publication of the American Society of Echocardiography)* 10:133–140, 1997.

17. von Ramm OT, Smith SW: Real time volumetric ultrasound imaging system. *J Digit Imag (Official journal of the Society for Computer Applications in Radiology)* 3:261–266, 1990.

18. von Ramm OT, Smith SW, Pavy HR: High-speed ultrasound volumetric imaging system. II. Parallel processing and image display. *IEEE Transac Ultrason Ferroelectr Freq Control* 38:109–115, 1991.

19. Hung Lang R, Flachskampf F, Shernan SK, et al: 3D echocardiography: A review of the current status and future directions. *J Am Soc Echocardiogr* 20:213–233, 2007.

20. Picard M: The time for 3D. *J Am Soc Echocardiogr* 20:A22–A23, 2007.

21. Lang RM, Badano LP, Tsang W, et al: Recommendations for image acquisition and display using three-dimensional echocardiography. *J Am Soc Echocardiogr* 25:3–46, 2012.

Integration of Three-Dimensional Echocardiography in Routine Clinical Practice

Lynn Weinert, Lissa Sugeng, and Edward A. Gill

INTRODUCTION

Two-dimensional echocardiography (2DE) has been one of the most established and ubiquitous diagnostic tools in cardiology over the past several decades. Echocardiography has come a long way from the early years of A and M modalities. Although transthoracic and transesophageal real-time three-dimensional echocardiography (RT3DE) is a significant advancement in technology, its values and limitations must be understood before using it on a daily basis.

Many advantages to using RT3DE have been shown by a large body of literature within the past 20 years. RT3DE accurately renders volumes that are more comparable with those of magnetic resonance imaging[1] because of its ability to obtain nonforeshortened images and semiautomated border detection unconstrained by geometry.[2] RT3DE is more accurate than 2DE for analysis of mitral stenosis, particularly the valve area determined by planimetry.[3]

RT3DE is more accurate because of its ability to visualize the very tips of the mitral leaflets and to document in an orthogonal plane when the measurement is being taken at that point. This ability to crop through a volume dataset, using the optimal cut plane, allows the precise assessment of pathology, such as mitral stenosis.

This chapter discusses ways to incorporate this technology into routine transthoracic echocardiography studies and help promote the promise that RT3DE imaging will someday be the "norm" in every echocardiography lab, not the exception.

THREE-DIMENSIONAL METHODOLOGY

In previous years, 3D methodology required data acquisition, offline image processing, reconstruction, display, and analysis. Currently, much of the image processing is performed online within the transducer; hence, the steps to achieve a 3D image necessitate data acquisition, image display, and analysis.

Data Acquisition

Several parameters must be considered before data acquisition:

1. Mode of acquisition
2. Acquisition beats
3. Volumetric size

There are three modes of data acquisition: (1) narrow-angled acquisition, (2) zoom acquisition, and (3) wide-angled acquisition. The choice of *acquisition mode* depends on the structure of interest. If the patient has mitral stenosis, a zoom acquisition is best to focus mainly on the mitral valve and reduce the chances of stitch artifacts and a higher frame rate. If left ventricular or right ventricular function were the object of interest, then a wide-angled acquisition would be preferable so that the entire ventricle could be acquired.

Acquisition beats pertain to the number of beats required to build a larger volume. Most systems allow a one-beat acquisition, for instance, of the left ventricle but also have the option of a lower frame rate with higher spatial resolution or a higher frame rate with lower spatial resolution. The most ideal acquisition is a one-beat acquisition with high frame rate and high spatial resolution. However, the physics of ultrasound does not allow this, so there is a tradeoff. The acquisition of valve pathology is best performed by using a one-beat acquisition since it avoids stitch artifacts. However, with a lower frame rate, fine structures may not be optimally visualized.

Image Display and Analysis

There are several methods of image display:

1. Volume-rendered imaging
2. Wire-frame image
3. Surface-rendered image
4. 2D slice planes

Most systems now acquire data and immediately display images on the ultrasound system without any delay in processing. A volume-rendered image is preferable for visualizing all anatomic structures. Endocardial tracing of a ventricle or chamber results in a wire-frame image, which then can be displayed as a surface-rendered image when a surface is placed over the wire-frame rendition of the structure. A 3D volume can also be displayed as 2D slices to demonstrate ventricular wall motion or measure an orifice such as atrial septal defect (ASD), ventricular septal defect (VSD), or the mitral valve area.

There are many approaches to RT3DE image display. However, after acquiring the data, the cut plane should be displayed so that it can be easily interrupted by the reader or others who are not familiar with RT3DE.

Transducer Technology

Several ultrasound vendors offer products with 3D imaging capabilities incorporated into a 2D imaging probe or an independent 3D imaging probe. With advanced electronics, significant miniaturization has resulted in a fully sampled 3D transesophageal echocardiography probe. Obviously, having one integrated 2D-3D transducer is key, particularly when trying to promote an imaging protocol with 3D imaging. However, in systems with separate 2D and 3D transducers, 3D imaging could be performed after the 2D standard protocol is obtained or even prior to the 2D exam (see Chapter 3). Essentially, the balance of spatial resolution and frame rate is more evident in 3DE compared with 2DE.

THREE-DIMENSIONAL IMAGING
Mitral and Aortic Valves

The parasternal long-axis or sagittal view usually is the starting point in most 2DE studies. After obtaining the 2D image, an RT3DE image can be obtained in the same view (**Figure 2-1**). Typically, adjustments of gain, time-gain compensation, and compression are used to optimize this image. This image can be acquired or used to prepare for zoom imaging of the mitral or aortic valve.

Zoom imaging of the mitral valve is shown in a multiplanar view in **Figure 2-2**. The RT3DE zoomed view of the mitral valve is displayed from the left atrial and left ventricular views. These views are acquired from one dataset and can be stored for later processing (**Figure 2-3**). In general, valve structures are shown as if visualized from a surgical perspective and also from a ventricular perspective. In the case of mitral stenosis and mitral valve prolapse, RT3DE imaging provides unique views of this pathology and enables the estimation of the mitral valve area (**Figures 2-4 to 2-6**).

The same imaging mode can be performed on the aortic valve. **Figure 2-7** zooms in on the aortic valve from the parasternal window. A multiplanar display

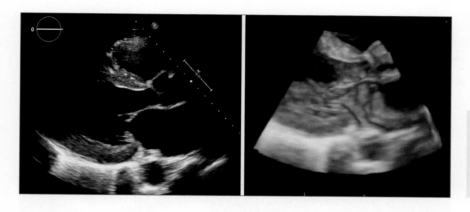

Figure 2-1   Two-dimensional and three-dimensional (3D) parasternal long-axis views, the standard starting point for 3D imaging in the lab. After acquiring this image, the next step is to prepare for zoom imaging of the mitral or aortic valve.

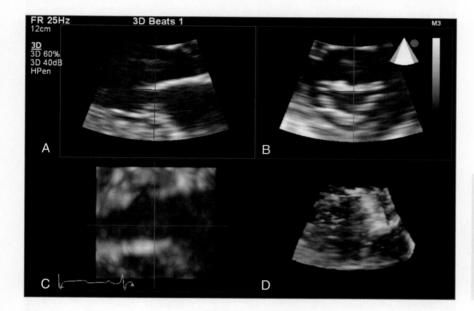

Figure 2-2   Zoom mitral valve view. From this parasternal long-axis view, a region of interest is placed over the mitral valve and aortic leaflets. The multiplanar display demonstrates a long-axis (**A**), short-axis view of the mitral valve (**B**), an orthogonal view of the parasternal long axis (**C**), and volume-rendered image of the valve from a left atrial perspective (**D**).

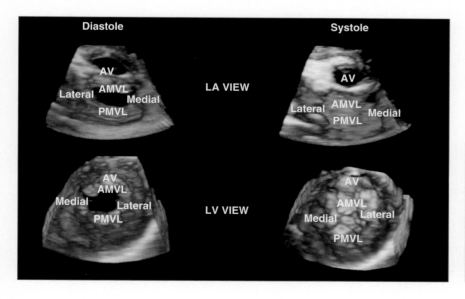

Figure 2-3   From this one real-time three-dimensional echocardiography zoomed dataset of the mitral valve, the valve can be displayed from the left atrial (*LA*) view in end diastole (*upper left*) and end systole (*upper right*) and the left ventricular (*LV*) view in end diastole (*lower left*), and end systole (*lower right*). AMVL, anterior mitral valve leaflet; AV, aortic valve; PMVL, posterior mitral valve leaflet.

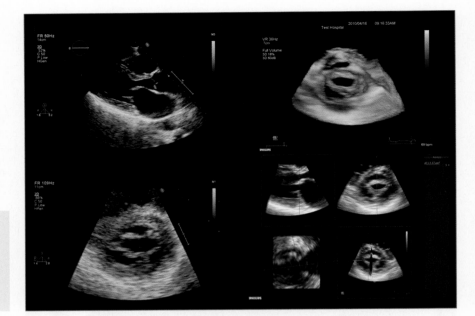

Figure 2-4 Mitral stenosis. The pathology in the mitral valve area is more accurately calculated by using three-dimensional echocardiography (*bottom right*). From the two-dimensional parasternal long axis (*left panels*), a zoomed volume of the mitral valve is captured (*upper right*).

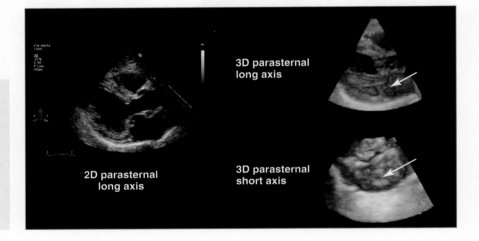

Figure 2-5 Two-dimensional (*2D*) parasternal long-axis view shows mitral valve prolapse. Three-dimensional (*3D*) echocardiography images from the parasternal long axis (*upper right*) indicate that the prolapse most likely involves the posterior leaflet. A zoom image on the mitral valve turns the dataset to view the leaflets from the left atrium (*lower right*). This image shows that the prolapse primarily involves the P2 segment.

Figure 2-6 Left atrial view of mitral valve prolapse (*MVP*). These zoomed images were acquired from the apical views. On the left is a patient with posterior MVP (*arrows*) involving most of the posterior segments. On the right is a patient with a flail P3 segment (*arrow*).

of the aortic zoomed dataset demonstrates the parasternal long-axis view (Figure 2-7, *upper left*), short-axis view (Figure 2-7, *upper right*), transverse cut (Figure 2-7, *lower left*), and the RT3DE volume-rendered image (Figure 2-7, *lower right*), which is cut to display the aortic valve from the aortic side. The aortic valve is displayed from the aortic and left ventricular perspectives (**Figure 2-8**). Similar views of the aortic and mitral valves may be obtained from an apical window (**Figure 2-9**).

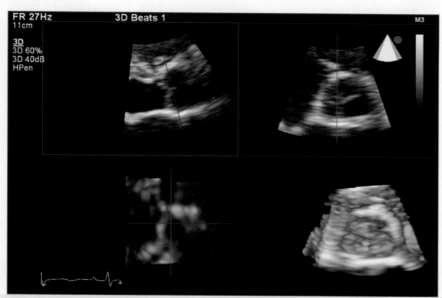

Figure 2-7   A zoomed aortic valve is shown from the parasternal long-axis view (*upper left*), short-axis view (*upper right*), transverse-cut view (*lower left*), and the real-time three-dimensional echocardiography volume dataset (*lower right*), which is cut to display the aortic valve from the aortic side.

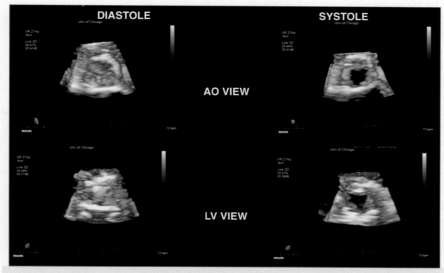

Figure 2-8   Images of a normal zoomed aortic valve seen in both diastole (*left panels*) and systole (*right panels*) as viewed from the aortic side (*AO, upper panels*) and from the left ventricular side (*LV, lower panels*).

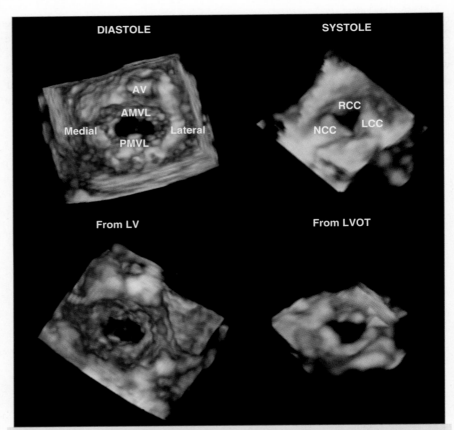

Figure 2-9 Both the aortic valve (*AV*) and the mitral valve can be assessed from the apical views. Examples of a zoomed mitral valve (*left*) and a zoomed aortic valve (*right*) are shown. AMVL, anterior mitral valve leaflet; LCC, left coronary cusp; LV, left ventricle; LVOT, left ventricular outflow tract; NCC, noncoronary cusp; PMVL, posterior mitral valve leaflet; RCC, right coronary cusp.

Tricuspid Valve

The tricuspid valve can be viewed either from the parasternal long-axis and short-axis views or from the apical view. Capturing the valve from the apical view makes it easier to ensure complete inclusion of the valve. In **Figure 2-10**, a zoomed image of the tricuspid valve from a parasternal window is shown in a multiplanar display. The tricuspid valve is then displayed from the right atrial and right ventricular views (**Figures 2-11 and 2-12**; see **Videos 2-1 and 2-2**).

Left Ventricle

Acquisition of the left ventricle (LV) could be used to display the volume-rendered images of valves and the anatomy of the LV, and to quantitate left ventricular function. Estimation of left ventricular volumes and function may be performed from multiple ventricular views deriving slice planes from the volume dataset (**Figure 2-13**). Currently, a wide-angled acquisition can be one beat to six beats. A pyramidal volume dataset, two orthogonal views (four-chamber and two-chamber views), and a short-axis view are shown in **Figure 2-14**.

After acquiring the 3D full volume of the LV, this dataset is processed by software to calculate the left ventricular ejection fraction (**Figure 2-15**). This analysis is demonstrated by two different systems. Note that with both Philips (Andover, MA) (Figure 2-15, *A*) and TomTec (Munich, Germany) (Figure 2-15, *B*) analyses of the same dataset, similar ejection fractions of approximately 31.23% (Philips) and 31.95% (TomTec, Inc.) are computed.

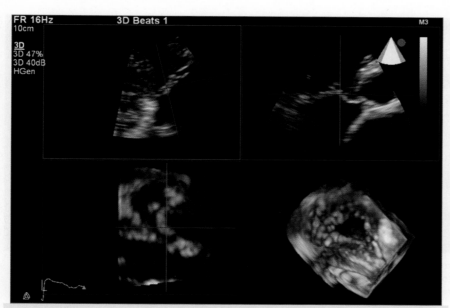

Figure 2-10 The tricuspid valve can be acquired either from the parasternal long-axis view or from apical views. In the zoomed image of the tricuspid valve, the long axis of the valve (*upper left*), the orthogonal view of the long axis (*upper right*), and the short axis of these views (*lower left*) with a volume-rendered image of the tricuspid valve from a ventricular orientation (*lower right*) are shown.

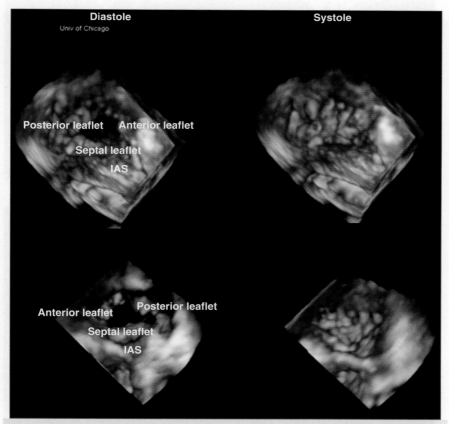

Figure 2-11 Normal tricuspid valve. The zoomed tricuspid valve is orientated with the interatrial septum (*IAS*) posteriorly. The anterior and posterior leaflets are labeled, and the valve is displayed from the right ventricle (*upper panels*) and the right atrium (*lower panels*).

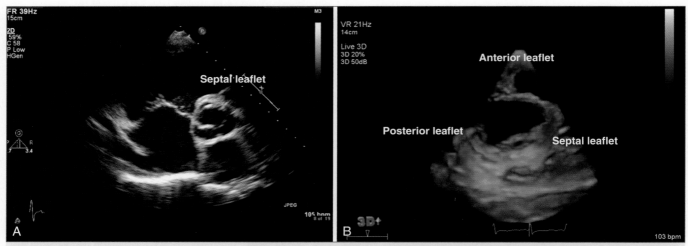

Figure 2-12 Tricuspid valve from the parasternal short-axis view. Two-dimensional (2D) view (**A**) and three-dimensional view (**B**). Note that with 2D imaging, it is difficult to distinguish the individual leaflets. Part of the septal leaflet is clearly seen attaching to the interventricular septum, but more laterally, part of the anterior and/or posterior leaflet is seen (see Videos 2-1 and 2-2).

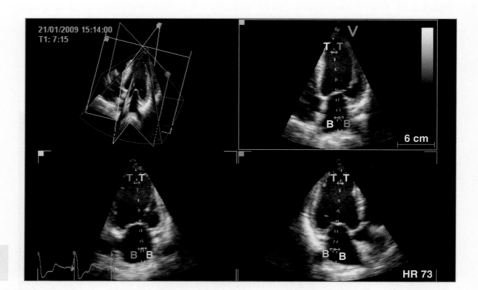

Figure 2-13 A triplanar view of the left ventricle acquired in one beat.

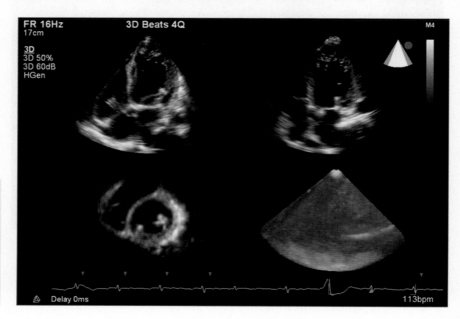

Figure 2-14 Left ventricular wide-angled acquisition. This apical left ventricular volume dataset was acquired over four cardiac cycles. The apical four-chamber view (*upper left*), the apical two-chamber view (*upper right*), the short-axis or cross-sectional view (*lower left*), and the rendered full-volume three-dimensional dataset (*lower right*).

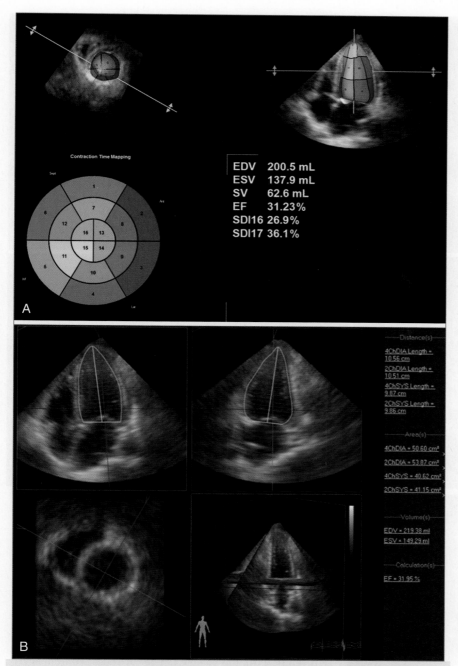

Figure 2-15   Left ventricular quantitation. Left ventricular analysis using a semiautomated border detection software (**A**) and an idealized biplane Simpson's method of disk volume analysis to derive ejection fraction (*EF*) and volumes (**B**). EDV, end-diastolic volume; ESV, end-systolic volume; SDI, systolic dyssynchrony index; SV, systolic volume.

From this apical 3D dataset of the LV (**Figure 2-16,** *A*), multiple views can be derived from one full-volume dataset, including a four-chamber view (Figure 2-16, *B*), two-chamber view (Figure 2-16, *C*), three-chamber view (Figure 2-16, *D*), and short-axis view at the level of the mitral valve (*lower right*, displayed from the left ventricular perspective).

Right Ventricle

The right ventricle (RV) is acquired slightly differently compared with the LV. It is important to ensure that the right ventricular outflow tract (RVOT) is acquired,

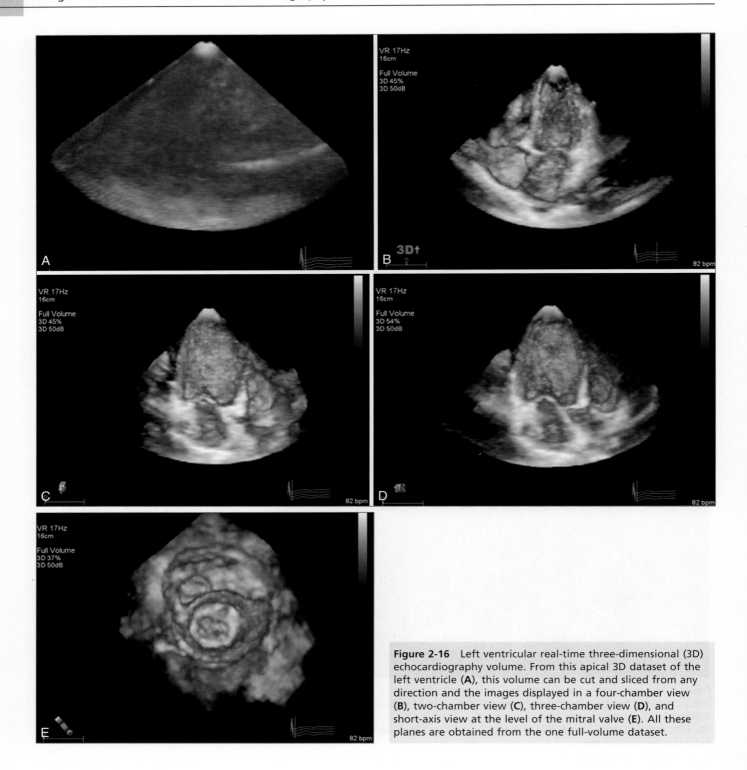

Figure 2-16 Left ventricular real-time three-dimensional (3D) echocardiography volume. From this apical 3D dataset of the left ventricle (**A**), this volume can be cut and sliced from any direction and the images displayed in a four-chamber view (**B**), two-chamber view (**C**), three-chamber view (**D**), and short-axis view at the level of the mitral valve (**E**). All these planes are obtained from the one full-volume dataset.

as seen in **Figure 2-17**. The right ventricular volume can be displayed from a four-chamber view. Using a cropping plane angled parallel to the tricuspid valve annulus from the apex, the tricuspid valve leaflets and the RVOT could be better visualized from the ventricular perspective (**Figures 2-18** and **2-19**).

Once a right ventricular volume is derived, quantitation of right ventricular function and volumes can be performed either online or offline.

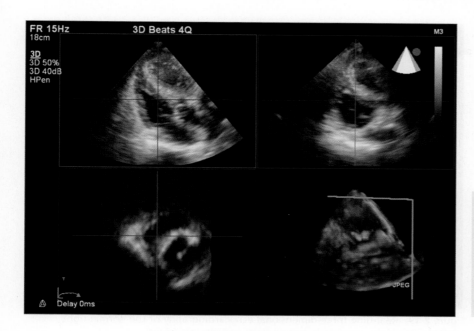

Figure 2-17 Right ventricular real-time three-dimensional echocardiography (RT3DE) volume. This is a full-volume acquisition of the right ventricle. The right ventricular apical view (*upper left*), the right ventricular outflow tract (*upper right*), the short axis (*lower right*), and the rendered RT3DE right ventricular volume (*lower right*).

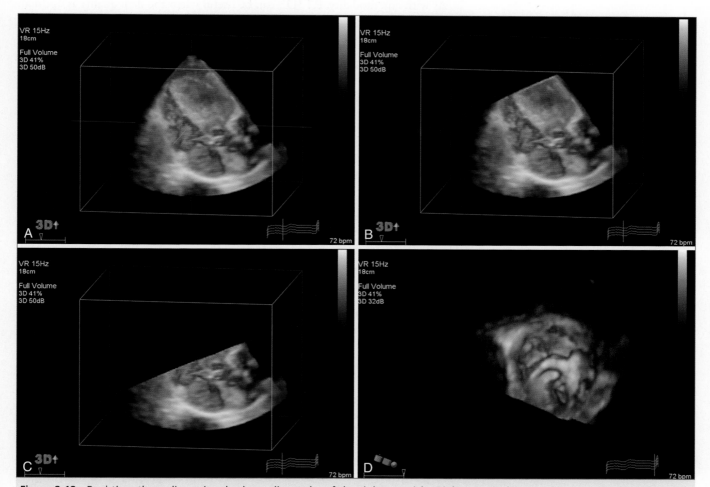

Figure 2-18 Real-time three-dimensional echocardiography of the right ventricle. Right ventricular cropping can subsequently be performed. Displayed is the right ventricular apical view (**A**); using a crop plane, the apex is sliced off (**B**), further cropping is done (**C**), and the tilted plane from the lower left panel is turned to the front to show the short axis of the right ventricle (**D**).

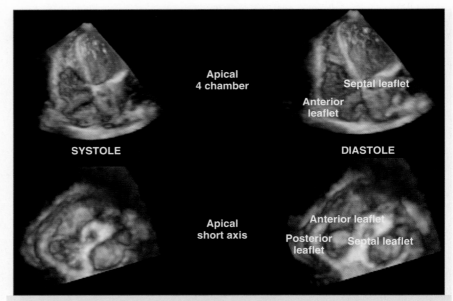

Figure 2-19   Real-time three-dimensional echocardiography of the normal right ventricle. The right ventricle in systole (*left*) and diastole (*right*).

As with any modality, RT3DE can be useful when the data quality is optimal. There is a learning curve in capturing and displaying the RT3DE images. This takes time and practice as well as dedication toward mastery of the technique.

Color Flow Imaging

RT3DE color flow imaging has been one of the more challenging aspects of 3DE. There have been efforts to quantitate the severity of mitral and tricuspid regurgitation; however, it has been more research focused and not used in clinical routine. In a patient with mitral regurgitation caused by perforation, RT3DE color flow demonstrates severe mitral regurgitation from the parasternal view in **Figure 2-20**. Using RT3DE color flow imaging in a patient with an ASD, the size and location of the ASD can be visualized by using a multiplanar display (**Figures 2-21** and **2-22**).

INTEGRATION OF THREE-DIMENSIONAL TECHNOLOGY IN A CLINICAL ROUTINE

The decision to purchase new technology may not be difficult; however, full utilization of this new technology necessitates certain considerations, as discussed below.

Acceptance by and Training of Sonographers and Physicians

There may be two approaches to successfully integrate 3DE into the clinical routine:

1. *"Champion" method:* Selection of sonographers and physicians who are seen as being the most knowledgeable and dedicated in performing 3DE. Once the selected members are well trained, their knowledge and skill are disseminated to the rest of the group.
2. *Group method:* Training, education, and implementation of 3DE technology are provided for the entire group.

Incorporation of Three-Dimensional Echocardiography into Imaging Protocol and Target Population

Integration of 3DE into a routine imaging protocol is essential. Although along with each standard 2DE image a 3DE image could be performed, RT3DE studies

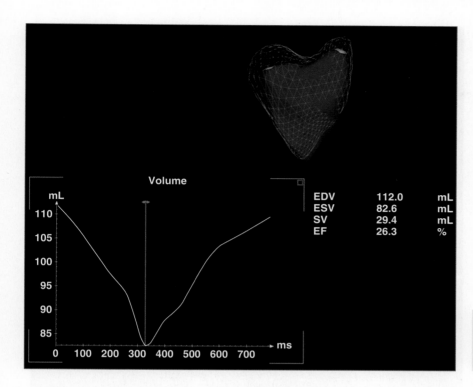

Figure 2-20 Right ventricular analysis. EDV, end-diastolic volume; EF, ejection fraction; ESV, end-systolic volume; SV, systolic volume.

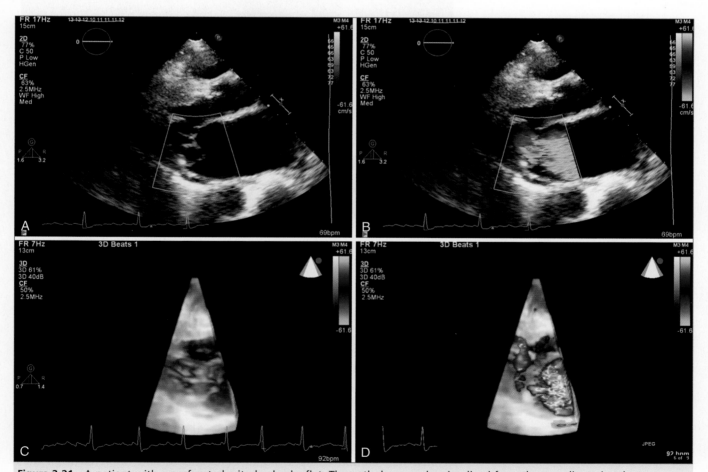

Figure 2-21 A patient with a perforated mitral valve leaflet. The pathology can be visualized from the two-dimensional echocardiography image (**A** and **B**). The real-time three-dimensional echocardiography images (**C** and **D**) show a perforation of the posterior mitral valve leaflet.

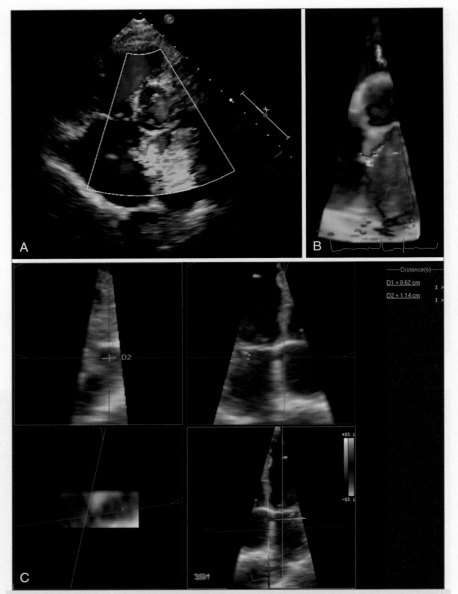

Figure 2-22 Patent foramen ovale (PFO) shown in two-dimensional color (*top left*) and in real-time three-dimensional echocardiography with color (*lower left*). From this full-volume color dataset, data were analyzed to measure the size of the PFO (*right*), which was 0.62 cm × 1.14 cm.

should be focused to better demonstrate and interrogate the patient's pathology. Because of the ease of acquisition and a strong body of evidence demonstrating better accuracy and reliability compared with 2DE, a 3DE left ventricular volume dataset with good image quality should be acquired in all patients. Right ventricular volume acquisition and analysis should depend on the availability of analysis software.

In every study, regardless of the pathology, a dedicated wide-angled acquisition of both the LV and the RV should be routinely acquired; ejection fractions and regional wall motion changes should be calculated and displayed from these volumes. (In our lab, the routine is parasternal long-axis view, parasternal short-axis view, and apical four-chamber view by 3DE. The apical four-chamber view is a full-volume acquisition dedicated to the LV.)

Determination of the target population should be done and included in the lab protocol. It could be applied to all patients with optimal-quality echocardiographic windows to quantitate left ventricular function or focused in patients with a particular pathology, such as congestive heart failure or valvular heart disease, or in those about to receive chemotherapy.

Management of Workflow

It is essential to determine the workflow with regard to 3DE. Once 3D technology has been acquired, display and analysis need to be performed. Depending on the existing 2DE workflow, this could mean a continuation on the ultrasound machine (on-cart) or offline on an image management system that has 3D software. 3D display of pathology or quantitation of ventricular volumes should be recorded as a loop or a still frame for immediate viewing on the image management system (picture archiving and communication system), with subsequent storage of 3D volume as native data for future use.

Although there have been major advances in ultrasound and computer technologies, RT3DE imaging has its limitations. Nonetheless, the developments have enabled more accurate estimation of ventricular function and improved and unique evaluation of valvular pathology. The integration of RT3DE into the clinical routine rests on these facts and the commitment of the leaders in echocardiography laboratories and sonographers.

References

1. Mor-Avi V, Jenkins C, Kuhl HP, et al: Real-time 3-dimensional echocardiographic quantification of left ventricular volumes: Multicenter study for validation with magnetic resonance imaging and investigation of sources of error. *JACC Cardiovasc Imag* 1:413–423, 2008.
2. Jenkins C, Moir S, Chan J, et al: Left ventricular volume measurement with echocardiography: A comparison of left ventricular opacification, three-dimensional echocardiography, or both with magnetic resonance imaging. *Eur Heart J* 30:98–106, 2009.
3. Zamorano J, Cordeiro P, Sugeng L, et al: Real-time three dimensional echocardiography for rheumatic mitral valve stenosis evaluation. *J Am Coll Cardiol* 43:2091–2096, 2004.

CHAPTER 3

Three-Dimensional Transesophageal Echocardiography Systems

Ivan S. Salgo

INTRODUCTION

Technologic advances continue to propel cardiac visualization forward. Advances in miniaturization, computer processing, and algorithms continue to have significant momentum. New acquisition technologies, coupled with the ability to process, display, and quantify enormous amounts of data, have pushed echocardiography forward into becoming a modality that will change cardiac intervention as well.[1-13] Today, three-dimensional transesophageal echocardiography (3DTEE) has generated near-optical cardiac images. An understanding of cardiac mechanical motion in all of its spatial and temporal dimensions is providing valuable general physiologic insight for echocardiography as well as precise diagnoses for patients.

It is expedient to address the technologic advances in terms of the operating sequence in an ultrasound system for echocardiography. This allows a framework consisting of transduction, beamforming, display, and quantification to be used. Echocardiographic instrumentation is unparalleled with respect to its portability, cost, lack of ionizing radiation, and ubiquitous presence.

TRANSDUCER TECHNOLOGY

Among imaging modalities, the defining aspect of echocardiography is the transducer. *Transduction* refers to the ability to convert one form of energy to another. Thus, an ultrasound transducer converts electrical energy into mechanical energy on "transmit" and acts as a microphone on "receive." All ultrasound transducers perform this operation, but what sets ultrasound advancements apart is the ability to steer in two or three dimensions. The earliest M-mode transducers created an image composed of one spatial dimension and one temporal dimension. The element is composed of specialized material that traditionally uses lead-zirconate-titanate. Newer single-crystal materials that contain homogeneous solid-state domains are more efficient in the transduction process and have higher bandwidth (more upper and lower frequency content). This creates a concomitant increase of echo penetration and resolution. Although the M mode was an advance over the stethoscope, it was limited by its lack of field of view. M mode used a "transmit-listen-wait" duty cycle to determine the distance of targets along an unsteered scanline, and the operator needed to point the transducer to examine different cardiac structures. The development of the phased-array paradigm allowed scan lines to be steered.

Conventional two-dimensional (2D) imaging, commonly used in echocardiography, uses transducers with several elements (**Figure 3-1**). Specifically, elements are oriented in a single row containing 48 to 128 elements, with each element electrically isolated from the others. Individual wavefronts are generated by firing elements in a certain sequence. Each element, constructively and destructively, adds and subtracts pulses, respectively, to generate a focused wave that has direction. This creates the radially propagated scan line. For example, if the farthest element on the right fires first and a timed sequence propagates along the element

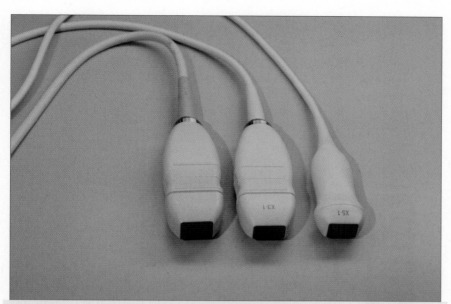

Figure 3-1 Transthoracic imaging transducers for three-dimensional echocardiography in the adult. Three generations of transducers from left to right: ×4, ×3-1 and ×5-1. Miniaturization is the key technological trend in the evolution of matrix array technology. The ×4 has 24 application-specific integrated circuits and the ×5 has one. This reduces power consumption and also allows a more ergonomic handle. Other changes that have evolved include changes to the physical and nose apertures to optimize acoustic coupling in intercostal spaces.

to the left, the beam will be steered to the left (**Figures 3-2** and **3-3**). Each element fires with a delay in phase with respect to a transmit initiation time. To further clarify this point, this one-dimensional array of elements can fire in two dimensions: *radially* and *azimuthally* (laterally). This spatiotemporal orientation of elements and their phase-timed firing sequence form the underpinning of any modern phased-array system.

Transducer material is cut, or "diced," by a diamond-tipped saw to create the checkerboard pattern. Elements are then electrically connected to a system. Early-generation systems were composed of sparsely sampled arrays, that is, arrays whose elements were not all electrically active. These sparse arrays created the first instantaneous 3D images; early clinical research was conducted using this type of transducer. It is advantageous to have every element independently active to control the ultrasound beam with more precision. The spacing, or pitch, of these elements depends on the desired frequency of operation (typically $\lambda/4$). Otherwise, undesirable diffraction effects such as grating lobes appear. This means that higher frequency transducers have finer pitches. Increased technologic challenges have emerged in the creation of these element connections. The major advance that allowed a fully sampled matrix array to be fabricated was the ability to develop electrical interconnections to every element.

The key aspects pertinent to 3D echocardiography (3DE) imaging involve imaging moving structures. If a static structure that is not moving in space needs to be visualized, a 2D imaging transducer could be swept if the third spatial dimension could be additionally registered within the coordinate space. By using electromagnetic trackers, early *gated* 3D methodologies exploited this paradigm. Naturally, the 2D images needed to be gated to the electrocardiogram (ECG). This could lead to error caused by movement or arrhythmias, and these lengthy scans could take tens of minutes, requiring a few hundred heart cycles. Ultimately, high-resolution cardiac imaging requires instantaneous imaging to overcome these limitations. The key difference between a 2D imaging transducer and an instantaneous 3D imaging transducer is the arrangement of elements

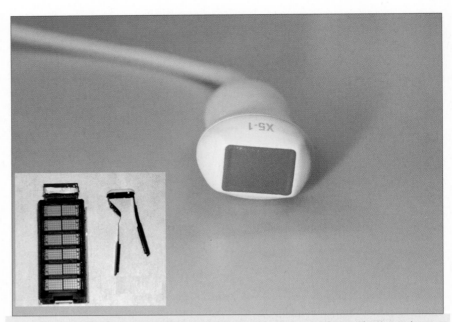

Figure 3-2   Integrated circuit miniaturization in the ×5-1 transducer. The *inset* shows previous technology using multiple application-specific integrated circuits (*left*). These perform the micro-beamforming and allow steering of acoustic lines in three-dimensional space both azimuthally and elevationally. *Inset at right,* These circuits have been condensed to one circuit whose dimensions are designed to match the aperture shown in red on the transducer face.

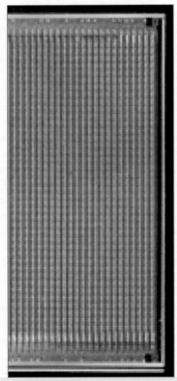

Figure 3-3   Portion of a three-dimensional beamforming application-specific integrated circuit (ASIC). Shown are electrical contact points that couple the transducer piezoelectric elements to the beamforming component circuitry. The ASIC is fully capable of performing M-mode, two-dimensional, and 3D imaging as well as spectral and color Doppler.

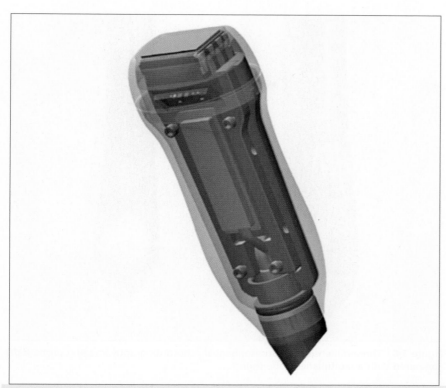

Figure 3-4 Internal component of a transthoracic three-dimensional imaging probe. Shown at the bottom is the cable coupling to the housing. The electrical cable connections to the main beamformer in the ultrasound system pass through the rectangular connector (shown in light green) in the middle of the handle. At the top is the beamforming application-specific integrated circuit and matching layer.

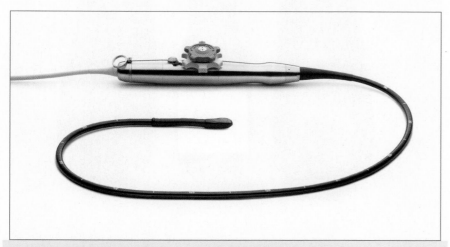

Figure 3-5 Three-dimensional transesophageal imaging transducer.

(**Figures 3-4** to **3-7**). Although a one-dimensional row is used for 2D imaging, a 2D matrix or checkerboard is used to steer an ultrasound scan line in the azimuthal as well as the elevational direction. A conventional 2D imaging transducer of one row steers energy in the azimuthal plane but unintentionally propagates elevational energy above and below the scanning plane. This checkerboard pattern allows phasic firing of elements to generate a radially propagated scan line that can be steered laterally and in elevation. Thus, the true 3D imaging transducer is born.

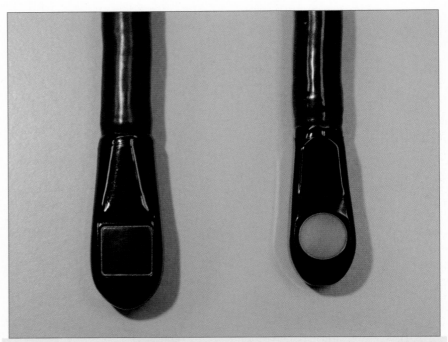

Figure 3-6 Three-dimensional transesophageal echocardiography imaging probe (*left*) compared with a multiplane probe (*right*).

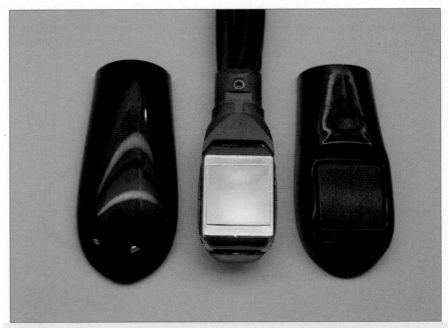

Figure 3-7 Three-dimensional transesophageal echocardiography (TEE) imaging probe tip with external housing removed. Shown is the matrix array in both azimuthal and elevational dimensions. Unlike a conventional multiplane TEE probe, there are no moving parts within the housing. Moreover, special shielding is built in to prevent electrical interference from external sources such as electrocautery.

Micro-beamforming is the process of using coarse and fine steering. This is implemented by putting fine-delay circuitry into special, application-specific integrated circuits (ASICs). The first commercial, fully sampled matrix array transducer used this methodology by placing 24 to 26 ASICs into the transducer handle. Approximately 3000 elements were electrically connected to these ASICs.

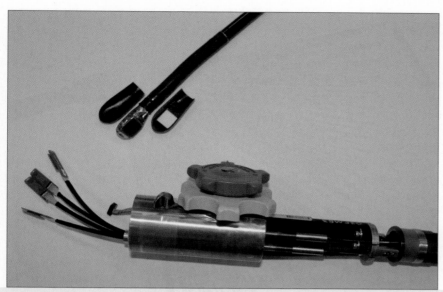

Figure 3-8 Three-dimensional transesophageal echocardiography transducer with probe handle components displayed. Shown are steering cables for the bending neck. The bending neck, which is proximal to the probe tip, allows anteroflexion and retroflexion within the esophagus. Four electrical connectors allow post–micro-beamformed acoustic information to pass within the cable.

Fine steering was performed using subsections of the element matrix known as *patches*. Coarse steering is performed within the system and through a conventional cable. Specially engineered ASICs allow an individual element to be electrically active but simultaneously keep the size of the transducer cable small, since a significant portion of beamforming has already taken place in the handle. Early transducers were specialized "3D-only probes," but it is now possible to perform all the transducer functions such as imaging, color flow, and spectral Doppler within the same transducer. Moreover, the transducer aperture should be large enough to allow sufficient lateral and elevational resolution but small enough to "fit" into the intercostals space. One of the most difficult aspects of transducer engineering is what is known as *thermal management*. The electronics generate heat, potentially more so at high mechanical indexes (e.g., higher waveform amplitudes). These issues need to be resolved if 3DE was to move to the operating room.

3DE depends on micro-beamforming miniaturization. By reducing the electronic substrate required to beamform onto a single chip, the transducer chip is miniaturized sufficiently to pass into the human esophagus. It also significantly reduces the power requirement and hence the amount of heat generated by live circuitry (**Figures 3-8** to **3-10**).

BEAMFORMING

3DE beamforming consists of steering and focusing of ultrasound energy both as transmitted and received scanlines. This creates useful signals that can be displayed or quantified. It is both advanced science and art. Significant advancements that maximize frame rate, scanning volume size, and resolution continue to occur. *Resolution* is defined as the ability to distinguish two point targets as distinct. The limiting item in current 3DE systems is the speed of sound, not computing power. Ultrasound image quality improves by firing more transmit lines with more closely associated line spacing. This slows the frame rate since there are many more duty cycles for the system to deal with.

Ultimately, the constraint of a system can be described by a triangle whose boundaries are defined by the number of transmit lines that can be fired. Lines

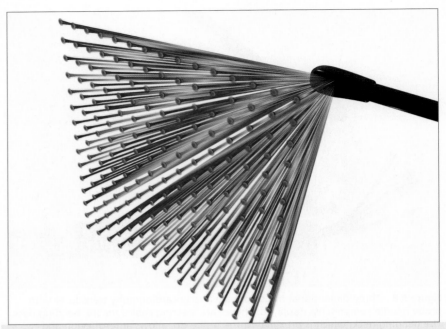

Figure 3-9 Three-dimensional (3D) steering acoustic lines in 3D space. By steering transmit lines, a fully functional matrix array can interrogate anatomy in 3D.

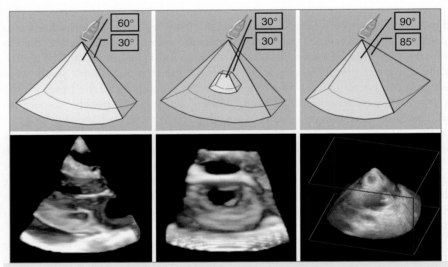

Figure 3-10 Three different volume scanning paradigms. At *left* is a volume used for live scanning. The *center* shows live scanning but in a smaller zoom fashion. At *right* is a larger volume with multiple gated slabs put together.

widely spaced can increase the volume size at the cost of lowering the resolution for a constant frame rate (**Figure 3-11**). Tight line spacing can be used in zoom modes to increase resolution, but at the price of a smaller volume. The number of transmit lines is a key determinant of frame rate; more lines increase the resolution but lower the frame rate.

Beamforming can be subdivided into a coarse stage that occurs in the system and a fine steering or micro-stage that occurs in the transducer. The act of combining element signals is known as *summing*. Summing of per-element pulses is what ultimately creates a scan line. The general sequence of events is as follows:

1. Compute (direction and aperture) and fire the transmit scanline.
2. Listen, or sense, the returning echoes and digitally sample and store them.

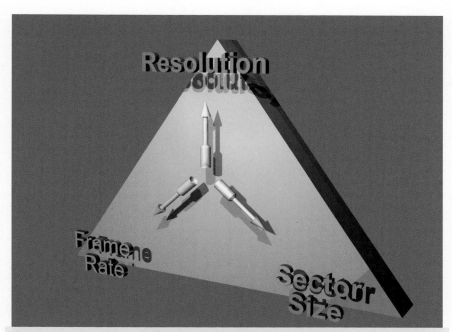

Figure 3-11   Relationship among frame rate, resolution, and sector size in three-dimensional beamforming. For a fixed number of lines, the sector size can be increased but at a tradeoff of resolution, which makes the point spread function more "blobby." Firing more scanning lines can increase resolution, sector size, or both (depending on line density), but firing more lines reduces frame rate.

3. Create multiple listening (after the fact) directions and foci (receive steering and dynamic focusing) from the digital data.
4. Compute the radiofrequency signal strength (envelope detection).
5. Scan to convert the 3D spherical system to the Cartesian (cubic) voxel system.

The most significant aspect of a 3D beamformer is the ability to steer both azimuthally (laterally) and elevationally. This creates a spherical coordinate system. The limits of resolution stem from lateral or elevational line spacing. Samples within a line are more finely spaced in the radial dimension (i.e., within a scan line) and are farther apart across scan lines in the lateral or elevational directions. Therefore, line spacing is a fundamental determinant of image quality.

Gating refers to the act of acquiring multiple acquisitions (timed to the ECG) to combine them at some later point. 3D acquisitions in the 1990s entailed acquiring 60 to 180 2D slices and interpolating them to create a 3D reconstructed volume. Since this process took several minutes, it was prone to misalignment and inferior resolution. Gating is still used today to overcome limitations in the speed of sound by combining only a few 3D slabs (e.g., 4 to 8) to create a larger volume. This process takes only seconds. Moreover, color Doppler techniques depend on analyzing multiple transmit events fired along a single line. The multiple returning pulses are compared or cross-correlated to infer velocity. Nevertheless, gating is prone to error in patients with irregular rhythms such as atrial fibrillation or multiple ventricular premature contractions.

3D ultrasound imaging is still subject to the laws of acoustic physics even though it is ungated or "live 3D." First, the aperture is an important determinant of image quality. Larger apertures allow better beamforming from a focus point of view. Unlike abdominal imaging, transthoracic echocardiography is limited by the ultrasound aperture that can fit between a rib space. In TEE, the aperture is limited by dimensions that can be accommodated within an adult esophagus. TEE generally uses higher frequencies compared with its transthoracic

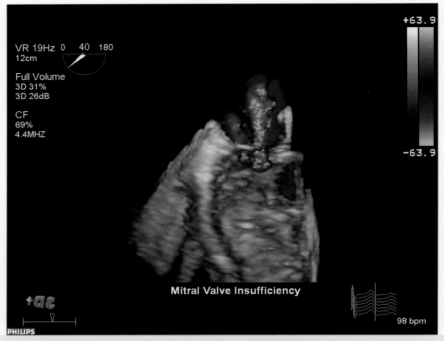

VR 19Hz 0   40 180
12cm

Full Volume
3D 31%
3D 26dB

CF
69%
4.4MHZ

+63.9

−63.9

Mitral Valve Insufficiency

98 bpm

PHILIPS

Figure 3-12 Three-dimensional (3D) volume rendering of mitral insufficiency. The left ventricle is shown, and color Doppler data have been scanned in 3D coordinates to the mitral valve leaking. Aliasing is also shown between red and blue pixels as the jet velocity exceeds the Nyquist sampling limit to quantify its true velocity.

counterparts. This allows better image resolution for a given aperture size. (The higher the frequency, the better the ultrasound beam can focus, but this comes at the loss of penetration.) Since TEE is not limited by significant chest wall acoustic aberration, the higher frequencies and better acoustic substrate allow higher resolution compared with transthoracic imaging (**Figures 3-11** and **3-12**).

Artifacts such as shadowing, reverberations, multipath transmission and aberration play a role in degrading the ultrasound image. As with 2DE, 3D ultrasound cannot image through metallic or highly calcified objects. One of the most significant issues pertains to the quality of the image as seen through chest wall windows versus the esophagus. This is due mainly to two phenomena: *aberration* and *multipath reflection*. Aberration stems from wavefronts traveling through different media with different velocities of sound. Fascial tissue layers create a distortion of the traveling wavefronts. This can be corrected for, in a limited way, by accounting for the varying speeds of sound. The layers of the chest wall contain varying degrees of adipose and connective tissues. This creates not only aberration but also multipath degradation. As ultrasound waves get diverted to altering paths of propagation, the superposition of transmitted and returning echo signals consists of wavefronts of both desired and nondesired targets. Unwanted, but real, signals are termed *clutter*. Since the esophagus represents a thin wall consisting of a stratified squamous epithelium and smooth muscle, these ultrasound effects do not occur in 3D-TEE. Hence, image quality is higher, and clutter is lower.

QUANTIFICATION FOR THREE-DIMENSIONAL ECHOCARDIOGRAPHY

Once 3D data are processed, they are "volume rendered" to create the appearance of three dimensions (**Figures 3-13** to **3-16**). 3D color voxels can be rendered as well (see Figure 3-12). The considerable advantage of 3DE in acquiring ultrasound images of the beating heart makes it especially useful for cardiac

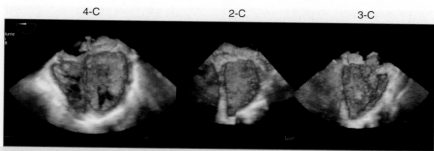

Figure 3-13 Transthoracic imaging showing apical four-, two-, and three-chamber views of the left ventricle. This is an example of volume rendering in which three-dimensional (3D) volume elements known as *voxels* are used to create the 3D appearance scanned by a 3D acoustic sweep. In addition, hue (color) is used to add to the visual effect of depth. Ultimately, these voxels are converted to two-dimensional (2D) picture elements (pixels) in a process known as *volume rendering*. Even though the picture is in 2D, real 3D data are used to create these images.

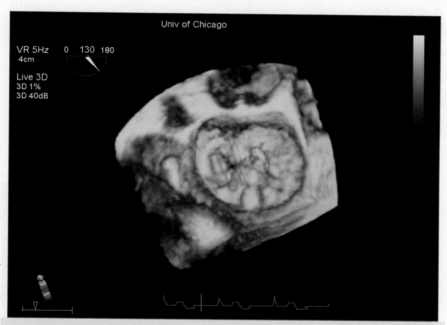

Figure 3-14 Three-dimensional transesophageal echocardiography of the mitral valve showing a flail segment near P2.

quantification. While the display of anatomy in its true 3D state is important, many physicians believe that the single most significant value that 3DE has is its ability to quantify. Myocardial and valvular motion occurs in three spatial dimensions. Traditional 2D scanning planes do not capture this entire motion, or the plane can "slip" during scanning. Quantifying requires segmenting or separating out structures of interest from the 3D image. Machine vision techniques use methods that define an interface, such as a left ventricular (LV)-endocardial border. This interface is generated as a mesh of points and lines and displayed by a process known as *surface rendering* (**Figure 3-17**).

The application of 3D beamforming in a TEE probe allows visualization of the beating mitral valve. The mitral valve can be segmented with significant accuracy by using this approach. The true 3D structure of the mitral annulus, leaflets, and chordal apparatus can be measured. This further allows sophisticated

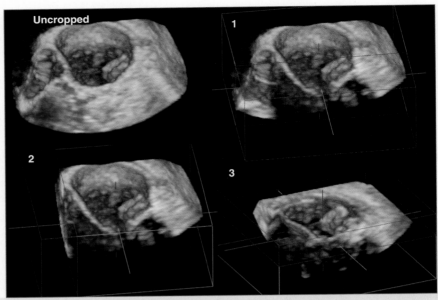

Figure 3-15   Three-dimensional transesophageal echocardiography image of the mitral valve showing the effect of cropping data. The *upper left panel* shows an uncropped image looking down from the left atrium. *1,* A cropping plane has been used to cut away data along the green axis. This allows better visualization of the anterior and posterior mitral leaflets. *2,* Another cropping pane, in this case along the red axis, has been used to cut away anterior anatomy as part of the aortic valve. In this case, since the cropping was at the side, there is not much benefit. *3,* A cropping plane along the blue axis has been used to crop away data from the left atrium toward the top of the image.

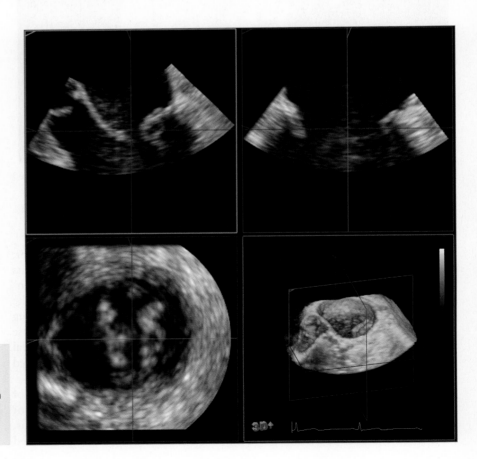

Figure 3-16   Multiplanar reformatting of two-dimensional (2D) slices taken from a three-dimensional (3D) dataset. Three orthogonal 2D views can be extracted from the 3D dataset (*lower left*). This allows any plane orientation of 2D views in displaying anatomy of interest.

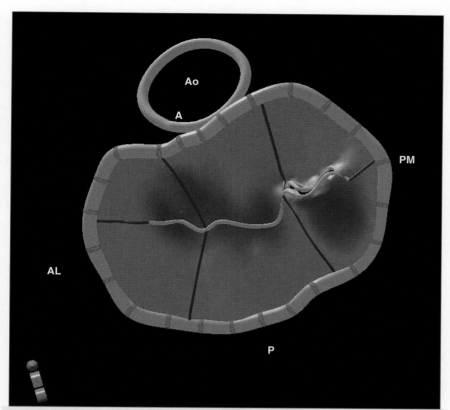

Figure 3-17 Surface rendering and segmentation of mitral leaflets. A prolapsed segment of P3 is shown in red. This portion of the leaflet extends above the annular surface into the left atrium. Also shown is the regurgitant orifice caused by malcoaptation of the leaflets. A, anterior; AL, anterolateral; Ao, aortic valve annulus; P, posterior; PM, posteromedial.

analyses of the nonplanar shape of the mitral annulus.[13-24] These 3D measurements include the following:

- Annular diameters
- Annular nonplanarity
- Commissural lengths
- Leaflet surface areas
- Aortic to mitral annular orientation

The ability to acquire structural data of the mitral valve allows advanced engineering techniques to examine the nature of fluid flow in three dimensions. For example, the *proximal isovelocity surface area (PISA) technique* is an important quantitative tool to estimate the degree of mitral regurgitation. It depends, however, on geometric assumptions, which must be respected.[25] By using actual echocardiographic data from a mitral valve that has been segmented after 3DTEE, the flow of blood through the orifice can be simulated to see the nature of converging isovelocity fluid zones. Near an irregularly shaped orifice, the zone is necessarily irregular and nonspherical. This indicates that care should be exercised in selecting the PISA aliasing velocity to select a near-hemispherical convergence zone (**Figure 3-18**).[26]

3D has a significant benefit over 2D in that if the entire LV chamber is encompassed in the acquisition volume, no foreshortening errors or assumption of LV volume are created. Biplane and triplane methods help avoid foreshortening errors and benefit from higher frame rates than 3D live acquisitions; however, if an aneurysmal dilation occurs between planes, the computed LV volumes will

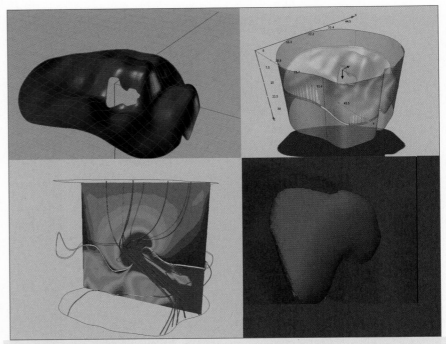

Figure 3-18 Three-dimensional (3D) computational fluid dynamics flow simulation of proximal isovelocity surface area using 3D transesophageal echocardiography segmentation of a regurgitant mitral orifice. *Upper left,* using similar technology as in Figure 3-17, a 3D mesh is created from 3D data and imported into a finite element environment (*upper right*). After setting initial pressure conditions, 3D stream lines pass through the regurgitant orifice from top to bottom (*bottom left*) (valve is upside down as from the left ventricular point of view). Close to the orifice, finite element simulation indicates that the proximal isovelocity convergence zone is not necessarily hemispherical (*bottom right*).

have some interpolation error. Surface rendering of the LV is used for chamber quantification. This can be used on all four chambers. Computer techniques allow calculation of volume, regional wall motion, and regional synchrony.[27-43] Specifically, a 3D deformable model is used to find the LV endocardial surface in three dimensions. This is the most accurate way to quantify LV volumes. Moreover, 3D LV remodeling can be parametrically displayed using differential geometry techniques.[44] This is done by calculating local curvatures around the LV endocardium (**Figure 3-19**). Since the normal LV is not a sphere, local radii of curvature vary around the segments of the LV. For example, the normal septum has different geometric characteristics from those of the apex. Quantification of LV synchrony is possible in 3D as well. The required frame rate depends on the questions being asked. Frame rates of 30 Hz (33 ms between frames) are inadequate to quantify intramyocardial motion; these are better suited to be studied by tissue Doppler or speckle tracking techniques. However, regional synchrony *can* be measured by 3D endocardial excursion because it assesses blood ejection, not tissue motion. 3DE provides a more complete assessment of 3D wall motion. Challenges in frame rate limitations, however, must be taken into account. Assessment of global function is more tolerant of lower frame rate acquisitions compared with that of regional function. That is, to find the ejection fraction, only accurate estimates of end-diastolic and end-systolic volumes are needed (**Figure 3-20**).

Acknowledgment

The author gratefully acknowledges the invaluable transducer engineering input from Michael Peszynski.

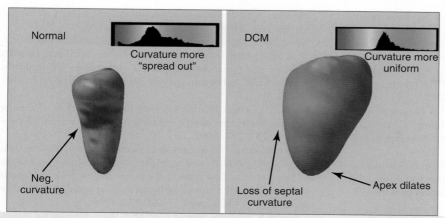

Figure 3-19 The left ventricular (LV) segmentation mesh technique (shown in Figure 3-19) can be used to create parametric displays of regional LV remodeling. At *left* is a normal patient with a smaller endocardial cavity and inward curvature of the LV septum. Patients with dilated cardiomyopathy (*DCM*) lose septal curvature and also have concomitant apical dilation (*right*). The histogram of curvatures has a smaller standard deviation and hence is more spherical in character. (A sphere has zero standard deviation since it has uniform radius.) Neg, negative.

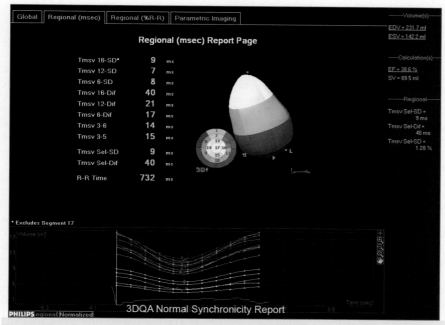

Figure 3-20 Three-dimensional segmentation of the left ventricle. The bull's-eye shows regional segmentation by anatomy. Both global and regional function without geometric assumptions can be made with this approach. Regional ejection curves for each segment can be computed over the cardiac cycle. All the regional waveforms appear similar (are correlated) and indicate synchronous ejection in this patient.

References

1. Lee AP-W, Lam YY, Yip GW, et al: Role of real time three-dimensional transesophageal echocardiography in guidance of interventional procedures in cardiology. *Heart* 96:1485–1493, 2010.

2. Lang RM, Mor-Avi V, Dent JM, et al: Three-dimensional echocardiography: Is it ready for everyday clinical use? JACC: *Cardiovasc Imag* 2:114–117, 2009.

3. Lodato JA, Cao QL, Weinert L, et al: Feasibility of real-time three-dimensional transoesophageal echocardiography for guidance of percutaneous atrial septal defect closure. *Eur J Echocardiogr* 10:543–548, 2009.

4. Perk GM, Lang R: Transesophageal echocardiography: Three-dimensional echocardiography, percutaneous interventions. Use of real time three-dimensional transesophageal echocardiography in

intracardiac catheter based interventions. *J Am Soc Echocardiogr* 22:865–882, 2009.

5. Perrin DP, Vasilyev NV, Novotny P, et al: Image guided surgical interventions. *Curr Prob Surg* 46:730–766, 2009.

6. Fischer GW, Salgo IS, Adams DH, et al: Real-time three-dimensional transesophageal echocardiography: The matrix revolution. *J Cardiothorac Vasc Anesth* 22:904–912, 2008.

7. Muller S, Feuchtner G, Bonatti J, et al: Value of transesophageal 3D echocardiography as an adjunct to conventional 2D imaging in preoperative evaluation of cardiac masses. *Echocardiography* 25:624–631, 2008.

8. Sugeng L, Shernan SK, Salgo IS, et al: Live 3-dimensional transesophageal echocardiography initial experience using the fully-sampled matrix array probe. *J Am Coll Cardiol* 52:446–449, 2008.

9. Vasilyev NV, Novotny PM, Martinez JF, et al: Stereoscopic vision display technology in real-time three-dimensional echocardiography-guided intracardiac beating-heart surgery. *J Thorac Cardiovasc Surg* 135:1334–1341, 2008.

10. Vasilyev NV, Melnychenko I, Kitahori K, et al: Beating-heart patch closure of muscular ventricular septal defects under real-time three-dimensional echocardiographic guidance: A preclinical study. *J Thorac Cardiovasc Surg* 135:603–609, 2008.

11. Suematsu Y, Marx GR, Stoll JA, et al: Three-dimensional echocardiography-guided beating-heart surgery without cardiopulmonary bypass: A feasibility study. *J Thorac Cardiovasc Surg* 128:579–587, 2004.

12. Cannon JW, Stoll JA, Salgo IS, et al: Real-time three-dimensional ultrasound for guiding surgical tasks. *Comp Aid Surg* 8:82–90, 2003.

13. Hung J, Guerrero JL, Handschumacher MD, et al: Reverse ventricular remodeling reduces ischemic mitral regurgitation: Echoguided device application in the beating heart. *Circulation* 106:2594–2600, 2002.

14. Chandra SM, Salgo ISMM, Sugeng LMM, et al: Characterization of degenerative mitral valve disease using morphologic analysis of real-time three-dimensional echocardiographic images: Objective insight into complexity and planning of mitral valve repair. *Circ Cardiovasc Imag* 4:24-32, 2011.

15. Otani K: Assessment of aortic valve annulus size and shape using real-time 3D transesophageal echocardiography: P3-47. *J Am Soc Echocardiogr* 23:B76–BB77, 2010.

16. Malagoli A, Bursi F, Modena MG, et al: Failure of mitral valve repair: Partial detachment of valvular ring by 3D transesophageal echocardiography reconstruction. *Echocardiography* 26:111–112, 2009.

17. Sugeng L, Chandra S, Lang R: Color flow Doppler, mitral regurgitation, three-dimensional echocardiography. Three-dimensional echocardiography for assessment of mitral valve regurgitation.[Miscellaneous Article]. *Curr Opin Cardiol* 24:420–425, 2009.

18. Valocik G, Kamp O, Mannaerts HF, et al: New quantitative three-dimensional echocardiographic indices of mitral valve stenosis: New 3D indices of mitral stenosis. *Int J Cardiovasc Imag* 23:707–716, 2007.

19. Messas E, Yosefy C, Chaput M, et al: Chordal cutting does not adversely affect left ventricle contractile function. *Circulation* 114:I524–I528, 2006.

20. Sugeng L, Coon P, Weinert L, et al: Use of real-time 3-dimensional transthoracic echocardiography in the evaluation of mitral valve disease. *J Am Soc Echocardiogr* 19:413–421, 2006.

21. Ton-Nu TT, Levine RA, Handschumacher MD, et al: Geometric determinants of functional tricuspid regurgitation: Insights from 3-dimensional echocardiography. *Circulation* 114:143–149, 2006.

22. Watanabe N, Ogasawara Y, Yamaura Y, et al: Quantitation of mitral valve tenting in ischemic mitral regurgitation by transthoracic

real-time three-dimensional echocardiography. *J Am Coll Cardiol* 45:763–769, 2005.

23. Watanabe N, Ogasawara Y, Yamaura Y, et al: Mitral annulus flattens in ischemic mitral regurgitation: Geometric differences between inferior and anterior myocardial infarction: A real-time 3-dimensional echocardiographic study. *Circulation* 112:I1458–I1462, 2005.

24. Salgo IS, Gorman JH, III, Gorman RC, et al: Effect of annular shape on leaflet curvature in reducing mitral leaflet stress. *Circulation* 106:711–717, 2002.

25. Schwammenthal E, Chunguang C, Giesler M, et al: New method for accurate calculation of regurgitant flow rate based on analysis of Doppler color flow maps of the proximal flow field: validations in a canine model of mitral regurgitation with initial application in patients. *J Am Coll Cardiol* 27:161–172, 1996.

26. Chandra S, Salgo IS, Sugeng L, et al: A three-dimensional insight into the complexity of flow convergence in mitral regurgitation: adjunctive benefit of anatomic regurgitant orifice area. *Am J Physiol Heart Circ Physiol* 301:H1015–H1024, 2011.

27. Caiani EG, Corsi C, Sugeng L, et al: Improved quantification of left ventricular mass based on endocardial and epicardial surface detection with real time three dimensional echocardiography. *Heart* 92:213–219, 2006.

28. Yang HS, Pellikka PA, McCully RB, et al: Role of biplane and biplane echocardiographically guided 3-dimensional echocardiography during dobutamine stress echocardiography. *J Am Soc Echocardiogr* 19:1136–1143, 2006.

29. Jacobs LD, Salgo IS, Goonewardena S, et al: Rapid online quantification of left ventricular volume from real-time three-dimensional echocardiographic data. *Eur Heart J* 27:460–468, 2006.

30. Jenkins C, Chan J, Hanekom L, et al: Accuracy and feasibility of online 3-dimensional echocardiography for measurement of left ventricular parameters. *J Am Soc Echocardiogr* 19:1119–1128, 2006.

31. Marsan NAMD, Bleeker GBMDP, Ypenburg CMD, et al: Real-time three dimensional echocardiography permits quantification of left ventricular mechanical dyssynchrony and predicts acute response to cardiac reynchrononization therapy. *J Cardiovasc Electrophysiol* 19:392–399, 2008.

32. Abraham TMD, Kass DMD, Tonti GMD, et al: Imaging cardiac resynchronization therapy. *J Am Coll Cardiol Imag* 2:486–497, 2009.

33. Marsan NAMD: Real-time three-dimensional echocardiography as a novel approach to quantify left ventricular dyssynchrony: A comparison study with phase analysis of gated myocardial perfusion single photon emission computed tomography. *J Am Soc Echocardiogr* 21:801–807, 2008.

34. Kapetanakis SM, Kearney MTMD, Siva AP, et al: Real-time three-dimensional echocardiography a novel technique to quantify global left ventricular mechanical dyssynchrony. *Circulation* 112:992–1000, 2005.

35. Agler DA, Adams DB, Waggoner AD, et al: Cardiac resynchronization therapy and the emerging role of echocardiography (part 2): The comprehensive examination. *J Am Soc Echocardiogr* 20:76–90, 2007.

36. Takeuchi M, Jacobs A, Sugeng L, et al: Assessment of left ventricular dyssynchrony with real-time 3-dimensional echocardiography: Comparison with Doppler tissue imaging. *J Am Soc Echocardiogr* 20:1321–1329, 2007.

37. Zamorano J, Perez DI, Roque C, et al: The role of echocardiography in the assessment of mechanical dyssynchrony and its importance in predicting response to prognosis after cardiac resynchronization therapy. *J Am Soc Echocardiogr* 20:91–99, 2007.

38. Pulerwitz T, Hirata K, Abe Y, et al: Feasibility of using a real-time 3-dimensional technique for contrast dobutamine stress echocardiography. *J Am Soc Echocardiogr* 19:540–545, 2006.

39. Mor-Avi V, Sugeng L, Weinert L, et al: Fast measurement of left ventricular mass with real-time three-dimensional echocardiography: Comparison with magnetic resonance imaging. *Circulation* 110:1814–1818, 2004.

40. Qin JX, Jones M, Travaglini A, et al: The accuracy of left ventricular mass determined by real-time three-dimensional echocardiography in chronic animal and clinical studies: A comparison with postmortem examination and magnetic resonance imaging. *J Am Soc Echocardiogr* 18:1037–1043, 2005.

41. Nishikage T, Nakai H, Mor-Avi V, et al: Quantitative assessment of left ventricular volume and ejection fraction using two-dimensional speckle tracking echocardiography. *Eur J Echocardiogr* 10:82–88, 2009.

42. Thomas JD, Popovi ZB: Assessment of left ventricular function by cardiac ultrasound. *J Am Coll Cardiol* 48:2012–2025, 2006.

43. Takeuchi M, Nishikage T, Mor-Avi V, et al: Measurement of left ventricular mass by real-time three-dimensional echocardiography: Validation against magnetic resonance and comparison with two-dimensional and m-mode measurements. *J Am Soc Echocardiogr* 21:1001–1005, 2008.

44. Salgo IS, Tsang W, Ackerman W, et al: Geometric assessment of regional left ventricular remodeling by three-dimensional echocardiographic shape analysis correlates with left ventricular function. *J Am Soc Echocardiogr* 25:80–88, 2012.

Evaluation of the Aortic Valve

Edward A. Gill

INTRODUCTION

The aortic valve is the third largest valve in the body, behind the tricuspid and mitral valves, and has a typical valve area of 3 to 4 cm^2. Despite its smaller size, it is arguably the most important because it lies between the high-resistance aorta and the high pressure–generating left ventricle. Like the pulmonary valve, the aortic valve is semilunar in nature; the major difference between the two semilunar valves is that the left and right coronary arteries arise from the aortic valve and from the left and right coronary sinuses of Valsalva, respectively. However, the aortic valve is also a more resilient valve than the pulmonic valve, as has been shown when the pulmonic valve has been switched into the aortic position in the Ross procedure.[1] The anatomy of the semilunar valves is unique in that a discrete, well-defined annulus, as in the mitral and tricuspid valves, is not present. That is, there is no well-formed fibrous band of tissue encircling the aorta, even though clinicians, especially surgeons, speak of this. Rather, there is a curvilinear attachment of the aortic valve cusps to the aortic wall. Real-time three-dimensional transesophageal echocardiography (RT3DTEE) has been used to reconstruct the aortic valve annulus, which has been shown to have significant variation depending on whether it is tricuspid, bicuspid, calcified, or quadricuspid (**Figure 4-1**).[2] In fact, the aortic annulus has the appearance of a crown and is well visualized in Figure 4-1. Furthermore, the valve cusps attach to tissue in both the aortic wall as well as the left ventricular arterial junction in a curvilinear fashion. The aortic valve cusps have a main core of tissue with endocardial lining present on each side. The individual leaflets meet at a central line of coaptation, the center of which is a thickened nodule called the *nodule of Arantius* (**Figure 4-2**). This nodule has important anatomic significance for RT3DE imaging because the extent of the nodule thickening often cannot be completely appreciated by two-dimensional echocardiography (2DE), and complete visualization is important in pathology of the valve leading to aortic regurgitation.[2-4] The body of the aortic valve leaflets is well seen by RT3DE, as opposed to 2DE (**Figure 4-3**).

AORTIC VALVE PATHOLOGY AND REAL-TIME THREE-DIMENSIONAL ECHOCARDIOGRAPHY

The evaluation of the aortic valve, including the sinuses of Valsalva and the aortic root, by both 2DE and 3DE has become even more important in modern-day cardiology because of the advent of the percutaneously delivered aortic valve and the ability to close defects in the aortic root and sinuses of Valsalva by using percutaneously placed vascular plugs.[5] The characteristic *Gerbode defect*, defined as right coronary sinus of Valsalva rupture into the right atrium, is just one example in which RT3DTEE can particularly perform well in terms of visualization of the many (right atrium, right coronary sinus of Valsalva, tricuspid valve, interatrial and interventricular septae) structures that are in proximity to each other (**Figure 4-4; Video 4-1**). The anatomic relationships of these structures are not trivial, and RT3DTEE can sort them out nicely in many, if not all, instances.[1,2] My own experience

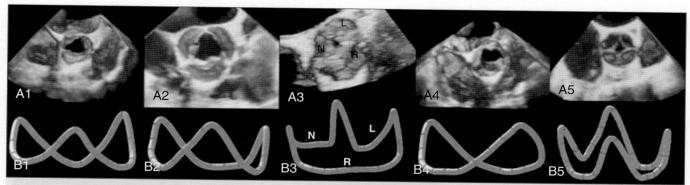

Figure 4-1 The varying shape of the aortic valve annulus reconstructed from real-time three-dimensional transesophageal echocardiography data. *A1,* normal trileaflet valve; *A2,* calcified tricuspid valve; *A3,* scalene tricuspid valve; *A4,* bicuspid aortic valve, and *A5,* quadricuspid aortic valve. (From Ren B, Tang H, Kang Y: Visualisation of the aortic annulus using the real-time three-dimensional transesophageal echocardiography. *Heart* 97:862–863, 2011.)

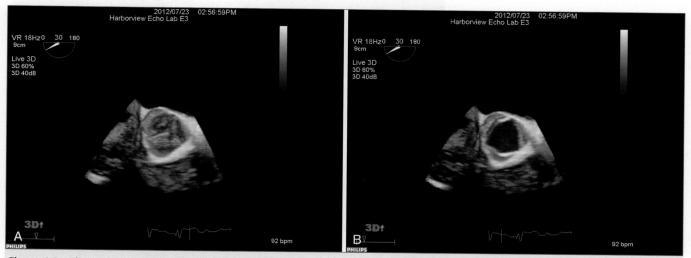

Figure 4-2 The center nodule of Arantius is prominent in this real-time three-dimensional transesophageal echocardiography short-axis view of the aortic valve.

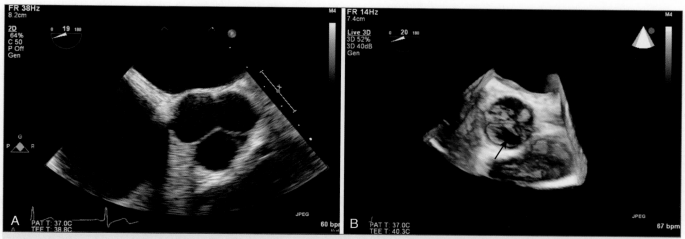

Figure 4-3 **A,** Short-axis two-dimensional transesophageal echocardiography (TEE) of normal aortic valve. **B,** Short-axis real-time three-dimensional (3D) TEE of a normal aortic valve. This case shows an advantage and disadvantage of real-time 3D echocardiography. The advantage is the ability to see the body of the aortic valve cusp. The disadvantage is that there is some dropout (*arrow*) of the leaflet rather than an actual hole in the leaflet. This problem is encountered more with the semilunar valves than the atrioventricular valves because the former are thinner.

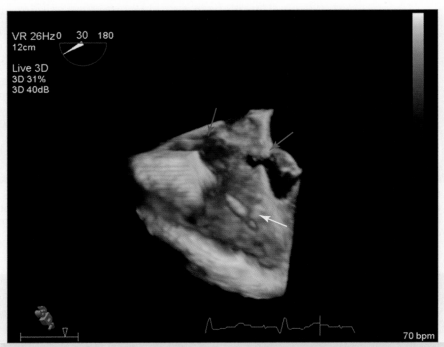

Figure 4-4   Gerbode defect. *Clockwise from top*, Right atrium (*red arrow*), interatrial septum, defect in right coronary sinus of Valsalva (*green arrow*), mitral valve, and right ventricle with pacemaker (*white arrow*) (see Video 4-1).

with closing the Gerbode defect with vascular plugs using RT3DTEE guidance has been extremely favorable.

The most common clinically significant aortic valve lesion is calcific aortic stenosis; this problem is becoming more and more common as the population ages. Significant hemodynamic effects develop with aortic stenosis when the valve area reaches roughly one fourth its normal value, depending on patient size. In young and middle-aged patients with aortic stenosis, the cause is frequently bicuspid aortic valve.[6] RT3DE of the aortic valve can produce quite satisfactory images, particularly of bicuspid aortic valves, although visualization of the valve leaflets typically is more challenging than that of the mitral valve because the leaflets are very thin in the former (**Figure 4-5; Videos** 4-2 to 4-8). The advantage of RT3DE over traditional 2DE is the ability to visualize the body of the valve leaflets as opposed to only the borders of the leaflets at the coaptation point and as they come together to form the commissures at the circumference of the aortic valve. This particular strength of RT3DE is shown in **Figure** 4-6 with direct comparison with 2DE imaging in the same patient. A step-by-step approach to acquisition of the RT3DTEE dataset, starting with the 2DTEE views and then moving to the 3D zoom mode, is described (**Videos** 4-9 to 4-14). Both RT3D transthoracic echocardiography (TTE) and RT3DTEE have been extensively used for evaluation of the disease of the cusp body. Because the most common cause of aortic stenosis is degenerative or calcific aortic stenosis, RT3DE is particularly useful because that type of aortic stenosis preferentially involves the body of the aortic cusps. The same is true for evaluation of the precursor of calcific aortic stenosis: aortic sclerosis (**Figure** 4-7; **Videos** 4-15 to 4-17). For aortic regurgitation, the second most common clinically significant aortic valve lesion, RT3DE can provide data about the degree of regurgitation, particularly by evaluating the 3D vena contracta of the regurgitation, especially with regard to the etiology of the aortic regurgitation.

One of the first reports specific for RT3DE imaging of the aortic valve, performed by Blot-Souleti,[12] looked at the accuracy of aortic stenosis quantitation

Text continued on page 66

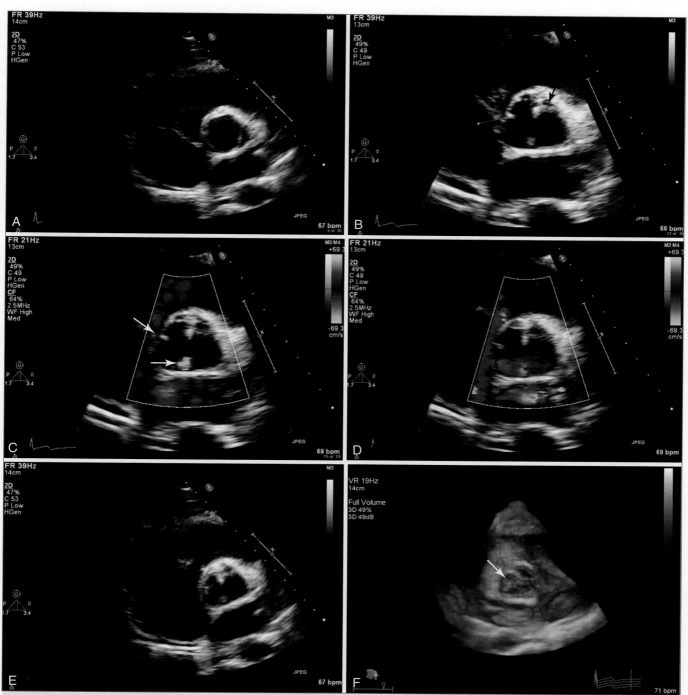

Figure 4-5 These figures are from the same patient and demonstrate two-dimensional (2D) and real-time (RT) three-dimensional (3D) echocardiography images of a bicuspid aortic valve. **A,** Bicuspid aortic valve by 2D transthoracic echocardiography (TTE) parasternal short-axis view. In this view, the valve has the typical "fish mouth" bicuspid look, and no raphe is clearly visible. **B,** 2DTTE parasternal short-axis view. In this image, the main closure of the bicuspid valve is shown from the 12:30 to 6:30 o'clock positions (*arrow*). There is also a small raphe shown at the 9:00 o'clock position, in the area where the right and noncoronary cusp would fuse if this were a trileaflet valve. **C,** 2DTTE, parasternal short-axis view. In this image, a small amount of aortic regurgitation is shown (*red arrow*). The raphe shown in **B** is seen again (*white arrow*). **D,** Image of the aortic regurgitation and the raphe shown in **C** (see Video 4-2). **E,** 2DTTE parasternal short axis view. The raphe seen in **C** is again seen, as well as the closure line of the bicuspid valve at the 1:00 and 6:30 o'clock positions (see Video 4-3). **F,** RT3D transesophageal echocardiography (TEE) image of the bicuspid aortic valve closed. The raphe seen by 2D in **C** is shown in 3D here. This emphasizes how the raphe is more complex and longer than appreciated by the 2D image.

Continued

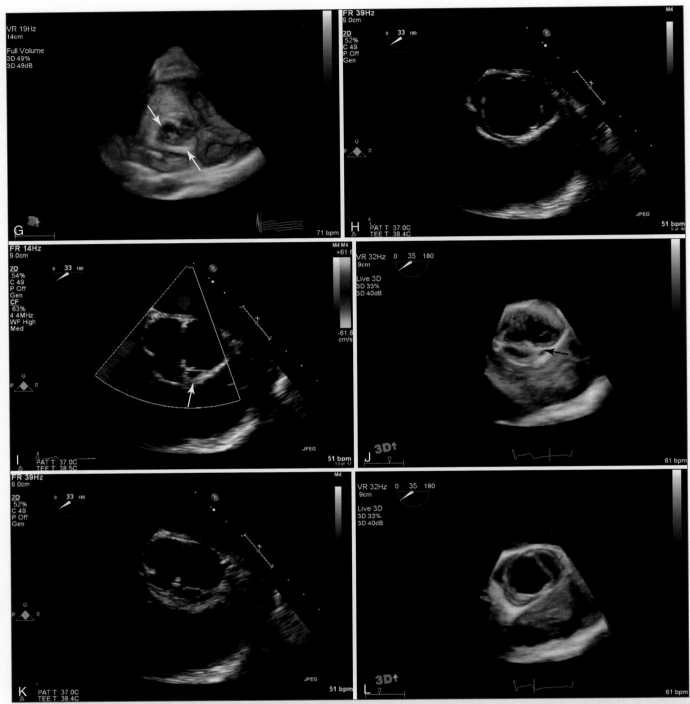

Figure 4-5, cont'd   G, RT3DTTE image showing that there are two raphes, one at approximately the 11:00 o'clock position and one at the 5:00 o'clock position. Again, the anatomy of the raphes is appreciated better than in 2D (see Video 4-4). **H,** 2DTEE image of the bicuspid aortic valve taken at an angle of 33 degrees. Note that with the aortic valve completely open in mid-systole, the raphes are not seen. **I,** 2DTEE image of the bicuspid aortic valve. Note the aortic regurgitation; the orientation of the valve is now opposite the transthoracic orientation, with the posterior at the top of the image. Note the complex raphe near the anterior opening of the valve (*arrow*). **J,** RT3DTEE of the bicuspid aortic valve. Note the additional raphes seen with RT3DE that were not seen in the 2DTEE images (*arrow*). **K,** 2DTEE of the bicuspid aortic valve. Note the raphes present, but the lack of perception of depth in the 2D image (see Video 4-5). **L,** RT3DTEE of the bicuspid aortic valve. Note the "fish mouth" appearance of the aortic valve opening as well as the depth perception of the aortic valve leaflets.

Continued

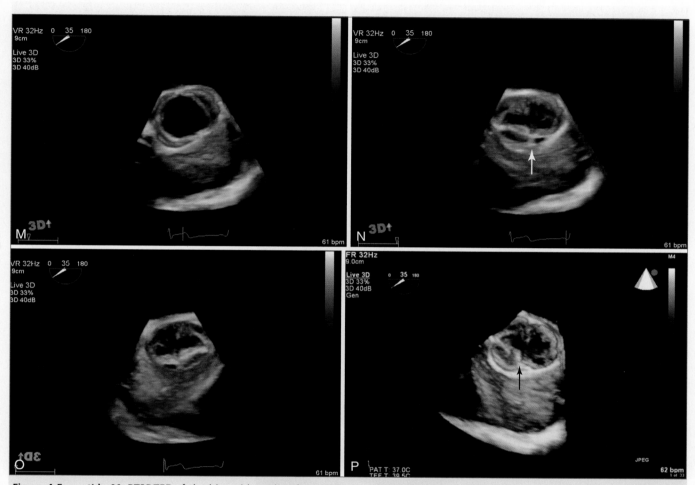

Figure 4-5, cont'd   M, RT3DTEE of the bicuspid aortic valve. As opposed to **L,** the valve is more open as it is captured in mid-systole. Note that this is frame 9 of the cardiac cycle. **N,** RT3DTEE showing raphe formation at the 9:00 and 6:00 o'clock positions in this bicuspid aortic valve (see Videos 4-6 and 4-7). **O,** RT3DTEE of the bicuspid aortic valve taken from the opposite side of the valve. In this case, the image is taken from the aortic side of the valve (see Video 4-8). **P,** RT3DTEE with the transducer at 35 degrees shows the closed bicuspid valve with raphes present at the 9:00 and 6:00 o'clock positions and thickening of the tissue associated with the raphe.

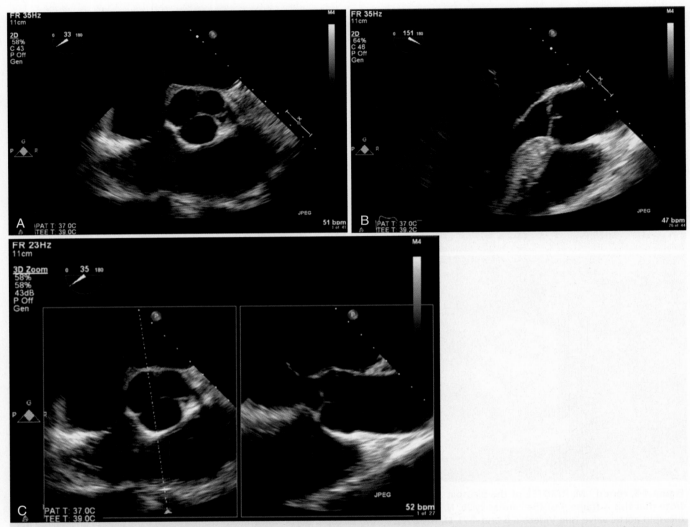

Figure 4-6 Two-dimensional (2D) transesophageal echocardiography (TEE) views of the aortic valve. **A,** Short-axis view of the aortic valve by RT3DTEE with the transducer at 35 degrees. **B,** Long-axis view of the aortic valve with the transducer at 150 degrees (see Videos 4-9 and 4-10). **C,** The setup for going to RT3DTEE in the 3D zoom mode. Image of the biplane, or "X-plane," view is shown at *left.* Note that the aortic valve is shown simultaneously in orthogonal views (35 degrees and roughly 150 degrees) (see Video 4-11).

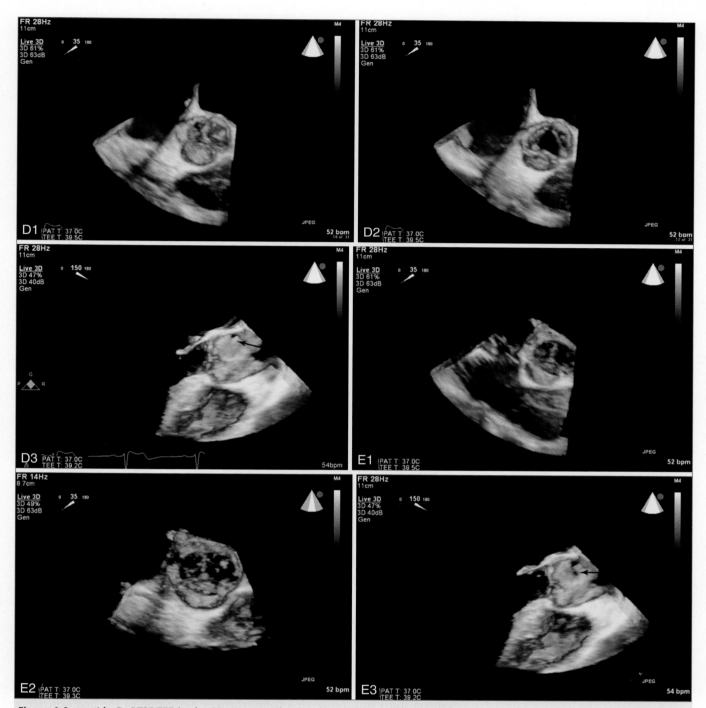

Figure 4-6, cont'd   D, RT3DTEE in the 3D zoom mode. *D1,* Short-axis view of the aortic valve (closed); *D2,* short-axis view of the aortic valve (open); *D3,* long-axis view of the aortic valve. Note the coronary artery shown coming off the sinus of Valsalva (*arrow*). **E,** RT3DTEE in the 3D zoom mode. *E1,* Short-axis view of the aortic valve (with right ventricular outflow tract more anterior and tricuspid valve); *E2,* short-axis view of the aortic valve (zoomed); *E3,* long-axis view of the aortic valve. Note the coronary artery shown coming off the sinus of Valsalva (*arrow*) (see Videos 4-12 to 4-14).

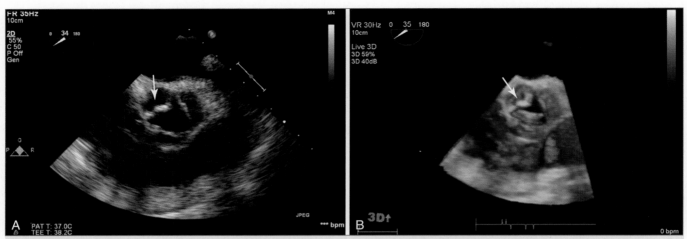

Figure 4-7   Aortic sclerosis shown by (**A**) two-dimensional (2D) transesophageal echocardiography (TEE) and (**B**) real-time three-dimensional (3D) TEE. In both cases, a short-axis view at an angle near 35 degrees is shown. There is particular sclerosis of the noncoronary cusp seen in both 2D and 3D (*arrows*). The extent of the sclerosis throughout the entire cusp is more readily apparent on the 3D image (see Videos 4-15 to 4-17).

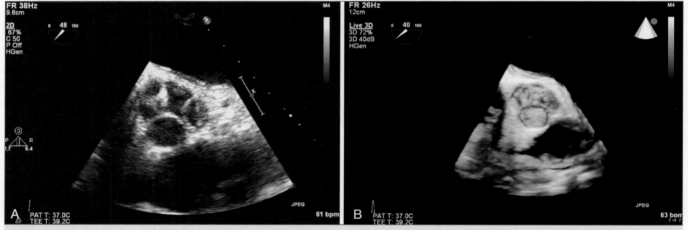

Figure 4-8   Quadricuspid valve. **A,** Two-dimensional transesophageal echocardiography (TEE) short-axis view of a quadricuspid valve. Note that the cusp at the 2 o'clock position is substantially smaller than the others. **B,** Real-time three-dimensional (RT3D) TEE short-axis view of the quadricuspid valve. The major difference and advantage appreciated in RT3DTEE is the ability to see the body of the aortic valve cusps. This also gives a more realistic perspective of the relative sizes of the cusps (see Videos 4-18 and 4-19).

using RT3DTTE. Previously, there had been multiple reports of the general use of RT3DTTE to visualize many structures, including the aortic valve.[7] Blot-Souleti's study was, however, a comprehensive evaluation of the first experience with RT3DTTE. Later, several case reports of imaging bicuspid aortic valves by RT3DTTE appeared. Imaging of a quadricuspid aortic valve by RT3DTTE was described by Aggarwal, Burri, and Chen, and that of the unicuspid aortic valve by Matsumoto.[8-11] In the first report, the right upper sinus of Valsalva ruptured into the right atrium, which was well visualized by RT3DTTE as well as color RT3DTTE. **Figure 4-8** shows a quadricuspid valve by 2DE and RT3DTEE (**Videos 4-18** and **4-19**).

As previously mentioned, the accuracy of imaging the aortic valve area in aortic stenosis by RT3DTTE has been compared with the 2D continuity equation and TEE planimetry, with a correlation of 0.82 and 0.94, respectively.[12] Furthermore, aortic stenosis imaging accuracy by RT3DTTE was compared with catheterization and planimetry by 2DTEE, and only very small absolute differences (between

0.01 and 0.15 cm) were noted.[13] Aortic annular motion is a significant pitfall in measuring the aortic valve area by 2DTEE planimetry. This seems to be at least partially overcome by using the volumetric data obtained by RT3DTEE.[14]

Aortic regurgitation severity has been evaluated by RT3DE using the 3D color vena contracta method. In this comparison, the vena contracta severity was favorably compared with a gold standard of magnetic resonance imaging phase contrast regurgitant volume and regurgitant fraction.

BICUSPID AORTIC VALVE PATHOLOGY AND REAL-TIME THREE-DIMENSIONAL ECHOCARDIOGRAPHY

Bicuspid aortic valves typically can be diagnosed with 2DTTE imaging, although in some patients transthoracic imaging is inadequate and 2DTEE is necessary. However, RT3DE imaging can visualize the presence or absence of a raphe between the fused cusps as well as the relationship of the raphe to the other cusps and the coronary arteries. This characterization is useful from a prognostic standpoint, since bicuspid aortic valves with an anterior or posterior orientation with the coronary arteries arising from the anterior cusp have more complications and less longevity than the right or left orientation. Furthermore, bicuspid valves with a raphe have a worse prognosis than those without.[15-17] Also, the presence or absence of a raphe as well as presence of a cleft have been reported to affect surgical repair in patients who have valve preservation surgery.[18] Hence, imaging of the bicuspid valve morphology by RT3DE becomes important because (1) bicuspid aortic valve is the most common congenital heart defect, present in 2% of the population; and (2) RT3DE is the imaging test of choice to evaluate for the presence and extent of a raphe. Examples of RT3DTEE views of bicuspid aortic valves are shown in **Figure 4-9** (**Videos 4-20** and **4-21.**)

ENDOCARDITIS OF THE AORTIC VALVE AND REAL-TIME THREE-DIMENSIONAL ECHOCARDIOGRAPHY

Endocarditis is a significant cause of aortic regurgitation in adult patients with trileaflet aortic valves. In addition, when an abscess cavity develops in endocarditis, the aortic valve is involved in 83% of the cases. Evaluation of endocarditis by RT3DE has been shown to improve the accuracy of vegetation size and morphology and also aid in the diagnosis of abscess cavity associated

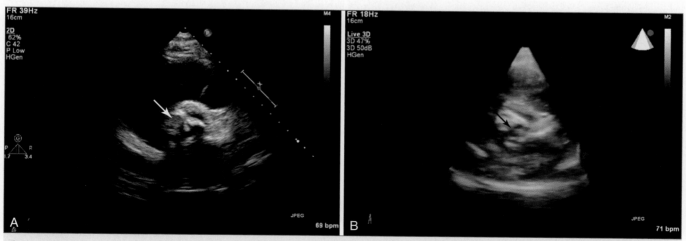

Figure 4-9   A bicuspid valve with a possible vegetation present. The two-dimensional transesophageal echocardiography (2DTEE) image (**A**) has a higher frame rate (38 Hz) compared with the corresponding three-dimensional (3D) image (18 Hz) (**B**). As a consequence, it is easier to see that the mass on the aortic valve is undulating and has movement and is independent of the aortic valve. The real-time 3DTEE image shows the body of the aortic valve cusp in more detail compared with the corresponding 2D image. As it turned out, the patient's blood cultures were negative and did not meet the Duke criteria for endocarditis despite having this mass (see Videos 4-20 and 4-21).

with the endocarditis process. For aortic valve endocarditis specifically, both RT3DTTE and RT3DTEE have been used extensively to determine aortic valve cusp integrity and to diagnose an abscess cavity associated with the aortic valve. **Figure 4-10** shows several examples of aortic valve endocarditis visualized by RT3DTEE (**Videos 4-22 to 4-26**).

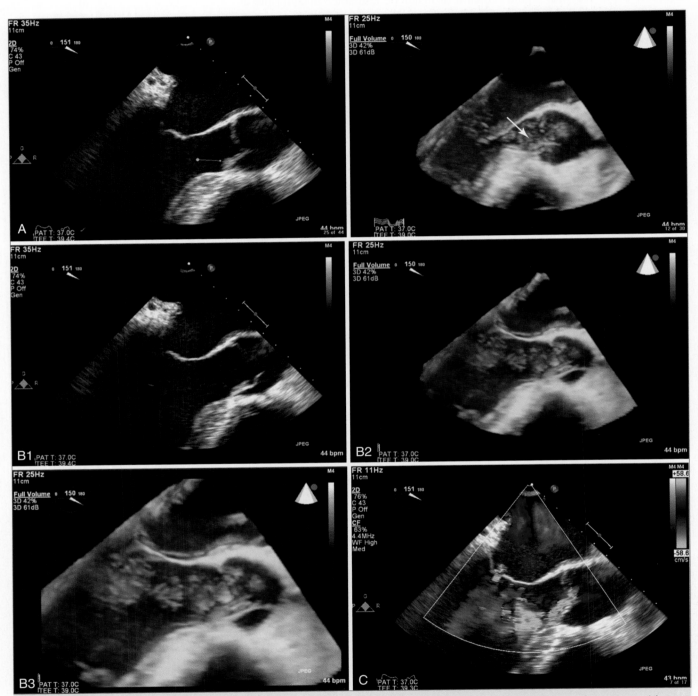

Figure 4-10 Endocarditis. Real-time (RT) three-dimensional (3D) transesophageal echocardiography (TEE) view of a patient with a vegetation on the aortic valve (*right, arrow*). The two-dimensional (2D) TEE view is shown for comparison (*left, blue line*). The 3D image reveals the actual shape of the vegetation to be papillary in nature. **B1,** 2DTEE with the transducer at 151 degrees showing the aortic valve vegetation (same view as **A**). **B2,** RT3DTEE image of a vegetation on the aortic valve. **B3,** A more zoomed RT3DTEE image of the vegetation on the aortic valve (see Videos 4-22 to 4-24). **C,** 2DTEE with the transducer at 151 degrees showing aortic regurgitation as a result of the vegetation on the aortic valve. Note that in this case aortic regurgitation is directed at the area where the aortic vegetation is located, possibly contributing to the reason that the vegetation was present in this location.

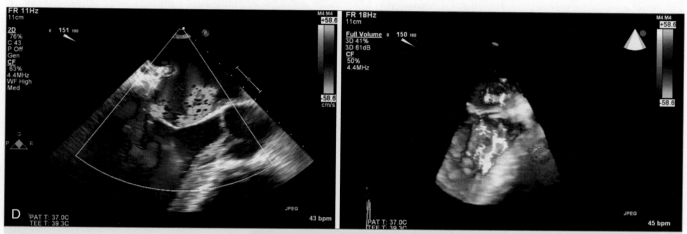

Figure 4-10, cont'd   **D,** 2DTEE (*left*) and RT3DTEE (*right*) of aortic regurgitation showing the aortic regurgitation jet hitting the area where the aortic vegetation is located. Hence, the aortic regurgitation jet is possibly contributing to why the vegetation was present in this location (see Videos 4-25 and 4-26).

INTERVENTIONAL PROCEDURES AND THE AORTIC VALVE BY REAL-TIME THREE-DIMENSIONAL ECHOCARDIOGRAPHY

Interventional procedures involving the aortic valve, including transcatheter aortic valve implantation, closure of paraaortic prosthetic aortic valvular leak, closure of sinus of Valsalva ruptured aneurysm, and closure of aortic root pseudoaneurysms have all been described with RT3DTTE or RT3DTEE guidance.[19] Closure of paraaortic prosthetic aortic valvular leak, in fact, is quite difficult to perform without RT3DTEE. **Figure 4-11** shows imaging of a transcatheter-placed aortic valve by RT3DTEE. Evaluation of the aortic annulus size has been shown to be more accurate by 3DTEE than by 2DTEE when compared with magnetic resonance imaging.

PROSTHETIC AORTIC VALVES

Although prosthetic valve imaging by RT3DE is covered in Chapter 8, it is important to mention RT3DE imaging specifically for the aortic position. The good news is that on the basis of my experience, there is less shadowing from the prosthetic valves with RT3DE than with traditional 2DE. This, however, is not easily explained, since RT3DE still uses ultrasound and shadowing artifact from prosthetic material remains a significant limitation. So, this is a small triumph. However, the unfortunate news is that compared with the mitral valve, the aortic valve remains much more difficult to image by any echocardiography modality. And, as in the 2D realm, although TEE helps dramatically with mitral imaging, TEE helps only to a certain extent for imaging the aortic valve. Finally, in the case of patients with mechanical prosthetic valves in both the mitral and aortic positions, aortic valve imaging remains a substantial challenge. **Figure 4-12** shows an example of imaging of a prosthetic aortic valve by RT3DTEE. Further aortic valve images of interest are shown in **Figures 4-13 to 4-18; Videos 4-27 to 4-34**).

SUMMARY

Aortic regurgitation, particularly aortic stenosis, is a frequent problem. RT3DE has been shown to be useful in a variety of settings in which the aortic valve is involved in the disease process. The elevation dimension of RT3DE has proved to be particularly useful for viewing the aortic cusps and has definite advantages over the use of standard 2DE imaging. In the future, it would be expected that color Doppler using RT3DE would improve and would further aid in the quantification of aortic regurgitation. Finally, for some interventional procedures involving the aortic valve, RT3DTEE has proved to be indispensable.

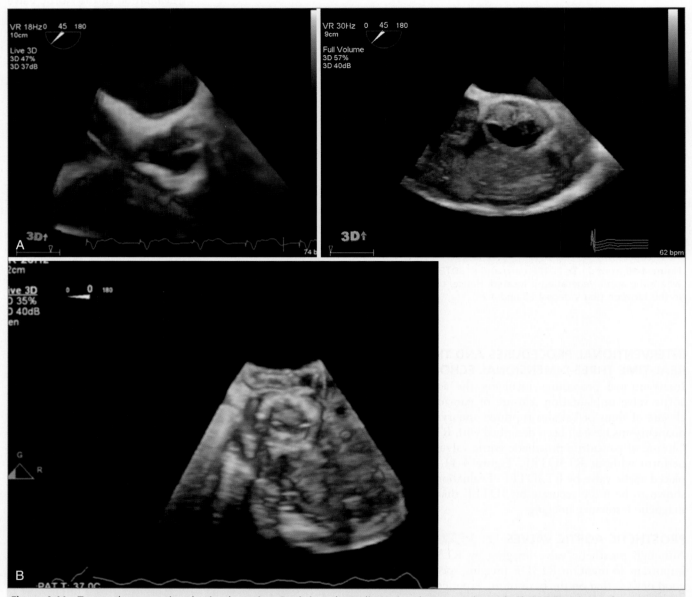

Figure 4-11 Transcatheter aortic valve implantation. Real-time three-dimensional transesophageal echocardiography of a properly positioned stent valve (**A**) and a stent valve that has prolapsed into the left ventricular outflow tract (**B**).

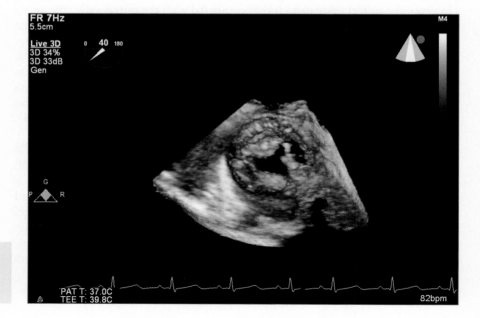

Figure 4-12 Real-time three-dimensional transesophageal echocardiography of a bioprosthetic valve, open, in the aortic position.

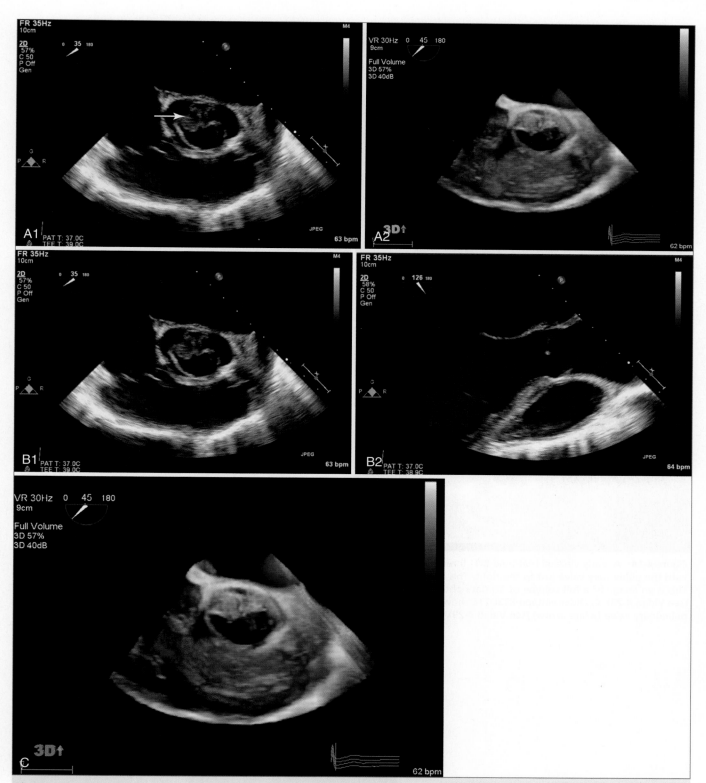

Figure 4-13   A, A bicuspid valve with a prominent nodule is seen by two-dimensional (2D) transesophageal echocardiography (TEE; *A1*) and real-time (RT) three-dimensional (3D) TEE (*A2*). The nodule seen in the 2D image (*arrow*) is seen also in RT3DTEE with added depth perception. **B,** Same patient as in **A.** *B1,* The same 2DTEE short-axis view is seen, again with the prominent nodule. *B2,* The 2DTEE long-axis view (125-degree view) is shown, with the nodule prolapsing into the left ventricular outflow tract. This lesion led to suspicion of endocarditis. The patient, however, did not have positive blood culture results for endocarditis and did not meet the Duke criteria for endocarditis (see Video 4-27). **C,** Repeat view of the RT3DTEE view of the nodule.

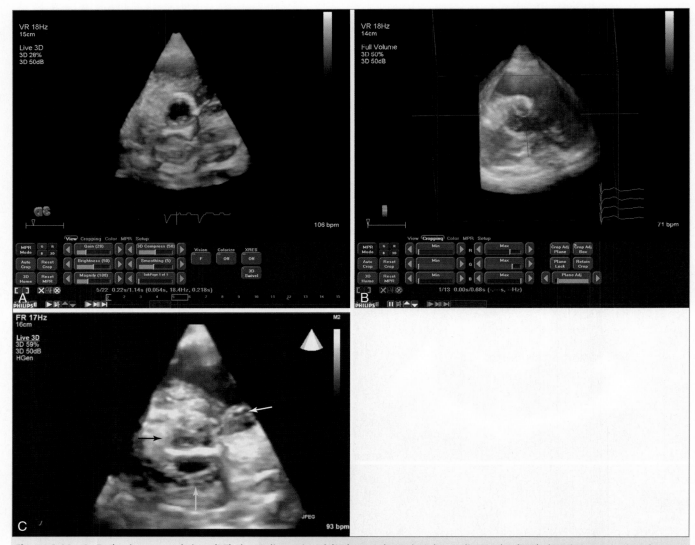

Figure 4-14   A, Early vintage real-time (RT) three-dimensional (3D) transthoracic echocardiography (TTE) showing an aortic valve with the pulmonary valve just to the right. This image was created via cropping in the software program QLab. **B,** Cropping in QLab. This is an image of a full volume of 3D data obtained by RT3DTTE. In this case, the volume set is cropped to show the aortic valve (see Video 4-28). **C,** Older vintage RT3DTTE showing simultaneous aortic valve (*black arrow*), mitral valve (*yellow arrow*), and pulmonary valve (*white arrow*) (see Video 4-29).

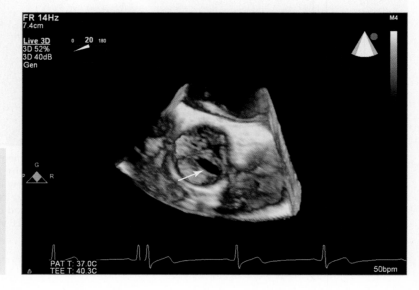

Figure 4-15   Real-time three-dimensional transesophageal echocardiography image of aortic valve showing the limitation of dropout. In this case, a notable dropout of the right coronary cusp (*arrow*) is seen (see Video 4-30). There is a tradeoff with the gain in these types of cases between showing increased gain to eliminate dropout but, at the same time, not being able to visualize the body of the aortic valve cusp.

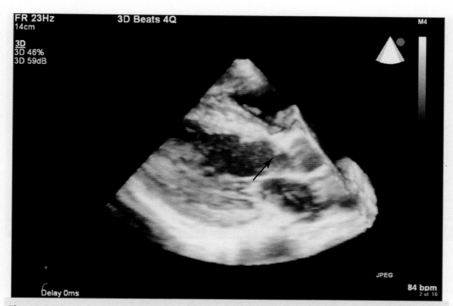

Figure 4-16 Subaortic membrane (*arrow*) by real-time three-dimensional transthoracic echocardiography (see Video 4-31).

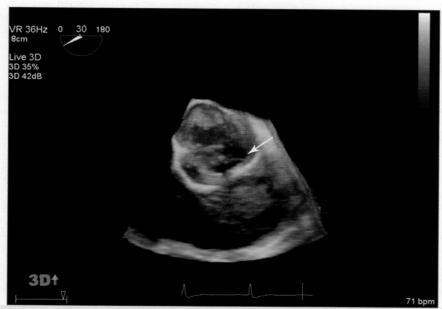

Figure 4-17 A patient with systemic lupus erythematosus has lack of cusp coaptation at the central point (*arrow*) (see Video 4-32).

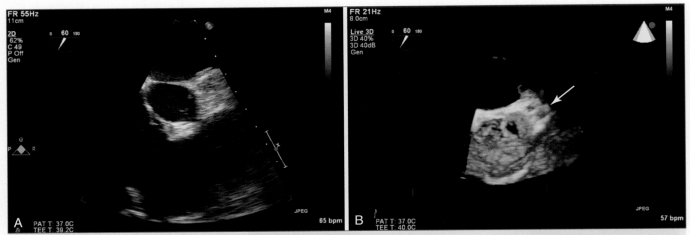

Figure 4-18 Two-dimensional (2D) transesophageal echocardiography (TEE) (**A**) and real-time (RT) three-dimensional (3D) TEE (**B**) of the aortic valve showing the coronary arteries. The 2DTEE image of the aortic valve shows the bifurcation of the left main artery into the left anterior descending (LAD) and circumflex (Cx) coronary arteries (*arrow*). The RT3DTEE view uses the elevation dimension to show the left main as well as the two bifurcating arteries (LAD and Cx). In the 2D image, the LAD and Cx arteries are seen, but the left main artery is into the plane and therefore not seen simultaneously (see Videos 4-33 and 4-34).

References

1. Hanke T, Charitos EI, Stierle U, et al: The Ross operation—a feasible and safe option in the setting of a bicuspid aortic valve? *Eur J Cardiothorac Surg* 38:333–339, 2010.
2. Ren B, Tang H, Kang Y: Visualisation of the aortic annulus using the real-time three-dimensional transesophageal echocardiography. *Heart* 97:862–863, 2011.
3. Janosi RA, Kahlert P, Plicht B, et al: Measurement of the aortic annulus size by real-time three-dimensional transesophageal echocardiography. *Minim Invasive Ther Allied Technol* 20:85–94, 2011.
4. Otani K, Takeuchi M, Kaku K, et al: Assessment of the aortic root using real-time 3D transesophageal echocardiography. *Circ J* 74:2649–2657, 2010.
5. Dvir D, Kornowski R: Percutaneous aortic valve implantation using novel imaging guidance. *Catheter Cardiovasc Interv* 76:450–454, 2010.
6. Subramanian R, Olson LJ, Edwards WD: Surgical pathology of pure aortic stenosis: A study of 374 cases. *Mayo Clin Proc* 59:683–690, 1984.
7. Pepi M, Tamborini G, Pontone G, et al: Initial experience with a new on-line transthoracic three-dimensional technique: Assessment of feasibility and of diagnostic potential. *Ital Heart J* 4:544–550, 2003.
8. Aggarwal SK, Lingan A, Reddy KK, et al: Quadricuspid aortic valve with ruptured sinus of valsalva aneurysm to the right atrium. *Echocardiography* 26:977–979, 2009.
9. Burri MV, Nanda NC, Singh A, Panwar SR: Live/real time three-dimensional transthoracic echocardiographic identification of quadricuspid aortic valve. *Echocardiography* 24:653–655, 2007.
10. Chen M, McRee D: An incidentally discovered quadricuspid aortic valve: Echocardiographic and clinical characteristics. *J Diagn Med Sonogr* 25:93–96, 2009.
11. Matsumoto K, Tanaka H, Hiraishi M, et al: A case of unicommissural unicuspid aortic valve stenosis diagnosed by real time three-dimensional transesophageal echocardiography. *Echocardiography* 28:E172–E173, 2011.
12. Blot-Souletie N, Hebrard A, Acar P, et al: Comparison of accuracy of aortic valve area assessment in aortic stenosis by real time three-dimensional echocardiography in biplane mode versus two-dimensional transthoracic and transesophageal echocardiography. *Echocardiography* 24:1065–1072, 2007.
13. Goland S, Trento A, Iida K, et al: Assessment of aortic stenosis by three-dimensional echocardiography: An accurate and novel approach. *Heart* 93:801–807, 2007.
14. Nakai H, Takeuchi M, Yoshitani H, et al: Pitfalls of anatomical aortic valve area measurements using two-dimensional transoesophageal echocardiography and the potential of three-dimensional transoesophageal echocardiography. *Eur J Echocardiogr* 11:369–376, 2010.
15. Schaefer BM, Lewin MB, Stout KK, et al: The bicuspid aortic valve: An integrated phenotypic classification of leaflet morphology and aortic root shape. *Heart* 94:1634–1638, 2008.
16. Guntheroth W: Risk of aortic dissection in patients with bicuspid aortic valves. *Am J Cardiol* 107:958, 2011.
17. Iqtidar AF, O'Rourke DJ, Silverman DI, et al: Predictors of rapid aortic dilatation in adults with a bicuspid aortic valve. *J Heart Valve Dis* 20:292–298, 2011.
18. Mangini A, Lemma M, Contino M, et al: Bicuspid aortic valve: Differences in the phenotypic continuum affect the repair technique. *Eur J Cardiothorac Surg* 37:1015–1020, 2010.
19. Hoffmayer KS, Zellner C, Kwan DM, et al: Closure of a paravalvular aortic leak: With the use of 2 AMPLATZER devices and real-time 2- and 3-dimensional transesophageal echocardiography. *Tex Heart Inst J* 38:81–84, 2011.

Normal Mitral Valve Anatomy and Measurements

Jennifer L. Dorosz and Ernesto E. Salcedo

The complexity of the mitral valve is such that two-dimensional (2D) imaging does not adequately describe its anatomy and function. Indeed, the mitral valve apparatus is a dynamic three-dimensional (3D) structure composed of the saddle-shaped annulus; two asymmetric leaflets; multiple chordae tendineae of various lengths, thicknesses, and points of attachment; the left ventricular wall and the attached papillary muscles; and parts of the left atrium (**Figure 5-1**). During normal function, this array of parts constantly shifts in a complex but defined pattern. Normal alignment of all aspects of this biologic machine is required to avoid dysfunction. Therefore, full understanding of the mitral valve anatomy is not ascertained without 3D imaging. Real-time 3D echocardiography (RT3DE) gives echocardiographers a rapid and easily accessible method of identifying the entire mitral valve apparatus in most patients. As a prominent structure in the posterior left heart, the mitral valve often can be displayed in 3D using either a transthoracic approach or a transesophageal approach. Furthermore, detailed volumetric and positional analysis of the various mitral valve components often is possible (Table 5-1). RT3DE, however, is a novel modality, and its use in mastering the analysis of the intricate mitral valve requires a substantial time commitment. This chapter highlights the use of RT3DE in imaging the normal mitral valve, demonstrating usual transthoracic and transesophageal views for each of its components. It also provides an overview of typical 3D quantitative analyses of the size and position of the mitral valve structures.

MITRAL VALVE ANNULUS

3DE has increased the understanding of the anatomy of the mitral valve annulus more than that of any other structure in the heart. 3D reconstructions identified the mitral valve annulus as a hyperbolic paraboloid or a saddle-shaped structure with curved planes parallel to the anteroposterior axis opening upward and orthogonal curved planes that open downward (**Figure 5-2**).[1] This complex shape is not appreciated on 2D imaging, which tends to simplify the annulus as a planar ring. In fact, the anterior and posterior portions of the mitral valve annulus are about 5 mm higher than the medial and lateral commissural points.[1] This height, along with the commissural diameter (the distance between the two low points) and the anteroposterior diameter (the distance between the two high points), can be easily measured with 3D imaging. The nonplanar shape of the mitral valve annulus is very important in reducing leaflet stress, which is increased when the annulus flattens.[2] As such, the hyperbolic paraboloid annular shape with a height/commissural width ratio of 15% to 20% is preserved in many mammalian species, including humans.[2-4]

RT3DE is fundamental to clarifying annular geometry. In fact, obtaining accurate annular dimensions is best done with 3D datasets because 2DE underestimates these values by 6% to 14%.[5] The mitral valve annulus is best seen using the large-sector (3D full volume) and wide-sector focused (3D zoom) formats. In particular, computer remodeling from large-sector datasets can quickly measure and display these changes without requiring the

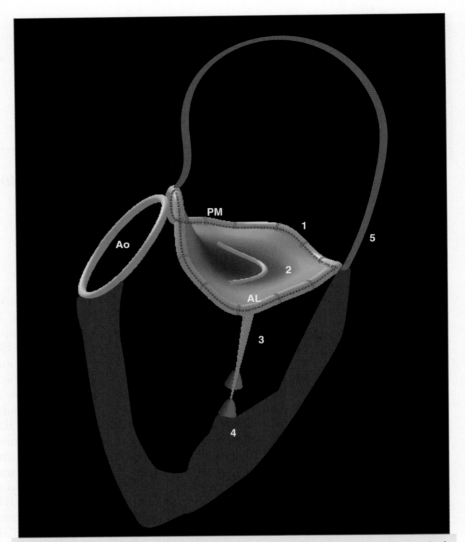

Figure 5-1 The mitral valve apparatus as it sits in the left ventricle. It is composed of the annulus (*1*), the leaflets (*2*), chordae (*3*), papillary muscles and ventricular wall (*4*), and atrium (*5*). *AL*, anterolateral commissure; *Ao*, aorta; *PM*, posteromedial commissure.

time-consuming reconstructions from multiple 2D images. 3D volume data can be obtained from either transthoracic or transesophageal exams. These models are obtained offline by tracing the mitral valve annulus contours in relation to other structures (such as the papillary muscles and aortic valve) in several 3D views (**Figure 5-3**). From these computer renditions, several annular dimensions, including circumference, anteroposterior (high-point) dimension, commissural (low-point) dimension, height, and annular area, can be measured (**Figure 5-4**).[6]

Recognizing the mitral valve annulus as a nonplanar structure is very important to understanding mitral valve function. For example, the complex shape of the mitral valve annulus has led to the overdiagnosis of mitral valve prolapse with 2DE. In certain 2D views, particularly the apical four-chamber view, which shows the mitral valve annulus in mediolateral directions, the leaflets appear to be on the atrial side of the mitral valve annulus, when, in fact, they are still inferior to the high anterior and posterior points. In 2DE imaging without fully realizing the nonplanarity of the mitral valve annulus, this normal anatomy can be mischaracterized as mitral valve prolapse.[1]

RT3DE has also shown that annular area significantly depends on body size and height.[7] The normal diastolic mitral valve area (which is a projection onto

Table 5-1 Key Normal Measurements Obtained by Real-Time Three-Dimensional Echocardiography for Each Mitral Valve Structure

Key Measurements	Normal Values	Reference
Mitral Valve Annulus		
Anteroposterior dimension	30.8 ± 4.4 mm	Sonne et al[7]
	24 ± 1 mm	Kwan et al[41]
Commissural dimension	35.1 ± 4.9 mm	Sonne et al[7]
	28 ± 1 mm	Kwan et al[41]
Circumference	10.5 ± 1.4 mm	Sonne et al[7]
	10.0 ± 0.8 mm	Watanabe et al[40]
Height	4.3 ± 2.1 mm	Sonne et al[7]
	3.0 ± 1.0 mm	Flachskampf et al[12]
	4.5 ± 1.1 mm	Watanabe et al[40]
Area/BSA (end diastole)	4.6 ± 1.3 cm^2/m^2	Qin et al[10]
	5.9 ± 1.2 cm^2/m^2	Flachskampf et al[12]
Area/BSA (mid systole)	5.1 ± 0.8 cm^2/m^2	Sonne et al[7]
Area/BSA (end systole)	3.8 ± 1.1 cm^2/m^2	Qin et al[10]
Area change	23.8% ± 5.1%	Flachskampf et al[12]
	15% ± 16%	Qin et al[10]
Linear systolic motion	16 ± 3 mm	Qin et al[10]
	10 ± 3 mm	Flachskampf et al[12]
Mitral Valve Leaflets		
Volume	4.5 ± 0.7 cm^3	Limbu et al[28]
Maximum tenting height	5.3 ± 2.4 mm	Sonne et al[7]
	3.1 ± 1.2 mm	Watanabe et al[40]
	5 ± 0.2 mm	Kalyanasundaram et al[5]
Mean tenting height	1.9 ± 1.5 mm	Sonne et al[7]
	0.7 ± 0.5 mm	Watanabe et al[40]
Tenting volume	1.5 ± 0.9 cm^3	Sonne et al[7]
	0.45 ± 0.29 cm^3	Watanabe et al[40]
Papillary Muscles (Indexed to BSA)		
AL papillary to annular distance	21.0 ± 5.8 mm/m^2	Sonne et al[7]
PM papillary to annular distance	22.3 ± 5.6 mm/m^2	Sonne et al[7]
Interpapillary muscle angle	17.6 ± 9.1 degrees/m^2	Sonne et al[7]
Interpapillary distance	10.5 ± 3.3 mm/m^2	Sonne et al[7]
Left Ventricle		
End-systolic volume	43.7 ± 10.7 mL	Chukwu et al[56]
	59 ± 18 mL	Corsi et al[69]
	43 ± 18 mL	Zeidan et al[70]
	47 ± 6 mL	Nosir et al[71]
End-diastolic volume	115 ± 22.6 mL	Chukwu et al[56]
	143 ± 30 mL	Corsi et al[69]
	108 ± 32 mL	Zeidan et al[70]
	113 ± 16 mL	Nosir et al[71]
Left Atrium		
End-diastolic volume	48.9 ± 25.1 cm^3	Azar et al[68]
End-systolic volume	62.3 ± 17.2 cm^3	Azar et al[68]

In some cases, values vary due to technique and studied population.
AL, anterolateral; *BSA*, body surface area; *PM*, posteromedial.

the least squares plane) is 5 to 6.5 cm^2 (indexed to body service area).[8] The mitral valve annulus, however, is a dynamic structure whose complex motion throughout the cardiac cycle has not been fully ascertained.[9-11] On the basis of early studies in 3DE from 2D renditions, it was believed that the mitral valve area decreases during systole by up to 24%, which is thought to occur as the anterior and lateral high points move closer together, increasing the height and eccentricity of the annulus.[8,12] In addition to a decrease in annular area, there is a significant apical displacement of the annulus during systole, with an average annular motion of 16 ± 3 mm in normal hearts.[10]

Recent investigations using RT3DE with volumetric reconstructions have further characterized this motion in both normal ventricles and those with

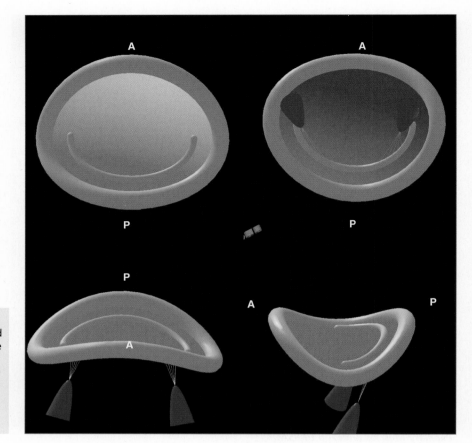

Figure 5-2 The mitral value annulus as a hyperbolic paraboloid with anterior (*A*) and posterior (*P*) peaks that are higher than the plane containing the commissures. In this figure, the papillary muscles are in red. The *top left image* shows the annulus from the left atrial side. The *top right image* demonstrates the annulus from the left ventricular view.

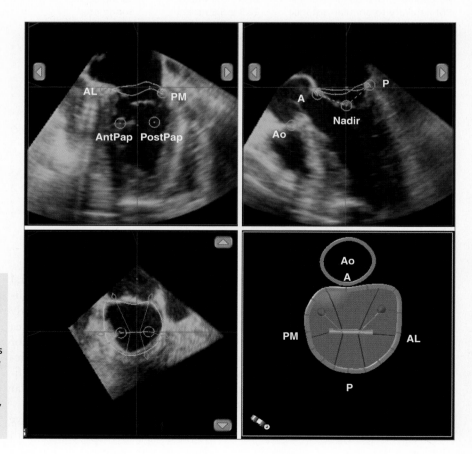

Figure 5-3 A computer rendition of the mitral value annulus (*bottom left*) obtained by identifying key annular structures on a three-dimensional full-volume dataset cropped to form several different views (two-chamber view at the *top left,* long-axis view on the *top right,* and a short-axis view on the *bottom left*). A, anterior; AL, anterolateral commissure; AntPap, anterior papillary muscle; Ao, aorta; P, posterior; PM, posteromedial commissure; PostPap, posterior papillary muscle.

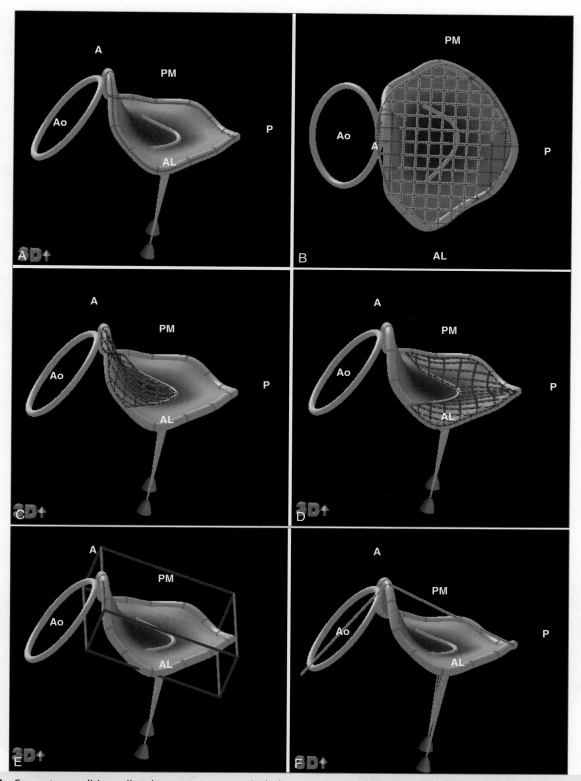

Figure 5-4   Computer renditions allow key measurements, including annular circumference (**A**); annular area (**B**); anterior leaflet area (**C**); posterior leaflet area (**D**); annular height, commissural distance, and anteroposterior distance (**E**); and aortic-mitral angle (**F**). A, anterior; AL, anterolateral; Ao, aortic valve; P, posterior; PM, posteromedial.

cardiomyopathy. In disease states, the shape and dynamic function of the mitral valve can change dramatically. For example, in dilated cardiomyopathy, especially with functional mitral regurgitation, the annulus flattens, dilates, and becomes more circular.[8] These annuli also demonstrate less dynamic variability. During systole, they may have less change in height and diameter, leading to a smaller change in the projected valve area.[12,13] Most significantly, those with cardiomyopathy have less apical excursion during systole. In fact, the degree of annular displacement correlates well with ejection fraction; a linear motion less than 12 mm accurately identifies those with an ejection fraction less than 50%.[10]

MITRAL VALVE LEAFLETS

Like the annulus, the attached mitral valve leaflets are 3D dynamic structures. The anterior leaflet covers two thirds of the orifice and is attached to the part of anterior annulus adjacent to the aortic valve near the right fibrous trigone, aortic-mitral fibrosa, and left fibrous trigone (**Figure 5-5**). The posterior leaflet, although smaller, covering only one third of the mitral orifice, is semicircular in shape and borders most of the annulus from one commissure to the other.[6] Figure 5-5 shows the mitral valve leaflets and related cardiac structures as seen from the left atrium (the surgeon's view) and the left ventricle. Each leaflet is composed of three scallops. Scallops A1 and P1 are the most lateral, located near the left atrial appendage; the middle scallops, A2 and P2, are the most posterior; and A3 and P3 are the most medial.

With 3DE, all six scallops of the mitral valve leaflets can be clearly visualized from either the left atrium or the left ventricle. These views can be obtained offline from cropping 3D full-volume (large-sector) datasets, which can be obtained by either a transthoracic or a transesophageal approach (**Figure 5-6** and **Video 5-1**). During transesophageal exams, the 3D zoom (wide-sector focused) format also is helpful, especially to obtain real-time information on leaflet function during surgery or catheter procedures. In this case, the images are obtained

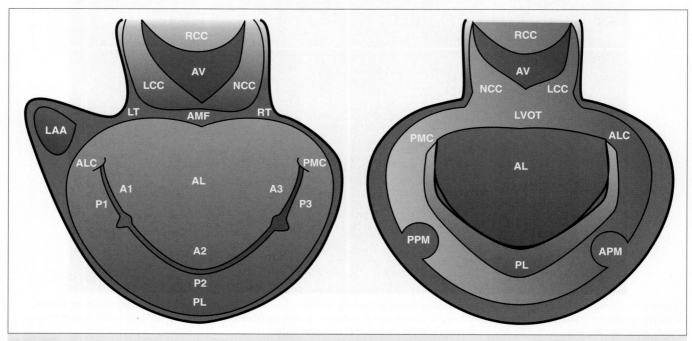

Figure 5-5 Mitral valve leaflets as viewed from the left atrium (the surgeon's view) on the *left* and as viewed from the left ventricle on the *right*. *AL*, anterior leaflet; *AMC*, anteromedial commissure; *AMF*, aortic-mitral fibrosa; *APM*, anterolateral papillary muscle; *AV*, aortic valve; *LAA*, left atrial appendage; *LCC*, left coronary cusp of aortic valve; *LT*, left trigone; *LVOT*, left ventricular outflow tract; *NCC*, noncoronary cusp of the aortic valve; *PMC*, posteromedial commissure; *PL*, posterior leaflet; *PPM*, posteromedial papillary muscle; *RCC*, right coronary cusp of the aortic valve; *RT*, right trigone.

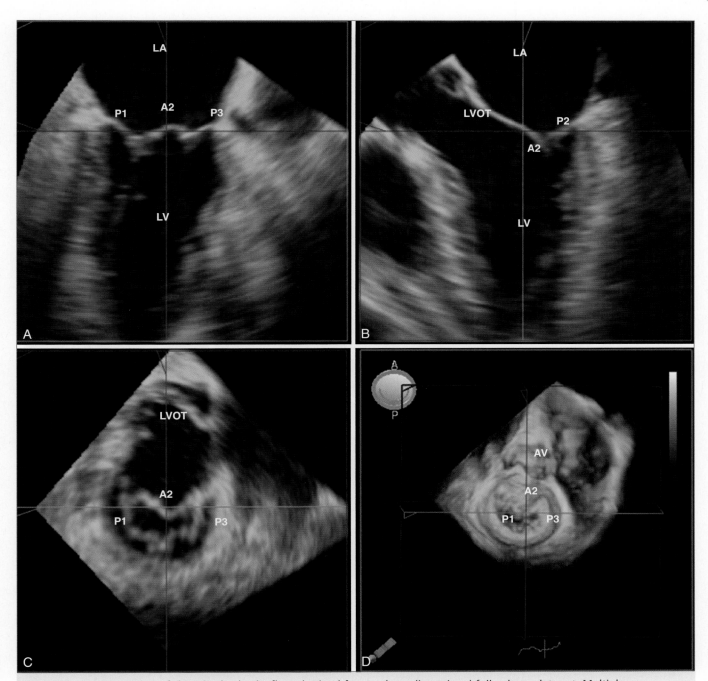

Figure 5-6 Demonstration of the mitral valve leaflets obtained from a three-dimensional full-volume data-set. Multiplane reconstructions are shown in **A** through **C.** The on-face view of the leaflets from the left atrium (*LA*) is shown in **D.** LV, left ventricle; LVOT, left ventricular outflow tract; A2, P1, P2, and P3, scallops of the mitral valve leaflets.

by identifying the entire mitral valve on orthogonal biplane 2D images. The resulting 3D zoom display is rotated with the aortic valve in the 12 o'clock position to obtain the surgeon's view from the left atrium. In this view, normal systolic bulging of the central part of the anterior leaflet can be visualized. When this image is flipped 180 degrees, the leaflet scallops are displayed as viewed from the left ventricle (**Figure 5-7**). In transthoracic exams, similarly detailed 3D images also can be obtained. **Figure 5-8** demonstrates how clearly the mitral valve leaflets can be displayed from a 3D full-volume dataset acquired during a transthoracic exam. In this case, the image is rotated and the vertical axis is cropped from the atrial side to obtain the surgeon's view. By flipping the image 180 degrees and

LA view   LV view

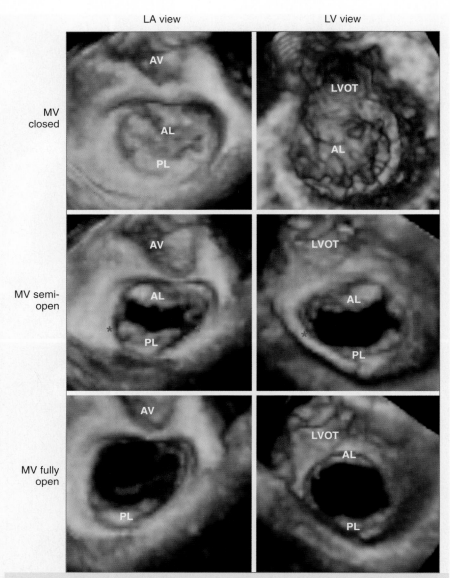

Figure 5-7   The mitral valve (*MV*) leaflets from three-dimensional wide-sector datasets obtained during a transesophageal exam. The leaflets are viewed from the left atrium (*LA*) on the *left* and from the left ventricle (*LV*) on the *right*. *Red asterisk*, anterolateral commissure; *green asterisk*, posteromedial commissure; *AL*, anterior leaflet; *AV*, aortic valve; *LVOT*, left ventricular outflow tract; *PL*, posterior leaflet.

cropping from the ventricular side, the valve leaflets can be seen as viewed from the apex in relation to the commissures and papillary muscles.

The commissures of the mitral valve are easily identified by RT3DE. The anterolateral commissure is located next to the left atrial appendage and the left fibrous trigone and represents the point of fusion between A1 and P1. The posteromedial commissure is located next to the right fibrous trigone and represents the point of fusion between A3 and P3. A short-axis view of the mitral valve using the narrow-sector format can clearly display both commissures from the atrium and the ventricle by either the transesophageal or the transthoracic approach (see Figures 5-7 and 5-8). In the transesophageal exam, the midesophageal view allows ideal visualization of both commissures. The anatomy of the commissures is of particular importance in patients with mitral valve stenosis before balloon valvuloplasty. In fact, commissural splitting is believed to be the primary mechanism of increasing valve area during balloon valvuloplasty. Thus,

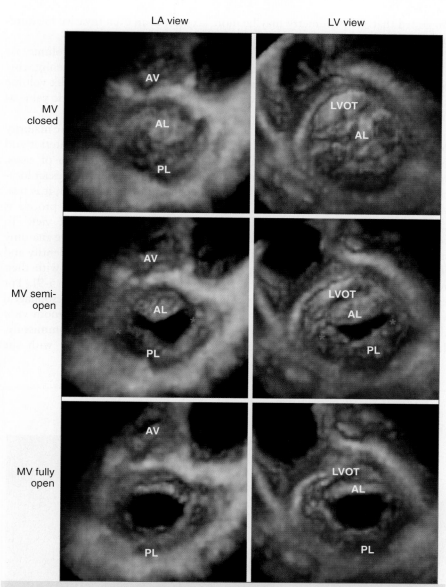

LA view   LV view

MV closed

MV semi-open

MV fully open

Figure 5-8 The mitral valve (*MV*) leaflets displayed from a cropped three-dimensional full-volume dataset obtained during a transthoracic exam. The leaflets are viewed from the left atrium (*LA*) on the *left* and from the left ventricle (*LV*) on the *right*. *Red asterisk*, anterolateral commissure; *green asterisk*, posteromedial commissure; *AL*, anterior leaflet; *AV*, aortic valve; *LVOT*, left ventricular outflow tract; *PL*, posterior leaflet.

the degree of noncalcified commissural fusion, as assessed by RT3DE, correlates with successful valvuloplasty and may be a better predictor of procedural success compared with traditional 2D scoring algorithms.[14-16] Heavily calcified commissures are unlikely to split during the procedure and should be identified before referral for valvuloplasty.[17,18]

In the evaluation of mitral stenosis, RT3DE can improve assessments of leaflet opening. In 2D, calculating valve area by planimetry is unreliable because it is difficult to determine if the traced plane intersects the valve at its smallest dimensions.[18] This limitation, however, is overcome with 3DE imaging because the entire valve can be imaged and the short-axis plane can be cropped at the smallest area.[17,19,20] As demonstrated in several studies, this method may be superior to estimating true mitral valve area when compared with 2D measurements by pressure half-time, proximal isovelocity surface area, and planimetry.[17,20-26] Some have suggested that 3D planimetry may be more accurate than even invasive measurements of mitral valve area.[21,22,27]

With RT3DE, it is also possible to ascertain mitral valve leaflet volume. As rheumatic disease progresses, the leaflets thicken. The degree of thickening correlates with complications such as atrial fibrillation and death.[28] Leaflet volume also can be assessed with RT3DE, which may have as much prognostic value as mitral valve area.[25]

RT3DE allows full assessment of the mitral valve leaflet motion in the majority of cases. Even during transthoracic exams, all three scallops of the anterior and posterior leaflets are completely visualized in up to 84% and 77% of cases, respectively.[29-32] This technology is of particular use in identifying the exact location of leaflet pathology. On transesophageal echocardiography (TEE), it is possible to see each individual scallop with 2D imaging alone, but this process is cumbersome because the entire leaflets cannot be seen in the same view. To reconstruct all six scallops, an excellent working memory of mitral valve anatomy is required, and it is necessary to rotate through the various views to identify and locate pathology. With 3D imaging, however, all six scallops, along with their relationships to other structures, can be visualized at once (**Figure 5-9**). For example, a fibroelastoma is shown in **Figure 5-10**. In the 2D transesophageal views, this tumor is easily seen on the posterior leaflet, but the 3D zoom view demonstrates its exact location on P1 very close to the anterolateral commissure. In addition, mitral valve prolapse can be easily identified in 3D with the

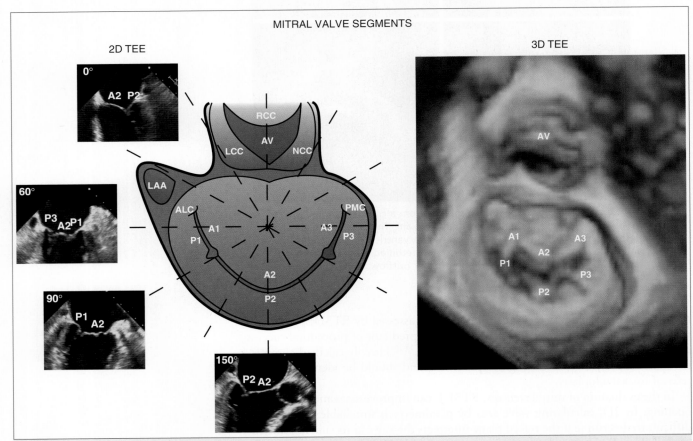

Figure 5-9 Two-dimensional (2D) imaging (*left*) shows only parts of the mitral valve leaflets in any given view. To mentally reconstruct the exact location of leaflet pathology during a 2D exam, one must have an excellent working knowledge of mitral valve anatomy. With three-dimensional imaging (*right*), the entirety of both leaflets can be seen in one view. ALC, anterolateral commissure; AV, aortic valve; LAA, left atrial appendage; LCC, left coronary cusp; NCC, noncoronary cusp; PMC, posteromedial commissure; TEE, transesophageal echocardiography; A1, A2, A3, P1, P2, and P3, scallops of the mitral valve leaflets.

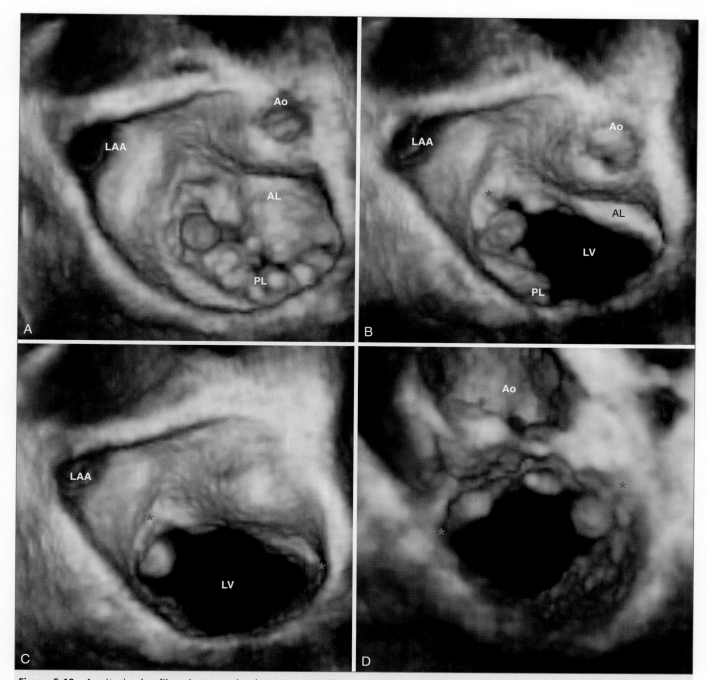

Figure 5-10   A mitral valve fibroelastoma clearly seen on P1 close to the anterolateral commissure (*red asterisk*) in this three-dimensional wide-sector view. **A** and **B** show the tumor from the surgeon's view in systole and diastole. It is also seen prolapsing into the ventricle from the left atrial view in **C.** In **D,** the tumor is seen in diastole as viewed from the apex. *Green asterisk*, posteromedial commissure. Ao, aortic valve; AL, anterior leaflet; LAA, left atrial appendage; LV, left ventricle; PL, posterior leaflet.

wide-sector focused view. As seen from the left atrium, the prolapsed segment is a bright bulge. From the ventricle, it is a spoon-shaped depression. Although 2DE may diagnose the presence of flail or prolapse in general, 3DE often is needed to identify the specific scallops involved.[32] In fact, myxomatous mitral valve disease highlights the usefulness of 3D techniques. Several studies have compared the accuracy of the various echo modalities in identifying the location of mitral valve prolapse (Table 5-2).[30,31,33-39] 3DE also can help visualize and quantify the location and size of the orifice regurgitant area that leads to mitral regurgitation. Color Doppler can be added to full-volume acquisitions. This

Table 5-2 Comparison of the Accuracy of Each Echo Modality in Identifying the Correct Location of Mitral Valve Prolapse (Validated by Surgical Inspection)

	N	2DTTE (%)	2DTEE (%)	3DTTE (%)	3DTEE (%)
Grewal et al[33]	42	—	90	—	98
Pepi et al[30]	112	77	87	90	—
Manda et al[34]	18	—	50	—	77
Muller et al[35]	74	—	86-97	—	97-100*
Fabricius et al[36]	42	—	97	—	91
Sharma et al[31]	39	82	96	—	94
Hirata et al[37]	42	97	100	—	100
Agricola et al[38]	59	—	92	94	—
Garcia-Orta et al[39]	54	67-94	89-100*	—	—

*Accuracy rates reported on each segment; entire range is given here.
2DTTE, two-dimensional transthoracic echocardiography; 2DTEE, two-dimensional transesophageal echocardiography; 3DTTE, three-dimensional transthoracic echocardiograpy; 3DTEE, three-dimensional transesophageal echocardiography.

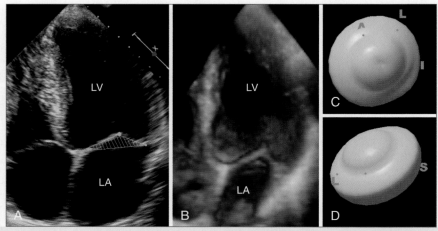

Figure 5-11 Mitral valve tenting. The tenting volume is shown in two-dimensions in **A** and is highlighted by the corresponding three-dimensional view (**B**). The tenting volume is calculated and shown in relation to the annulus in **C** and **D**. L, lateral; LA, left atrium; LV, left ventricle; S, septal.

increased level of visualization shows the regurgitation as a column or plane. Especially in eccentric mitral regurgitation, 3D allows visualization beyond a 2D "jet," thus better characterizing its severity. In planning mitral valve surgery, the increased level of detail proved by RT3DE is helpful to the surgeon and may increase repair rates.[33]

In addition to prolapse, RT3DE has been helpful in quantifying leaflet tethering associated with functional mitral regurgitation. Normally, the mitral valve leaflets are nearly level with the annulus (with a mean tenting height of 1.9 ± 1.5 mm).[7] **Figure 5-11** demonstrates mitral valve tenting in a normal mitral valve. In ischemic mitral regurgitation, the mitral valve leaflets may be pulled toward the ventricle by increased tension of the chordae. In extreme cases, with bileaflet restriction, the valve can form a funnel shape, allowing free central regurgitation. Several laboratories have developed methods of quantifying leaflet tethering using datasets from RT3DE.[13,40-42] With these models, information on the mechanism of ischemic mitral regurgitation is ascertained. For example, Kwan and colleagues[41] showed that an inferior infarct caused asymmetric tethering on the medial side of the valve.

CHORDAE TENDINEAE

Because they are not seen clearly on 2DE, the chordae tendineae are not well studied and often are overlooked as an important part of mitral valve function.

They are, however, an integral part of the mitral valve apparatus because chordae fusion or shortening can lead to subvalvular stenosis and leaflet tenting.

Approximately 140 individual leaflet chordae originate from the six heads of the papillary muscles and end at the mitral valve leaflets.[43] On average, each papillary muscle gives rise to 12 first-order chordae (two for each of the six heads). These divide to form an average of two second-order chordae, of which many further divide into two or three third-order chordea.[44] The majority of these chordae are marginal and insert into the rough zone of the leaflets' free edge. The purpose of these is to maintain leaflet coaptation and aid in mitral valve closure; rupture of primary chordae gives rise to mitral regurgitation.[4] Approximately 20 basal chordae insert into the ventricular free surface on the posterior leaflet and a few millimeters inward on the anterior leaflet at the junction of the smooth and rough zones. Among the basal chordae are several particularly thick fibrous "strut chordae," which insert in the central portion of the leaflets.[6,45,46] The purpose of these chordae is to support the left ventricular wall and maintain the aortic-mitral annular angle.[4] Each papillary muscle supplies chordae to both leaflets, but the anterolateral papillary muscle supports the structures on the left (the anterolateral commissure, A1 and P1 scallops, and the left half of A2 and P2 scallops). Likewise, the posteromedial papillary muscle supports the rightward structures (the posteromedial commissure, A3 and P3 scallops, and the right half of A2 and P2 scallops).[45,47]

The chordae are best seen in the wide-angle focused segments oriented from the ventricular side, where both the leaflet and papillary muscle attachments are visualized. In transesophageal exams, the transgastric long-axis view gives the best look at the subchordal apparatus (**Figure 5-12**).

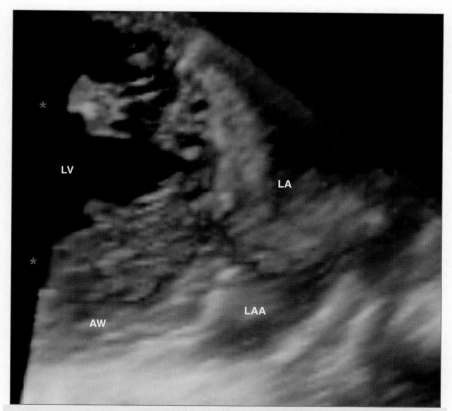

Figure 5-12 The mitral valve chordae as seen in the wide-sector three-dimensional format in a transgastric view. Both the origin of the chordae at the papillary muscle head and the termination at the rough zone of the valve leaflets are seen. *Red asterisk*, posteromedial papillary muscle; *green asterisk*, anterolateral papillary muscle; AW, anterior wall; LA, left atrium; LAA, left atrial appendage; LV, left ventricle.

In the past, information about the chordae has come from autopsy studies. As 3D investigations and techniques progress, more information will be obtained about how the chordae function in the setting of disease states that may cause rupture, thickening, and shortening of these structures. RT3DE has already proven to be better than 2DE in identifying chordal rupture in infectious endocarditis, aiding effective repair during surgery.[48,49]

PAPILLARY MUSCLES AND LEFT VENTRICULAR WALL

The importance of the papillary muscles and the associated left ventricular free wall to mitral valve function was first recognized in the 1960s. Autopsy data showed that ischemic mitral regurgitation often was associated with fibrosis and necrosis of the papillary muscles.[43,44] In general, the papillary muscles are attached to the left ventricular wall with a broad base larger than the area of the muscle itself. The papillary muscles are attached to the middle third of the left ventricular wall and oriented along the axis of the left ventricle and perpendicular to the mitral valve leaflets.[4] The width of the papillary muscles is nearly the same as the left ventricular wall. Each papillary muscle is composed of about six muscular heads that give rise to one or two primary chordae.[43] The anterolateral papillary muscle is connected to the mid-portion of the lateral free wall and usually is larger than the posteromedial one, which is attached to the mid-septum. **Figure 5-13** compares 2D biplane and 3D wide-sector views of the papillary muscles.

During systole, the papillary muscle shortens to maintain a fixed chordal distance from the tips to the leaflets, preventing prolapse of the leaflets into the atrium.[50] Their thickening also occupies space beneath the mitral valve (in the area of left ventricular inflow), directing blood toward the left ventricular outflow and the aortic valve.[4]

Using RT3DE, much more information about the location of the papillary muscles in the live heart has been ascertained. With computer reconstructions, the distance of the papillary muscle tips to the mitral valve annulus and their angle of orientation can easily be measured. The point of reference to make this measurement on the mitral valve annulus is the relatively stationary aortic-mitral fibrosa (at the junction of the anterior annulus and the aortic valve, as shown in Figure 5-5). The interpapillary angle is the angle of intersection of the two lines that connect each papillary muscle to this point on the mitral valve annulus. The interpapillary distance also is measured (**Figure 5-14**).

Annular to anterolateral papillary distance, annular to posteromedial papillary distance, and interpapillary distance depend on left ventricular remodeling and dilation, which increase in dilated cardiomyopathy. As such, 3D measurements of end-diastolic volume are also very important in this analysis, and normal left ventricular and papillary measurements depend on body size (see Table 5-1).[7] As discussed in more detail in other chapters, numerous studies have demonstrated the usefulness of RT3DE over 2D biplane measurements for assessing left ventricular volumes because 2DE tends to underestimate true volumes.[51-56] Normal values of left ventricular volumes and papillary muscle distances are provided in Table 5-1.

These measurements are very important in functional mitral regurgitation, in which chordal tethering of the leaflets occurs after left ventricular remodeling. In fact, the distance from the papillary muscle to the annulus is one of the best predictors of mitral regurgitation severity in models of dilated cardiomyopathy.[50,57,58] These models also have highlighted the necessity for maintaining a constant papillary to annular distance throughout the cardiac cycle.[50] Therefore, taking this measurement in real time during mitral valve surgery may be useful because increasingly complicated surgeries involve papillary muscle repositioning and chordal cutting.[57,59-61]

In ischemic mitral regurgitation, regional left ventricular wall motion abnormalities are directly associated with the degree of mitral regurgitation.[62] This is especially true in a posterior infarct, where posterolateral hypokinesis results in

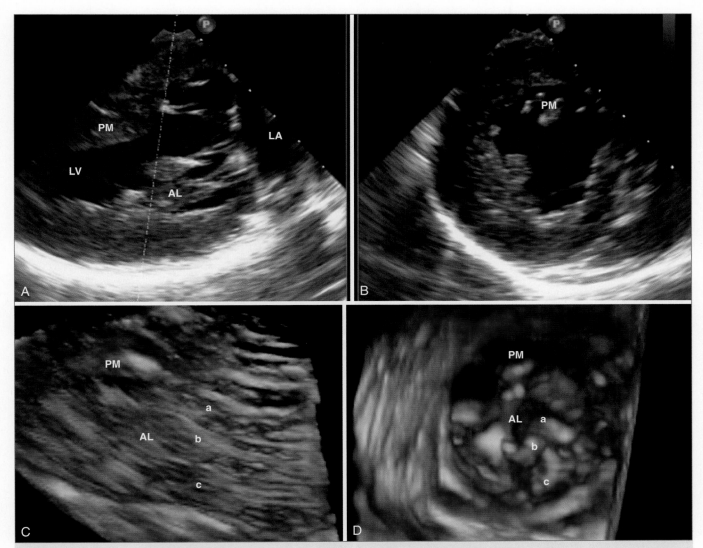

Figure 5-13 **A** and **B** show two-dimensional biplane images of the papillary muscles. The three-dimensional wide-sector views in **C** and **D** provide more detail, demonstrating three visible heads of the anterolateral papillary muscle (*a, b, c*) and the origins of the chordae. AL, anterolateral papillary muscle; LA, left atrium; LV, left ventricle; PM, posteromedial papillary muscle.

asymmetrical tethering of the posterior leaflet.[41] In these cases, it is still unclear how much of a role left ventricular focal wall motion abnormalities play.[58] RT3DE with segmental volumetric analysis quantifies wall motion abnormalities and may determine the mechanism of mitral valve dysfunction in ischemic disease.

LEFT ATRIUM

The left atrium influences mitral valve anatomy because the mitral valve leaflets can be characterized as a continuation of the left atrial walls and serve as the floor of the left atrium.[6,63] In particular, the lateral and posterior walls of the left atrium extend to form the posterior leaflet, whereas the anterior atrial wall extends to form the anterior leaflet.[6]

This interconnection between the atrial wall and the mitral valve can be appreciated on 3DE. The atrium can be best be visualized with full-volume datasets. In transesophageal exams, the mid-esophageal views also allow real-time imaging of the atrium with the 3D wide-sector format (**Figure 5-15**). In this view, the left atrial appendage (on the lateral wall of the atrium), the aortic valve (on the anterior wall), and fossa ovalis (on the medial wall) serve as important

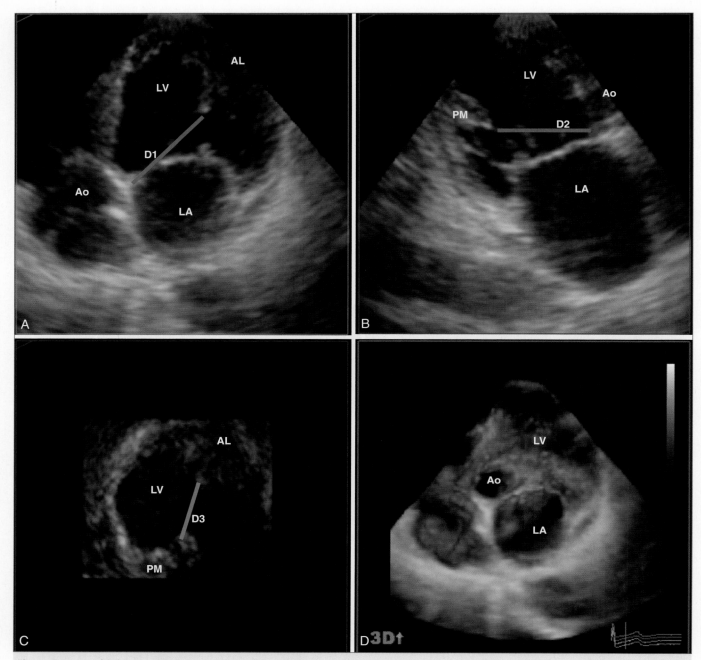

Figure 5-14 Multiplane reconstruction of the left ventricle, mitral valve, and papillary muscles obtained from a three-dimensional full-volume dataset. The distance from the annulus to each papillary muscle (*D1* and *D2*) and the interpapillary muscle distance (*D3*) are shown. The reference on the annulus for these measurements is the aortic-mitral fibrosa. AL, anterolateral papillary muscle; Ao, aortic valve; LA, left atrium; LV, left ventricle; PM, posteromedial papillary muscle.

landmarks. During transesophageal studies, the five-chamber deep gastric view also is helpful to view the entire left atrium, with a better view of the superior portions to assess volumes.

The importance of left atrial anatomy in mitral valve function may become clear in disease states, particularly in functional mitral regurgitation, in which increased atrial flow leads to impressive atrial dilation and decreased compliance. Like ventricular deformation, atrial enlargement also may, in turn, lead to further mitral valve dysfunction, creating a vicious cycle of remodeling and regurgitation.[63] Indeed, left atrial volume is associated with severity and outcomes in

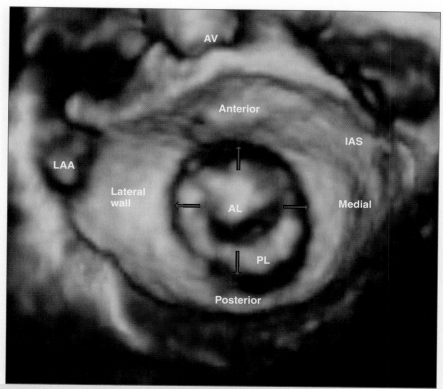

Figure 5-15   The mitral valve leaflets serve as the floor of the left atrium and are an extension of the atrial walls. AL, anterior leaflet; AV, aortic valve; LAA, left atrial appendage; IAS, interatrial septum; PL, posterior leaflet.

patients with a variety of disease states, including mitral regurgitation.[64] Whether this is a marker or a cause of the disease process is still unclear. 3DE may help elucidate the role of the left atrium. 3DE already has helped by allowing more accurate measures of left atrial volume.[65-68]

Although not formally part of the left atrium, the relationship of the coronary sinus to the mitral valve annulus has become important as new technologies, such as transcatheter mitral valve repair, use this structure. The usual position of the coronary sinus in the atrioventricular groove, just posterior to the mitral valve annulus, provides an ideal location for synch devices, which can be inserted into the coronary sinus. These devices hug the posterior annulus, decreasing the annular circumference and reducing functional mitral regurgitation. An example of the location of the coronary sinus with respect the mitral valve annulus is shown in **Figure 5-16**. In this case, RT3DE shows that the coronary sinus is located superior to the annulus, likely rendering it unusable as a conduit for transcatheter mitral valve repair.

CONCLUSION

Even with normal anatomy, the mitral valve is the most complex structure in the heart. It is composed of many parts, from the atrium at the base to the papillary muscles toward the apex, with the annulus, leaflets, and chordae between. Its intricate design is only fully appreciated with 3D imaging. With RT3DE, the normal positioning and size of each structure have been ascertained. In fact, RT3DE allows a more thorough evaluation of the individual valve structures, leading to a better understanding of their entire anatomy and function. As this technology improves and grows, it will become a routine part of all echocardiographic exams, especially when evaluating the mitral valve.

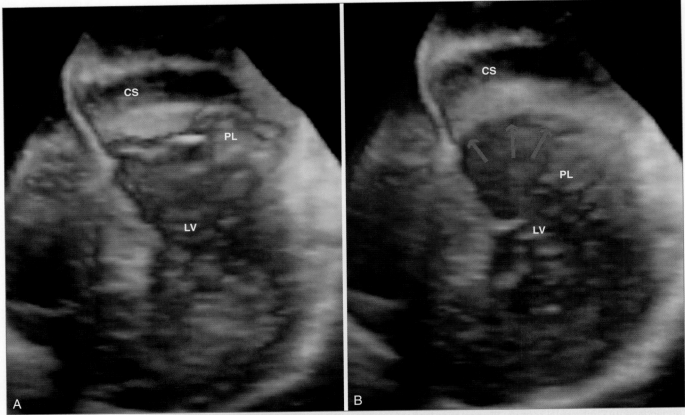

Figure 5-16 An example of the location of the coronary sinus (*CS*) with respect the mitral valve annulus. In this case, real-time three-dimensional echocardiography shows that the coronary sinus is located superior to the annulus (*red arrows*), making it unusable as a conduit for transcatheter mitral valve repair. *LV*, left ventricle; *PL*, posterior leaflet.

References

1. Levine RA, Handschumacher MD, Sanfilippo AJ, et al: Three-dimensional echocardiographic reconstruction of the mitral valve, with implications for the diagnosis of mitral valve prolapse. *Circulation* 80(3):589–598, 1989.
2. Salgo IS, Gorman JH, Gorman RC, et al: Effect of annular shape on leaflet curvature in reducing mitral leaflet stress. *Circulation* 106(6):711–717, 2002.
3. Solis J, Sitges M, Levine RA, Hung J: Three-dimensional echocardiography. New possibilities in mitral valve assessment. *Revista Española de Cardiología (English Edition)* 62(2):188–198, 2009.
4. Silbiger JJ, Bazaz R: Contemporary insights into the functional anatomy of the mitral valve. *Am Heart J* 158(6):887–895, 2009.
5. Kalyanasundaram A, Qureshi A, Nassef LA, Shirani J: Functional anatomy of normal mitral valve-left ventricular complex by real-time, three-dimensional echocardiography. *J Heart Valve Dis* 19(1):28–34, 2010.
6. Salcedo EE, Quaife RA, Seres T, Carroll JD: A framework for systematic characterization of the mitral valve by real-time three-dimensional transesophageal echocardiography. *J Am Soc Echocardiogr* 22(10):1087–1099, 2009.
7. Sonne C, Sugeng L, Watanabe N, et al: Age and body surface area dependency of mitral valve and papillary apparatus parameters: Assessment by real-time three-dimensional echocardiography. *Eur J Echocardiogr* 10(2):287–294, 2009.
8. Kaplan SR, Bashein G, Sheehan FH, et al: Three-dimensional echocardiographic assessment of annular shape changes in the normal and regurgitant mitral valve. *Am Heart J* 139(3):378–387, 2000.
9. Kwan J, Qin JX, Popović ZB, et al: Geometric changes of mitral annulus assessed by real-time 3-dimensional echocardiography: Becoming enlarged and less nonplanar in the anteroposterior direction during systole in proportion to global left ventricular systolic function. *J Am Soc Echocardiogr* 17(11):1179–1184, 2004.
10. Qin JX, Shiota T, Tsujino H, et al: Mitral annular motion as a surrogate for left ventricular ejection fraction: Real-time three-dimensional echocardiography and magnetic resonance imaging studies. *Eur J Echocardiogr* 5(6):407–415, 2004.
11. Kwan J, Jeon M-J, Kim D-H, et al: Does the mitral annulus shrink or enlarge during systole? A real-time 3D echocardiography study. *J Korean Med Sci* 24(2):203–208, 2009.
12. Flachskampf FA, Chandra S, Gaddipatti A, et al: Analysis of shape and motion of the mitral annulus in subjects with and without cardiomyopathy by echocardiographic 3-dimensional reconstruction. *J Am Soc Echocardiogr* 13(4):277–287, 2000.
13. Watanabe N, Ogasawara Y, Yamaura Y, et al: Geometric deformity of the mitral annulus in patients with ischemic mitral regurgitation: A real-time three-dimensional echocardiographic study. *J Heart Valve Dis* 14(4):447–452, 2005.
14. Sutaria N, Shaw TRD, Prendergast B, Northridge D: Transoesophageal echocardiographic assessment of mitral valve commissural morphology predicts outcome after balloon mitral valvotomy. *Heart* 92(1):52–57, 2006.

15. Langerveld J, Valocik G, Plokker HWT, et al: Additional value of three-dimensional transesophageal echocardiography for patients with mitral valve stenosis undergoing balloon valvuloplasty. *J Am Soc Echocardiogr* 16(8):841–849, 2003.

16. Gill EA, Kim MS, Carroll JD: 3D TEE for evaluation of commissural opening before and during percutaneous mitral commissurotomy. *JACC Cardiovasc Imag* 2(8):1034–1035, 2009.

17. Chen Q, Nosir YF, Vletter WB, et al: Accurate assessment of mitral valve area in patients with mitral stenosis by three-dimensional echocardiography. *J Am Soc Echocardiogr* 10(2):133–140, 1997.

18. Martin RP, Rakowski H, Kleiman JH, et al: Reliability and reproducibility of two dimensional echocardiographic measurement of the stenotic mitral valve orifice area. *Am J Cardiol* 43(3):560–568, 1979.

19. Binder TM, Rosenhek R, Porenta G, et al: Improved assessment of mitral valve stenosis by volumetric real-time three-dimensional echocardiography. *J Am Coll Cardiol* 36(4):1355–1361, 2000.

20. Sugeng L, Weinert L, Lammertin G, et al: Accuracy of mitral valve area measurements using transthoracic rapid freehand 3-dimensional scanning: Comparison with noninvasive and invasive methods. *J Am Soc Echocardiogr* 16(12):1292–1300, 2003.

21. de Agustin JA, Nanda NC, Gill EA, et al: The use of three-dimensional echocardiography for the evaluation of and treatment of mitral stenosis. *Cardiol Clin* 25(2):311–318, 2007.

22. Pérez de Isla L, Casanova C, Almería C, et al: Which method should be the reference method to evaluate the severity of rheumatic mitral stenosis? Gorlin's method versus 3D-echo. *Eur J Echocardiogr* 8(6):470–473, 2007.

23. Binder TM, Rosenhek R, Porenta G, et al: Improved assessment of mitral valve stenosis by volumetric real-time three-dimensional echocardiography. *J Am Coll Cardiol* 36(4):1355–1361, 2000.

24. Zamorano J, Cordeiro P, Sugeng L, et al: Real-time three-dimensional echocardiography for rheumatic mitral valve stenosis evaluation: An accurate and novel approach. *J Am Coll Cardiol* 43(11):2091–2096, 2004.

25. Valocik G, Kamp O, Mannaerts HFJ, Visser CA: New quantitative three-dimensional echocardiographic indices of mitral valve stenosis: New 3D indices of mitral stenosis. *Int J Cardiovasc Imag* 23(6):707–716, 2007.

26. Xie M-X, Wang X-F, Cheng TO, et al: Comparison of accuracy of mitral valve area in mitral stenosis by real-time, three-dimensional echocardiography versus two-dimensional echocardiography versus Doppler pressure half-time. *Am J Cardiol* 95(12):1496–1499, 2005.

27. Zamorano J, de Agustín JA: Three-dimensional echocardiography for assessment of mitral valve stenosis. *Curr Opin Cardiol* 24(5):415–419, 2009.

28. Limbu YR, Chen H, Shen X, et al: Assessment of mitral valve volume by quantitative three-dimensional echocardiography in patients with rheumatic mitral valve stenosis. *Clin Cardiol* 21(6):415–418, 1998.

29. Godoy IE, Bednarz J, Sugeng L, et al: Three-dimensional echocardiography in adult patients: Comparison between transthoracic and transesophageal reconstructions. *J Am Soc Echocardiogr* 12(12):1045–1052, 1999.

30. Pepi M, Tamborini G, Maltagliati A, et al: Head-to-head comparison of two- and three-dimensional transthoracic and transesophageal echocardiography in the localization of mitral valve prolapse. *J Am Coll Cardiol* 48(12):2524–2530, 2006.

31. Sharma R, Mann J, Drummond L, et al: The evaluation of real-time 3-dimensional transthoracic echocardiography for the preoperative functional assessment of patients with mitral valve prolapse: A comparison with 2-dimensional transesophageal echocardiography. *J Am Soc Echocardiogr* 20(8):934–940, 2007.

32. Sugeng L, Coon P, Weinert L, et al: Use of real-time 3-dimensional transthoracic echocardiography in the evaluation of mitral valve disease. *J Am Soc Echocardiogr* 19(4):413–421, 2006.

33. Grewal J, Mankad S, Freeman W, et al: Real-time three-dimensional transesophageal echocardiography in the intraoperative assessment of mitral valve disease. *J Am Soc Echocardiogr* 22(1):34–41, 2009.

34. Manda J, Kesanolla SK, Hsuing MC, et al: Comparison of real time two-dimensional with live/real time three-dimensional transesophageal echocardiography in the evaluation of mitral valve prolapse and chordae rupture. *Echocardiography* 25(10):1131–1137, 2008.

35. Müller S, Müller L, Laufer G, et al: Comparison of three-dimensional imaging to transesophageal echocardiography for preoperative evaluation in mitral valve prolapse. *Am J Cardiol* 98(2):243–248, 2006.

36. Fabricius AM, Walther T, Falk V, Mohr FW: Three-dimensional echocardiography for planning of mitral valve surgery: Current applicability? *Ann Thorac Surg* 78(2):575–578, 2004.

37. Hirata K, Pulerwitz T, Sciacca R, et al: Clinical utility of new real time three-dimensional transthoracic echocardiography in assessment of mitral valve prolapse. *Echocardiography* 25(5):482–488, 2008.

38. Agricola E, Oppizzi M, Pisani M, et al: Accuracy of real-time 3D echocardiography in the evaluation of functional anatomy of mitral regurgitation. *Int J Cardiol* 127(3):342–349, 2008.

39. García-Orta R, Moreno E, Vidal M, et al: Three-dimensional versus two-dimensional transesophageal echocardiography in mitral valve repair. *J Am Soc Echocardiogr* 20(1):4–12, 2007.

40. Watanabe N, Ogasawara Y, Yamaura Y, et al: Quantitation of mitral valve tenting in ischemic mitral regurgitation by transthoracic real-time three-dimensional echocardiography. *J Am Coll Cardiol* 45(5):763–769, 2005.

41. Kwan J, Shiota T, Agler DA, et al: Geometric differences of the mitral apparatus between ischemic and dilated cardiomyopathy with significant mitral regurgitation: Real-time three-dimensional echocardiography study. *Circulation* 107(8):1135–1140, 2003.

42. Otsuji Y, Handschumacher MD, Schwammenthal E, et al: Insights from three-dimensional echocardiography into the mechanism of functional mitral regurgitation: Direct in vivo demonstration of altered leaflet tethering geometry. *Circulation* 96(6):1999–2008, 1997.

43. Roberts WC, Cohen LS: Left ventricular papillary muscles. Description of the normal and a survey of conditions causing them to be abnormal. *Circulation* 46(1):138–154, 1972.

44. Silverman ME, Hurst JW: The mitral complex. Interaction of the anatomy, physiology, and pathology of the mitral annulus, mitral valve leaflets, chordae tendineae, and papillary muscles. *Am Heart J* 76(3):399–418, 1968.

45. Degandt AA, Weber PA, Saber HA, Duran CMG: Mitral valve basal chordae: Comparative anatomy and terminology. *Ann Thorac Surg* 84(4):1250–1255, 2007.

46. Da Col U, Ramoni E, Di Lazzaro D: Posterior mitral leaflet: New anatomical insight and review of nomenclature (mitral valve anatomy). *J Cardiovasc Med (Hagerstown)* 11(11):820–826, 2010.

47. Kumar N, Kumar M, Duran CM: A revised terminology for recording surgical findings of the mitral valve. *J Heart Valve Dis* 4(1):70–75, 1995.

48. Hansalia S, Biswas M, Dutta R, et al: The value of live/real time three-dimensional transesophageal echocardiography in the assessment of valvular vegetations. *Echocardiography* 26(10):1264–1273, 2009.

49. Ma N, Li Z-an, Meng X, Yang Y: Live three-dimensional transesophageal echocardiography in mitral valve surgery. *Chin Med J* 121(20):2037–2041, 2008.

50. Komeda M, Glasson JR, Bolger AF, et al: Papillary muscle-left ventricular wall "complex." *J Thorac Cardiovasc Surg* 113(2):292–301, 1997.

51. Jenkins C, Moir S, Chan J, et al: Left ventricular volume measurement with echocardiography: A comparison of left ventricular opacification, three-dimensional echocardiography, or both with magnetic resonance imaging. *Eur Heart J* 30(1):98–106, 2009.

52. Bicudo LS, Tsutsui JM, Shiozaki A, et al: Value of real time three-dimensional echocardiography in patients with hypertrophic cardiomyopathy: Comparison with two-dimensional echocardiography and magnetic resonance imaging. *Echocardiography* 25(7):717–726, 2008.

53. Jenkins C, Bricknell K, Chan J, et al: Comparison of two- and three-dimensional echocardiography with sequential magnetic resonance imaging for evaluating left ventricular volume and ejection fraction over time in patients with healed myocardial infarction. *Am J Cardiol* 99(3):300–306, 2007.

54. Gutiérrez-Chico JL, Zamorano JL, Pérez de Isla L, et al: Comparison of left ventricular volumes and ejection fractions measured by three-dimensional echocardiography versus by two-dimensional echocardiography and cardiac magnetic resonance in patients with various cardiomyopathies. *Am J Cardiol* 95(6):809–813, 2005.

55. Chuang ML, Hibberd MG, Salton CJ, et al: Importance of imaging method over imaging modality in noninvasive determination of left ventricular volumes and ejection fraction: Assessment by two- and three-dimensional echocardiography and magnetic resonance imaging. *J Am Coll Cardiol* 35(2):477–484, 2000.

56. Chukwu EO, Barasch E, Mihalatos DG, et al: Relative importance of errors in left ventricular quantitation by two-dimensional echocardiography: Insights from three-dimensional echocardiography and cardiac magnetic resonance imaging. *J Am Soc Echocardiogr* 21(9):990–997, 2008.

57. Hung J, Chaput M, Guerrero JL, et al: Persistent reduction of ischemic mitral regurgitation by papillary muscle repositioning: Structural stabilization of the papillary muscle-ventricular wall complex. *Circulation* 116(11 Suppl):I259–I263, 2007.

58. Otsuji Y, Handschumacher MD, Liel-Cohen N, et al: Mechanism of ischemic mitral regurgitation with segmental left ventricular dysfunction: Three-dimensional echocardiographic studies in models of acute and chronic progressive regurgitation. *J Am Coll Cardiol* 37(2):641–648, 2001.

59. Messas E, Guerrero JL, Handschumacher MD, et al: Chordal cutting: A new therapeutic approach for ischemic mitral regurgitation. *Circulation* 104(16):1958–1963, 2001.

60. Hung J, Guerrero JL, Handschumacher MD, et al: Reverse ventricular remodeling reduces ischemic mitral regurgitation: Echo-guided device application in the beating heart. *Circulation* 106(20):2594–2600, 2002.

61. Liel-Cohen N, Guerrero JL, Otsuji Y, et al: Design of a new surgical approach for ventricular remodeling to relieve ischemic mitral regurgitation: Insights from 3-dimensional echocardiography. *Circulation* 101(23):2756–2763, 2000.

62. Pecini R, Hammer-Hansen S, Dalsgaard M, et al: Determinants of exercise-induced increase of mitral regurgitation in patients with acute coronary syndromes. *Echocardiography* 27(5):567–574, 2010.

63. Schmitto JD, Lee LS, Mokashi SA, et al: Functional mitral regurgitation. *Cardiol Rev* 18(6):285–291, 2010.

64. Le Tourneau T, Messika-Zeitoun D, Russo A, et al: Impact of left atrial volume on clinical outcome in organic mitral regurgitation. *J Am Coll Cardiol* 56(7):570–578, 2010.

65. Russo C, Hahn RT, Jin Z, et al: Comparison of echocardiographic single-plane versus biplane method in the assessment of left atrial volume and validation by real time three-dimensional echocardiography. *J Am Soc Echocardiogr* 23(9):954–960, 2010.

66. de Groot NMS, Schalij MJ: Imaging modalities for measurements of left atrial volume in patients with atrial fibrillation: What do we choose? *Europace* 12(6):766–767, 2010.

67. Badano LP, Pezzutto N, Marinigh R, et al: How many patients would be misclassified using M-mode and two-dimensional estimates of left atrial size instead of left atrial volume? A three-dimensional echocardiographic study. *J Cardiovasc Med (Hagerstown)* 9(5):476–484, 2008.

68. Azar F, Pérez de Isla L, Moreno M, et al: Three-dimensional echocardiographic assessment of left atrial size and function and the normal range of asynchrony in healthy individuals. *Rev Esp Cardiol* 62(7):816–819, 2009.

69. Corsi C, Lang RM, Veronesi F, et al: Volumetric quantification of global and regional left ventricular function from real-time three-dimensional echocardiographic images. *Circulation* 112(8):1161–1170, 2005.

70. Zeidan Z, Erbel R, Barkhausen J, et al: Analysis of global systolic and diastolic left ventricular performance using volume-time curves by real-time three-dimensional echocardiography. *J Am Soc Echocardiogr* 16(1):29–37, 2003.

71. Nosir YF, Lequin MH, Kasprzak JD, et al: Measurements and day-to-day variabilities of left ventricular volumes and ejection fraction by three-dimensional echocardiography and comparison with magnetic resonance imaging. *Am J Cardiol* 82(2):209–214, 1998.

CHAPTER 6

Mitral Stenosis

Edward A. Gill

INTRODUCTION

Mitral stenosis is quite uncommon in Western countries, yet it still is a frequent problem worldwide, particularly in developing countries. The low incidence in the United States, in particular, is largely because rheumatic fever resulting in rheumatic heart disease has been largely eradicated; nevertheless, occasional outbreaks do occur. The occurrence of rheumatic fever in Utah in the mid-1980s and early 1990s is notable.[1,2] That particular outbreak had two unusual aspects. First, as opposed to previous history of outbreaks typically appearing in lower socioeconomic groups, this outbreak seemed to affect the middle class. Second, there was a distressingly low incidence of a symptomatic streptococcal infection in the group developing rheumatic fever.

Rheumatic heart disease preferentially affects the mitral valve, with the order of involvement being (1) mitral, (2) aortic, (3) tricuspid, and (4) pulmonic. The mitral valve is involved in virtually all cases, whereas the aortic valve is affected in 20% to 25% of cases. Pulmonary valve involvement in rheumatic heart disease is exceedingly rare. Even though the tricuspid valve frequently is involved, tricuspid valvular disease often is clinically silent.[3] From a functional standpoint, however, approximately 25% of patients with rheumatic heart disease have pure mitral stenosis and 40% have a combination of mitral stenosis and mitral regurgitation.[4] Two thirds of all patients with rheumatic mitral stenosis are female[5]; however, in my experience, it is almost 90%. In the United States and other Western countries, mitral stenosis develops over a period of decades, with a mean age of onset of 45 years. However, for reasons that are not entirely understood, individuals in developing countries such as India, in Africa, and in Alaskan Inuits, the time from rheumatic fever to onset of clinically significant mitral stenosis can be as little as 10 years. The factors for this rapid onset, however, appear to be more socioeconomic than necessarily related to specific medical care.[6,7]

CARDIAC IMAGING AND REAL-TIME THREE-DIMENSIONAL ECHOCARDIOGRAPHY

From the standpoint of cardiac imaging, echocardiography is clearly the mainstay for evaluation of mitral stenosis. The extent of mitral valvular deformity traditionally has been evaluated by two-dimensional (2D) echocardiography and graded based on a score of 0 to 4 for each of four factors: (1) valvular thickening, (2) valvular mobility, (3) degree of leaflet calcification, and (4) extent of subvalvular thickening and calcification.[8] The Wilkins scoring system does have several drawbacks, however. In particular, some patients with a high Wilkins score still respond well to percutaneous mitral valvuloplasty (PMV). Three-dimensional (3D) echocardiography provides incremental information regarding the status of rheumatic involvement of the mitral valve, particularly regarding the fusion of the commissures. Determination of the status of commissural fusion, particularly the *symmetry* and *length* of commissural fusion, is critical information to predict the success of treatment of mitral stenosis with PMV.[9] That is, mitral valvuloplasty is most effective when *extensive symmetric* commissural fusion is present and when such fusion is alleviated at the time of the procedure. 3D echocardiography (3DE) has a particular strength for visualizing the mitral commissures and commissural fusion because of the added dimension of elevation (**Figures 6-1 to 6-5; Videos 6-1 to 6-9**). The elevation dimension allows clearer assessment of the degree and

Text continued on page 101

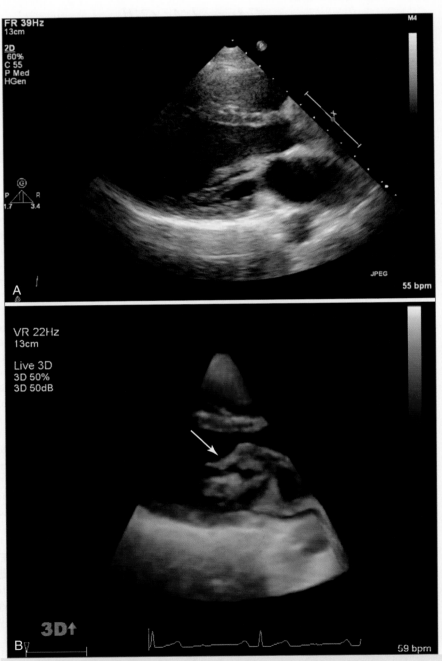

Figure 6-1   A and **B,** Two-dimensional (2D) and three-dimensional (3D) parasternal long-axis views of the mitral valve in a patient with mitral stenosis. Both show the characteristic "doming" or "hockey stick" appearance of the anterior mitral valve leaflet (*arrow*). The 3D details the subvalvular apparatus not appreciated on the 2D image (see Videos 6-1 and 6-2).

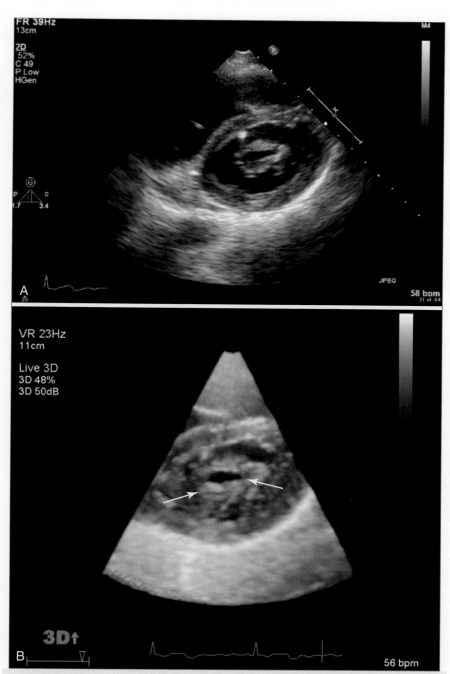

Figure 6-2 Two-dimensional (**A**) and three-dimensional (3D) (**B**) short-axis views of mitral stenosis. Both images show bilateral commissural fusion, with the lateral commissure more fused than the medial commissure. The 3D image allows superior visualization of the thickening of the mitral leaflets, particularly the commissures.

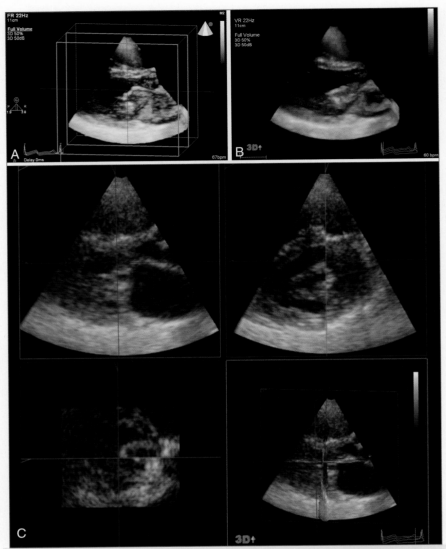

Figure 6-3   A, QLAB (Phillips Healthcare, Andover, MA) evaluation of the mitral valve area. This is the first step in using a transthoracic three-dimensional (3D) full-volume acquisition of the mitral valve to quantify the degree of mitral stenosis by measuring the mitral valve area. This is the starting point, with the full volume acquired and initial autocropping performed automatically by the software. The autocropping shows the mitral valve in the parasternal long-axis view. Here, the parasternal long-axis view has been acquired in full-volume mode and has been stored to an Xcelera (Phillips Healthcare) page. From here, the operator activates the QLAB icon (*pyramid*) to move into the cropping function and the 3DQ quantification package. **B,** Quantification step 2. The operator is now within the QLAB software. This particular view shows the full volume within QLAB, with the crop box turned off. From here, the operator enters the 3DQ quantification package. **C,** Quantification step 3 is the multiplanar reconstruction mode of QLAB. Here, the mitral valve is shown in parasternal long axis (*upper left*), parasternal short axis (*upper right*), a composite (*lower left*), and the entire volume of the heart (*lower right*). Placing the red plane cursor so the mitral valve is cut in cross-section (*upper right*) at the very tip of the mitral valve leaflets allows the mitral valve area to be measured at the most optimal angle.

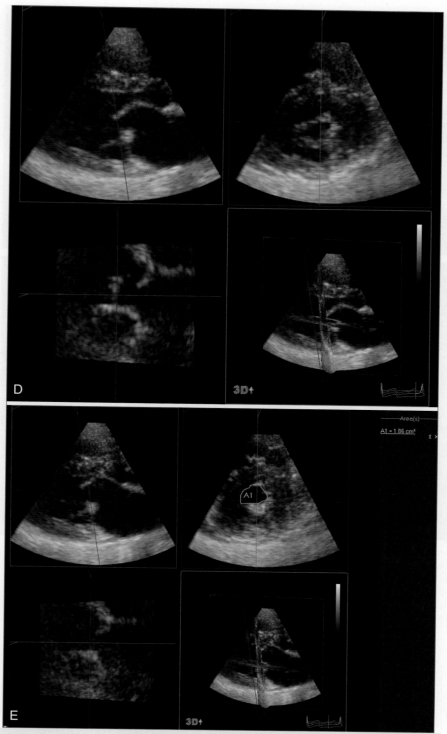

Figure 6-3, cont'd   D, Quantification step 4. Here, the red plane is positioned at the tips of the mitral leaflets (*upper left*) so that the operator can be certain that the orifice is in the true en face view in the upper right plane. The *lower right* image is a view of the entire volume that can be manipulated to see how the red plane is being moved relative to the entire mitral valve apparatus. **E,** Quantification final step. The mitral valve area is traced, resulting in a mitral valve area of 1.86 cm in this case.

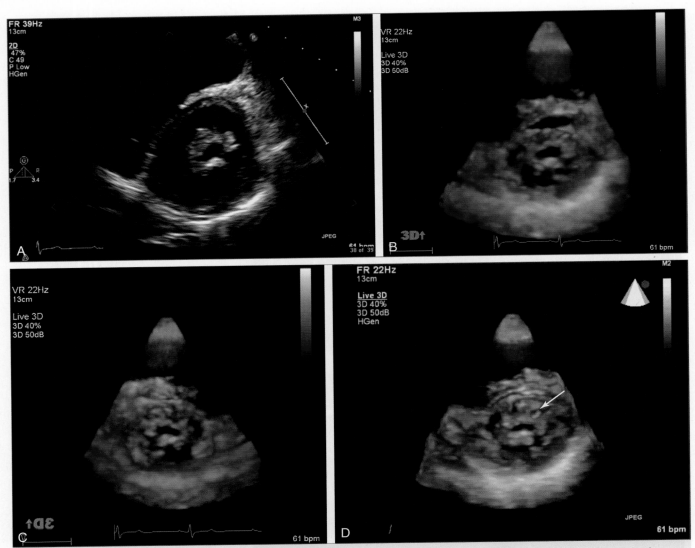

Figure 6-4 A, Two-dimensional (2D) transthoracic image of mitral stenosis. Note the marked thickening of the anterior mitral leaflet. **B,** The same patient as viewed by parasternal three-dimensional (3D) transthoracic echocardiography from the left ventricular side of the valve. Note the rheumatic nodules that are noted by 3D echocardiography that were not appreciated in 2D. Also note the details of commissural fusion shown in this swivel display and the asymmetric fusion of the commissures. The same patient viewed from the left atrial side (**C**) and ventricular side (**D**) with a slight tilt toward the anterior leaflet so that the extensive rheumatic disease, accentuated by the nodules (*arrow*), is seen (see Videos 6-6 to 6-9).

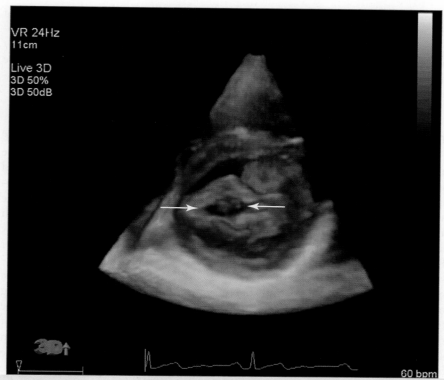

Figure 6-5 A patient 3 years after percutaneous mitral valvuloplasty. The splitting of the commissures is seen on both sides (*arrows*). In this case, the lateral commissure is more open; the three-dimensional view shows this in more detail (see Video 6-5).

length of commissural fusion as well as the presence of structures that could inhibit the process, such as rheumatic nodules and subvalvular (typically chordal) thickening. Although in mitral stenosis symmetric commissural fusion is the optimal morphology for PMV success, evidence indicates that if the commissural fusion is accompanied by significant calcification, results are not as satisfactory, which is a predictable finding.[10-12]

MITRAL VALVE AREA DETERMINATION

The severity of mitral stenosis can be determined by several echocardiographic measures: peak and mean pressure gradient by Doppler and mitral valve area by (1) Doppler pressure half-time, (2) Doppler-based continuity equation, and (3) direct planimetry of the mitral valve area by 2DE or 3DE. Direct planimetry of the mitral valve orifice by real-time 3DE (RT3DE) has now emerged as the gold standard, thanks to several investigations and publications.[13-20] RT3DE quantification of the mitral valve orifice begins with a full-volume RT3D transthoracic echocardiography (RT3DTTE) acquisition obtained in the parasternal long-axis orientation. From this full-volume dataset, the mitral valve can be cropped to obtain an en face view of the mitral orifice. A precise en face image of the stenotic mitral valve is crucial for accurate measurement of the mitral valve area. In addition to being lined up with the tips of the mitral valve leaflets using the orthogonal plane, the en face view can be panned above and below the valve and viewed from the atrial and ventricular sides. The cropping function markedly enhances the confidence in the accuracy of valve area quantification because multiple plane cropping ensures that the orifice area is traced in a plane that is (1) at the tips of the mitral valve and (2) perpendicular to the inflow through the valve. The progression shown in Figure 6-3 demonstrates the sequential plan for procurement of an accurate mitral valve area using planimetry of an RT3DE dataset. Note that such a dataset could be obtained using either RT3DTTE or RT3D transesophageal echocardiography (RT3DTEE).

TREATMENT: PERCUTANEOUS MITRAL VALVULOPLASTY

PMV is the current state-of-the-art treatment when valve morphology is favorable and mitral regurgitation is no worse than mild. Previously, Applebaum[21] had suggested the use of 3DE during PMV, although this was prior to the development of RT3DE. RT3DTTE and RT3DTEE have drastically changed the approach to PMV at some centers. PMV is a unique procedure that, along with a few others, has advanced the term "interventional echocardiography" to a new level. Echocardiography guidance of PMV can be performed with either RT3DTTE or RT3DTEE. RT3DTEE, however, provides benefits to the interventional cardiologist from the transseptal puncture, to positioning the Inoue balloon, to avoiding the left atrial appendage, and finally to assessing the splitting of the commissures on both the atrial and ventricular sides of the valve. The transseptal puncture is theoretically safer using RT3DTEE guidance because of the use of biplane or "X-plane" to view two orthogonal 2D views of the septum simultaneously. Classically, the two orthogonal planes that are used are (a) the bicaval view at 110 degrees and (b) the four-chamber view at the aortic valve area, roughly 30 degrees (**Figure 6-6; Video 6-12**). The bicaval view guides the interventionalists to the superior portion versus the inferior portion of the septum, and the four-chamber view is useful to avoid damaging the aortic valve and root during the transseptal puncture (see Figure 6-6; **Videos 6-10 to 6-12**). Visualization of the fossa ovalis is also safer by RT3DTEE by both X-plane orthogonal views as well as 3D zoom mode (to visualize the entire fossa ovalis en face in real time and the catheter relationship to the superior vena cava [SVC] and the inferior vena cava [IVC] as it traverses the interatrial septum) (see Figure 6-6; **Video 6-13**). RT3DTEE has the advantage of providing particularly vivid images of the interatrial septum, the left atrium, the left atrial appendage, and the mitral orifice. All four of these structures are important anatomic landmarks used during the procedure, so optimal visualization also is crucial to the success or failure of the procedure.[9,22,23]

Although severe mitral regurgitation can be a complication of PMV, the development of some minor mitral regurgitation actually can be viewed as a sign of success. That is because the mechanism of mitral regurgitation is typically related to the splitting of the mitral commissures during the procedure.[24] Further examples of RT3DTEE and RT3DTTE use during the course of PMV are shown in **Figures 6-7 to 6-15** (**Videos 6-14 to 6-24**).

CASES

CASE 1

A 22-year-old man presented with increasing dyspnea 9 years after having had a PMV. His symptoms were brought on by playing basketball; he was able to play for 10 minutes before developing severe dyspnea and having to stop. His 2D echocardiogram and Doppler showed moderate mitral stenosis with a valve area of 1.3 cm^2 and a mean gradient of 8 mm Hg. The Wilkins valvuloplasty score was believed to be 9 to 10. The mitral valve commissures, however, were fused. 3DTTE showed significant fusion of the mitral commissures and nodular formation, with neither sign readily apparent by 2DTTE. The patient underwent PMV

Text continued on page 109

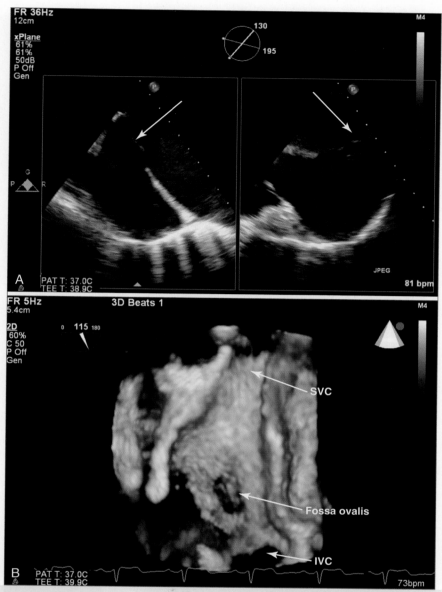

Figure 6-6   A, Transesophageal echocardiography (TEE) performed during percutaneous mitral valvuloplasty using biplane (X-plane) technology. Although the images are two-dimensional (2D), there are two simultaneously acquired 2D images. This is made possible by the three-dimensional (3D) TEE probe. That is, the matrix array transducer allows simultaneous display of two orthogonal planes. In this case, two orthogonal planes are displayed during the transseptal needle puncture portion of the procedure. The *arrows* point out "tenting" of the interatrial septum. The two orthogonal planes allow two perspectives on the septum. In particular, on the right image, the operator can tell how superior or inferior they are on the septum, given the relationship to the superior vena cava (*SVC*), and also, most importantly, avoid the aortic root. **B,** SVC and fossa ovalis shown by real-time 3DTEE. In the transseptal puncture procedure, the Brockenbrough needle is positioned to puncture the center of the fossa ovalis and then enter the left atrium (see Videos 6-12 and 6-13). IVC, inferior vena cava.

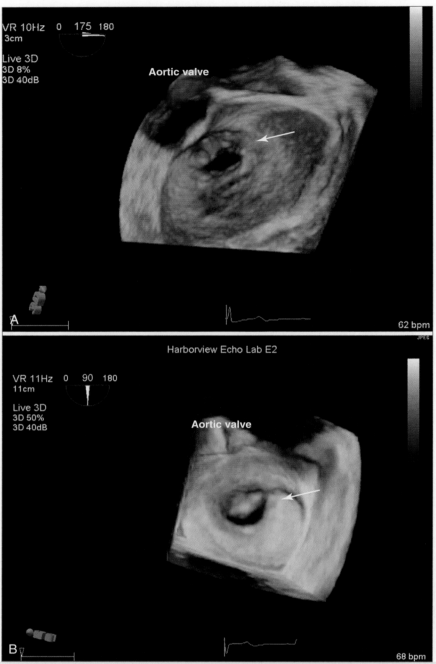

Figure 6-7 Three-dimensional transesophageal echocardiography of the mitral valve in two different patients with mitral stenosis are shown viewing the mitral orifice (*arrow*) from the left atrial side. The aortic valve is shown for orientation. This image display is shown in the surgeon's view. Mitral stenosis (**A**) is more severe with fusion of both the lateral (*arrow*) and medial commissures; in this case, the medial commissure is more fused. Note the more restricted orifice compared with that in **B** with a larger mitral orifice grossly and a much smoother orifice that is relatively early in the disease process (see Videos 6-14 and 6-15).

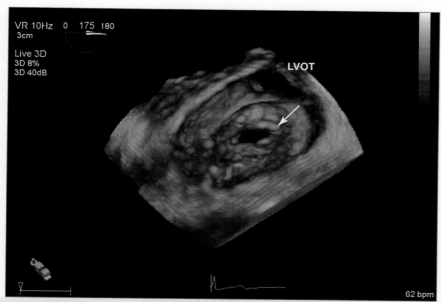

Figure 6-8   Real-time three-dimensional transesophageal echocardiography of a patient with mitral stenosis, showing an oval-shaped, restricted orifice with commissural fusion bilaterally. The orifice is viewed from the ventricular side. The commissural fusion is more severe with the medial commissure (*arrow*). The left ventricular outflow tract (*LVOT*) is shown for orientation (see Video 6-16).

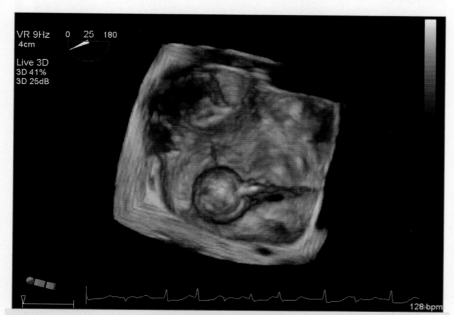

Figure 6-9   A three-dimensional transesophageal echocardiography image showing the Inoue balloon initially expanded across the mitral valve and then deflated (see Video 6-17).

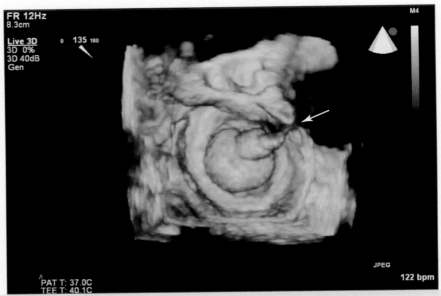

Figure 6-10 Three-dimensional transesophageal echocardiography image of a patient with mitral stenosis acquired during percutaneous mitral valvuloplasty. The site of the transseptal puncture is clearly seen (*arrow*). The balloon is being inflated across the mitral orifice (see Video 6-18).

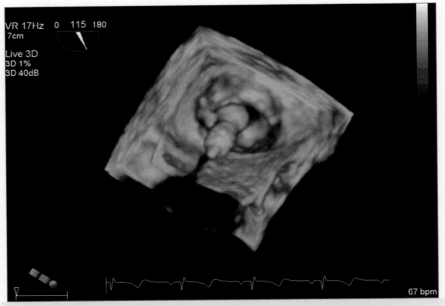

Figure 6-11 Unsuccessful attempt at crossing the mitral orifice by the balloon valvuloplasty catheter. In this three-dimensional transesophageal echocardiography view of a stenotic mitral valve, the interventional cardiologist is attempting to cross the orifice with the Inoue balloon. This particular attempt illustrates the importance of ruling out the left atrial appendage prior to percutaneous mitral valvuloplasty; in this case, the catheter lodged in the left atrial appendage (see Video 6-19).

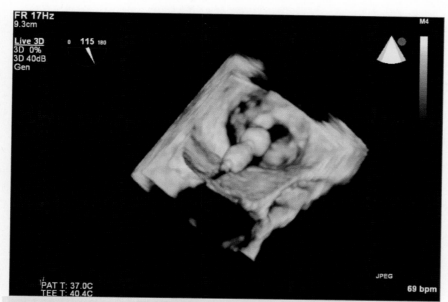

Figure 6-12   An example of successful crossing of the mitral orifice using three-dimensional transesophageal echocardiography guidance in percutaneous mitral valvuloplasty (see Video 6-20).

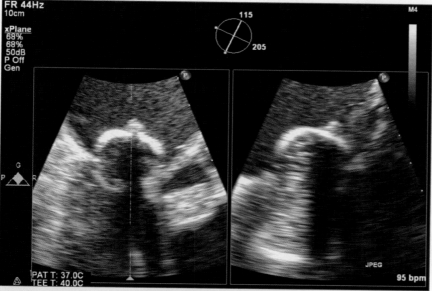

Figure 6-13   Transesophageal echocardiography (TEE) view of the Inoue balloon expanded across the mitral orifice. Once again, the matrix TEE probe is used to show two orthogonal two-dimensional views simultaneously; in this case, the Inoue balloon expanded across the mitral orifice (see Video 6-21).

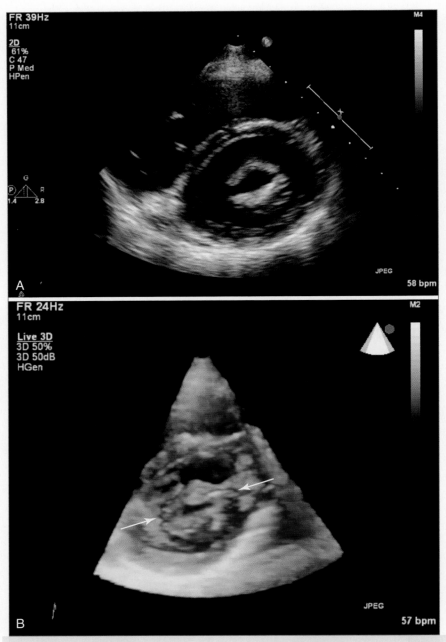

Figure 6-14   A successful percutaneous mitral valvuloplasty after the procedure. The commissures have been successfully split. **A,** The splitting by two-dimensional (2D) and three-dimensional (3D) echocardiography. The considerable commissural splitting is shown in the 3D view (**B**) to have considerable depth in a way that cannot be appreciated by the 2D image (*arrows*) (see Videos 6-22 and 6-23).

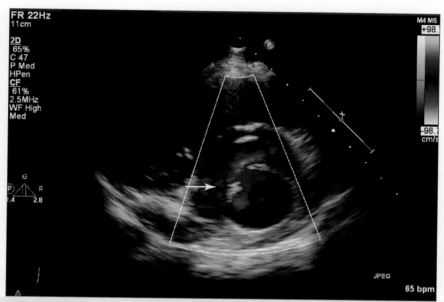

Figure 6-15 Evaluation of mitral regurgitation after mitral valvuloplasty. A two-dimensional color view of the mitral orifice and mitral regurgitation. A very small jet of mitral regurgitation is present along the medial commissure. This jet has developed as a result of the percutaneous mitral valvuloplasty and the commissural splitting. There clearly is a tradeoff between going too far with the valvuloplasty and causing significant regurgitation versus not going far enough and not relieving the mitral stenosis (see Video 6-24).

with a satisfactory result. The mitral valve area increased to 1.8 cm², and the mean gradient also decreased. 3DE showed bilateral commissural splitting. Four years after his procedure, the patient continues to do well.

CASE 2

A 48-year-old woman presented to the cardiology clinic reporting the presence of a heart murmur but also having symptoms of palpitations and dyspnea. The symptoms necessitated obtaining an echocardiogram that showed moderate mitral stenosis. The patient was gravida 3 para 3 and had not had any significant problems during her pregnancy with dyspnea, palpitations, or known arrhythmia. However, her most recent pregnancy was 7 years ago. The mitral valve area was 1.2 cm² by 3D planimetry and 1.3 cm² by Doppler pressure half-time. Pulmonary artery pressure was 45 mm Hg but increased to 60 mm Hg with bicycle exercise. Hence, the patient was deemed a candidate for PMV. A few challenges with the procedure were clearly aided by RT3DTEE. The first was a potential thrombus in the left atrial appendage, identified using standard 2DTEE (Figure 6-16, *A*). However, with the use of the biplane or X-plane feature, when viewing this structure in the orthogonal plane, the structure was clearly a trabeculation of the left atrial appendage wall rather than a thrombus (see Figure 6-16, *B*). This also was demonstrated using the RT3DTEE mode of 3D zoom. The second was the positioning of the catheter. It was difficult to cross the valve, and use of the RT3DTEE to steer the Ionue balloon dramatically hastened the procedure (see Figures 6-10 and 6-11; see also Videos 6-17 to 6-19). After successfully navigating these potential hurdles, the procedure had a successful result, increasing the mitral valve area to 1.7 cm² and decreasing the transmitral gradient to 5 mm Hg.

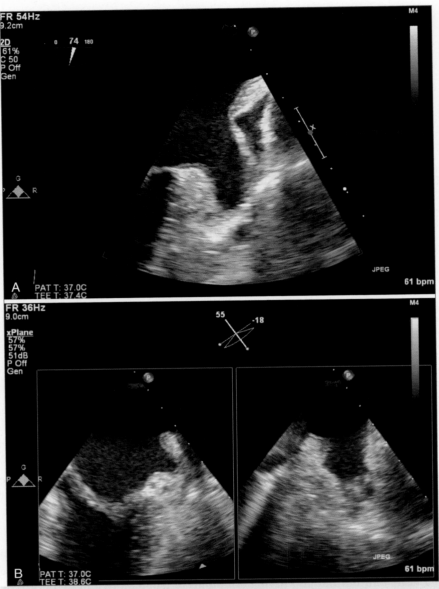

Figure 6-16   Possible thrombus in the left atrial appendage. The biplane, or X-plane, view shows that the possible thrombus in **A** is clearly a trabeculation seen in the orthogonal plane in **B**.

References

1. Veasy LG, Tani LY, Hill HR: Persistence of acute rheumatic fever in the intermountain area of the United States. *J Pediatr* 124:9–16, 1994.
2. Tani LY, Veasy LG, Minich LL, Shaddy RE: Rheumatic fever in children younger than 5 years: Is the presentation different? *Pediatrics* 112:1065–1068, 2003.
3. Meira ZM, Goular EM, Colosimo EA, Mota CC: Long term follow up of rheumatic fever and predictors of severe rheumatic valvular disease in Brazilian children and adolescents. *Heart* 91:1019, 2005.
4. Bono RO, Carabello BA, Chatterjee K, et al: ACC/AHA 2006 guidelines for the management of patients with valvular heart disease. *Circulation* 114:e84, 2006.
5. Rahimtoola SH, Durairaj A, Mehra A, et al: Current evaluation and management of patients with mitral stenosis. *Circulation* 106:1183, 2002.
6. Vijayaraghavan G, Cherian G, Krishnaswami S, et al: Rheumatic aortic stenosis in young patients presenting with combined aortic and mitral stenosis. *Br Heart J* 39:294, 1977.
7. Davidson M, Bulkow LR, Gellin BG: Cardiac mortality in Alaska's indigenous and non-Native residents. *Int J Epidemiol* 22:62–71, 1993.
8. Wilkins GT, Weyman AE, Abascal VM, et al: Percutaneous balloon dilatation of the mitral valve: An analysis of echocardiographic variables related to outcome and the mechanism of dilatation. *Br Heart J* 60:299, 1988.

9. Gill EA, Kim MS, Carroll JD: 3D TEE for evaluation of commissural opening before and during percutaneous mitral commissurotomy. *J Am Coll Cardiol Imag* 2:1034–1035, 2009.

10. Hernandez R, Banuelos C, Alfonso F: Long-term clinical and echocardiographic follow-up after percutaneous mitral valvuloplasty with the Inoue balloon. *Circulation* 99:1580, 1999.

11. Lung B, Garbarz E, Michaeud P, et al: Late results of percutaneous mitral commissurotomy in a series of 1024 patients. Analysis of late clinical deterioration: Frequency, anatomic findings, and predictive factors. *Circulation* 99:3272, 1999.

12. Cannon CR, Nishimura RA, Reeder GS, et al: Echocardiographic assessment of commissural calcium: A simple predictor of outcome after percutaneous mitral balloon valvotomy. *J Am Coll Cardiol* 29:175, 1997.

13. Chen Q, Hosir YF, Vletter WB, et al: Accurate assessment of MVA in patients with mitral stenosis by three-dimensional echocardiography. *J Am Soc Echocardiogr* 10:133–150, 1997.

14. Singh V, Nanda NC, Agrawal G, et al: Live three-dimensional echocardiographic assessment of mitral stenosis. *Echocardiography* 20:43–50, 2003.

15. Zamorano J, Cordeiro P, Sugeng L, et al: Real-time three dimensional echocardiography for rheumatic mitral valve stenosis evaluation. *J Am Coll Cardiol* 43:2091–2096, 2004.

16. Xie MX, Wang XF, Cheng TO, et al: Comparison of accuracy of mitral valve area in mitral stenosis by real-time, three-dimensional echocardiography versus two-dimensional echocardiography versus Doppler pressure half-time. *Am J Cardiol* 95:1496–1499, 2005.

17. Zamorano J, Perez de Isla L, Sugeng L, et al: Non-invasive assessment of mitral valve area during percutaneous balloon mitral valvuloplasty: Role of real-time 3D echocardiography. *Eur Heart J* 25:2086–2091, 2004.

18. Perez de Isla L, Casanova C, Almeria C, et al: Which method should be the reference method to evaluate the severity of rheumatic mitral stenosis? Gorline's method versus 3D echo. *Eur J Echocardiogr* 8(6):470–273, 2007.

19. Mannaerts HF, Kamp O, Visser CA: Should mitral valve area assessment in patients with mitral stenosis be based on anatomical or on functional evaluation? A plea for 3D echocardiography as the new clinical standard. *Eur Heart J* 25:2073–2074, 2004.

20. Zamorano J, Cordeiro P, Sugeng L, et al: Real-time three-dimensional echocardiography for rheumatic mitral valve stenosis evaluation: An accurate and novel approach. *J Am Coll Cardiol* 43:2091, 2004.

21. Applebaum RM, Kasliwal RR, Kanojia A, et al: Utility of three-dimensional echocardiography during balloon mitral valvuloplasty. *J Am Coll Cardiol* 32:1405–1409, 1998.

22. Gill EA, Bhola R, Carroll J, et al: Three dimensional echocardiography predictors of percutaneous balloon mitral valvuloplasty success. *Eur J Echocardiogr* 1:S32, 2001.

23. Gill EA, Bhola R, Carroll JD, et al: Live 3D echo and biplane evaluation of mitral stenosis for prediction of mitral valvuloplasty success. *J Am Soc Echocardiogr* 17:499, 2004.

24. Kim MJ, Song JK, Song JM, et al: Long-term outcomes of significant mitral regurgitation after percutaneous mitral valvuloplasty. *Circulation* 114:2815, 2006.

CHAPTER 7

Planning and Guiding Mitral Valve Repair

Gary S. Mak and Judy Hung

INTRODUCTION

Mitral valve prolapse is the most common structural cause of chronic mitral regurgitation leading to surgery in developed countries. The prevalence of mitral valve prolapse has been reported to be 2.5%.[1] Mitral valve repair is the clear treatment choice for symptomatic severe mitral regurgitation and now asymptomatic mitral regurgitation in many cases. An important advance in assessing mitral valve disease has been the development and application of real-time three-dimensional echocardiography (RT3DE), particularly RT3D transesophageal echocardiography (RT3DTEE), which allows accurate localization of segmental anatomy and pathology of the mitral valve. This chapter provides an overview of the pathophysiology, anatomy, variants, and natural history of mitral valve prolapse and the clinical applications of RT3DE for mitral valve repair.

BACKGROUND

Mitral valve prolapse is defined echocardiographically as superior displacement of the mitral leaflets into the left atrium by at least 2 mm beyond the mitral annular plane. Histologically, there is myxomatous degeneration of the leaflets, resulting in excessive and redundant leaflet tissue with elongated or ruptured chordae. The result is leaflet prolapse beyond the mitral annular plane during systole, causing regurgitation. This may lead to annular dilation and further progression of mitral regurgitation over time. There is a wide spectrum of mitral valve prolapse based on leaflet morphology. In the classic and more common form of mitral valve prolapse, the leaflets are diffusely thickened and redundant as a result of myxomatous degeneration. Such myxomatous changes may be localized to a single segment or involve the entire valve. The latter situation is known as *Barlow disease*, in which there is generalized thickening and billowing of the leaflets. In the less common, nonclassic form, the leaflets are normal in thickness. *Fibroelastic deficiency* is a term used when the disease is localized to isolated areas of the valve. Repair of Barlow disease can be challenging, with mitral valve repair techniques ranging from excision of excessive leaflet tissue to chordal manipulation and retention of leaflet tissue.[2] RT3DTEE has provided quantitative and mechanistic analysis of Barlow's disease versus fibroelastic deficiency, confirming the annular size and leaflet height in Barlow's disease.[3] Mitral valve prolapse appears to be both sporadic as well as familial. The familial cases appear to be inherited in an autosomal dominant fashion with variable expression. Mitral valve prolapse has been mapped to three genetic loci.[4,5]

The natural history of mitral valve prolapse is heterogeneous but largely determined by the severity of mitral regurgitation. Although most patients remain asymptomatic and may have a near-normal life expectancy, approximately 5% to 10% eventually develop severe mitral regurgitation.[6,7] Without surgical treatment, mitral valve prolapse with severe mitral regurgitation results in left ventricular dysfunction, heart failure, atrial fibrillation, and pulmonary hypertension. Other serious complications include spontaneous rupture of the chordae, endocarditis, and stroke. Patients with mitral valve prolapse and severe mitral regurgitation have mortality rates of 6% to 7% per year if left unoperated, and approximately 10% per year progress to meeting clear surgical indications.[8,9]

Unlike mitral valve prolapse, functional mitral regurgitation is caused by geometric ventricular remodeling without any valve leaflet pathology. This condition typically is secondary to ventricular dilation from chronic ischemic mitral regurgitation or dilated cardiomyopathy. In chronic ischemic mitral regurgitation, the valve leaflets and chordae appear relatively normal, without chordal elongation or rupture. Closure of the mitral valve leaflets is restricted by tethering of the leaflets caused by papillary muscle displacement.[10]

Mitral valve repair frequently is performed for both degenerative disease and functional disease. However, repair rates have been disappointingly low. Only 44% of patients in the United States and 46% of patients in Europe who required surgery for mitral regurgitation received mitral valve repair, but the rates of repair have been increasing over time.[11,12] Repair rates are lowest among patients with multiple comorbidities, those in New York Heart Association (NYHA) class III to IV, and those whose surgery is emergent.[12] The listed rates of 44% and 46% in the United States and Europe, respectively, were published in 2003 and hence represent surgical practices in the late 1990s. In the decade starting in 2010, the standard for mitral valve repair is approaching 75% in some institutions.[13] RT3DTEE has clearly played a role in this improvement, but there are many factors involved.

USE OF TWO-DIMENSIONAL AND THREE-DIMENSIONAL ECHOCARDIOGRAPHY IN MITRAL VALVE REPAIR

Noninvasive imaging, particularly echocardiography, plays a critical role in the initial and serial assessment of patients with chronic mitral regurgitation. A comprehensive echocardiographic examination is essential to a thorough understanding of the etiology and pathology of mitral regurgitation.[14] A systematic approach has been previously described to interrogate the mitral valve with two-dimensional TEE (2DTEE).[15] By using a standard approach to obtain four midesophageal views (four-chamber, bicommissural, two-chamber, and long-axis views) and the transgastric basal short-axis view, both mitral leaflets and their corresponding segments are carefully interrogated to determine the underlying pathophysiology of mitral regurgitation. The severity of mitral regurgitation can be determined by qualitative or quantitative Doppler assessment. The left ventricular end-systolic dimensions and ejection fraction can be accurately assessed by 2D and 3D techniques, although the assessment is more accurate by 3D volumes. With RT3DTEE, the mitral valve can be easily obtained in an anatomically correct orientation. The surgeon's view also can be easily displayed by rotating the aortic valve to the 11 o'clock position. Compared with 2DTEE, 3DTEE is able to provide more accurate assessment of the annular dimensions and height, the leaflet length and surface area, and the coaptation area. The distances between the commissures and papillary muscles also can be measured. Such measurements are important for understanding the mechanism of mitral regurgitation and improving surgical planning of mitral valve repair. In a large cohort of patients undergoing mitral valve repair, 3DTEE has provided an objective means of predicting repair complexity in mitral regurgitation with a range of etiologies.[16] The most predictive model for complex mitral valve repair includes multisegment pathology, prolapsing height, and posterior leaflet angle. These simple parameters are suggested to be objective indicators to guide surgical decisions about mitral valve repair. 3DTEE also has been shown to have the best agreement in identifying anterior leaflet prolapse compared with other echocardiographic techniques.[17]

WHY MITRAL VALVE REPAIR?

Despite the major limitation of a finite incidence of recurrence of mitral regurgitation, mitral valve repair results in significant improvement in long-term survival compared with mitral valve replacement.[18] The goals of mitral valve repair are to obtain an adequate surface of coaptation of both leaflets in systole and to preserve or repair leaflet mobility and the subvalvular annulus. In addition, an annuloplasty ring or band should be placed to reinforce the repair to correct and prevent progressive annular dilation.[19,20] Carpentier's technique remains the most common approach and is associated with excellent long-term results. It generally involves resection of abnormal or pathologic tissue, followed by precise reconstruction to restore normal valve anatomy.[21] In patients with isolated prolapse of the posterior middle scallop (P2), the most common cause of degenerative mitral regurgitation, repair usually is treated with limited quadrangular or triangular leaflet resection and the removal of the elongated or ruptured chordae and supporting apparatus. The remaining scallops of the posterior leaflet are then reapproximated. To correct excessive posterior leaflet tissue, a sliding annuloplasty is performed to reduce the height of the posterior leaflet, followed by reapproximation of the free edges.[22] Finally, the dilated or distorted annulus is stabilized with an annuloplasty ring or band. The ultimate goals are to restore the normal height and shape of residual leaflet segments and the normal relationship of the surface areas of the anterior and posterior leaflets to the annular size in a given patient. To prevent systolic anterior motion (SAM) of the anterior mitral leaflet, it is important to keep the coaptation point of the leaflets from being too close to the ventricular septum and causing left ventricular outflow tract obstruction.[22-24]

To resolve SAM of the anterior leaflet intraoperatively, volume loading, increasing afterload, and stopping inotropic drugs may help. In some cases, repeat repair or replacement of the mitral valve with a prosthetic valve may be necessary. SAM has been reported in as many as 14% of patients with myxomatous disease after valve repair, but it affects fewer than 10%.[25] The need for complex sliding annuloplasty or other reconstruction is reduced with the use of new large-diameter rings that accommodate larger leaflets and move the coaptation point farther away from the septum.[26]

Isolated anterior leaflet repair or concomitant repair of anterior and posterior leaflets traditionally has been considered more complex. However, the experiences and approaches to repair of the anterior leaflet continue to evolve and improve. The major challenge to anterior leaflet repair is created by the anterior portion of the mitral annulus sharing tissue with the aortic valve. This makes the anterior leaflet less amenable to the quadrangular resection because of increased rigidity. There are multiple approaches to anterior leaflet repair, including limited triangular resection of the anterior leaflet, chordal shortening and transposition, artificial chordal replacement, and edge-to-edge repair.[27,28] However, there has not been a consensus or scientific evidence of a preferred approach. There is substantial variability from institution to institution in the approach to anterior leaflet repair and combined repair of the anterior and posterior leaflets.

Intraoperative 2DTEE and RT3DTEE should be routinely performed in mitral valve repair. Evaluation of the mitral leaflets by 3DTEE has been shown to be superior to 2DTEE, and the complexity of the repair can be predicted.[17,29,30] When planning mitral valve repair, the following are important determinants of the complexity: (1) severity of mitral regurgitation, (2) the mechanism of mitral regurgitation, (3) the anatomic lesions, (4) the underlying degenerative etiology (Barlow disease vs. fibroelastic deficiency), (5) segmental leaflet pathology, (6) subvalvular pathology and calcification, (7) left ventricular size and function, (8) left atrial size and presence of thrombus, (9) other concomitant valve lesions, (10) presence of a patent foramen ovale, and (11) right ventricular function.[15,31] Measurements, including the mitral annular diameter, anterior and posterior mitral leaflet dimensions, and the distance from the coaptation point of the mitral leaflets to the septum, can be made with intraoperative TEE to predict the likelihood of SAM developing after mitral valve repair.[23] A short anterior mitral leaflet, a long posterior leaflet, or a short distance from the coaptation point to the septum is associated with higher likelihood of SAM developing after repair. The chance of SAM after repair can be minimized with knowledge of these echocardiographic parameters. After completion of the repair and removal of the patient from cardiopulmonary bypass, the valve should be reassessed for any residual mitral regurgitation, mitral gradient, and SAM. Ventricular function and any residual intracardiac air also can be assessed. A finding of more than mild mitral regurgitation should lead to consideration of reexploration of the mitral valve to identify the etiology of residual regurgitation, such as uncorrected prolapse, separation of a leaflet cleft, a defect in a leaflet-to-leaflet coaptation, or a perforation of a leaflet from a ring suture near the leaflet hinge. For persistent SAM with residual mitral regurgitation and a significant outflow tract gradient, reoperative correction should be considered. The main surgical approaches to address SAM are leaflet shortening or the use of a short neochordae to displace the posterior leaflet of excess leaflet height into the ventricle and out of the orifice.[24] A larger mitral ring annuloplasty device can also be placed if there is a question about inappropriate sizing of the annulus during the initial repair.[26]

Patients who have undergone mitral valve repair should have a follow-up transthoracic echocardiography (TTE) prior to discharge to assess the mitral regurgitation under normal loading and pressure conditions. The presence of residual moderate or severe mitral regurgitation should lead to strong consideration of repeat valve exploration for additional repair or replacement. Quantification of mitral regurgitation can be assessed by RT3DTTE with 3D vena contracta methods.[32]

DATA ON CHORDAL PRESERVATION

RT3DTEE has been shown to be superior to 2DTEE for assessment of chordal rupture.[33,34] Although RT3DTEE has not yet been evaluated for surgical replacement of chordae, an emerging paradigm is based on the use of polytetrafluoroethylene (PTFE) neochordae to reconstruct the support of the free edge of prolapsing segments and to ensure a good leaflet coaptation surface, thereby preserving the valve without SAM of the anterior leaflet.[35,36] A common technique is to anchor the neochordae into the papillary muscle heads in the fibrous portion and attach the branches to the free edges to prevent excess tension on the leaflet margins.[37] With significant excess posterior leaflet height, the neochordae are sufficiently short to displace the prolapsing segment into the left ventricle to maintain a large surface of coaptation for the anterior leaflet while preventing SAM of the anterior leaflet. The surgery is significantly more complex with the placement of artificial chordae. On one hand, residual mitral valve prolapse and residual regurgitation may occur when chordae are too long. On the other hand, leaflet restriction and residual mitral regurgitation may occur when chordae are too short.

Chordal transfer to the free margin within the same segment or chordal transposition from one segment to another may be considered if residual prolapse remains after resection of abnormal tissue. In cases of mitral valve prolapse without redundant leaflet tissue, limited resection or artificial chordal replacement may be performed, followed by reinforcement with an annuloplasty ring or band. Diffuse mitral annular calcification can pose a special challenge to valve reconstruction.[38] With the presence of calcification of the chordae, papillary muscles, leaflets, and annulus, careful debridement of calcified tissue often is required to restore normal leaflet motion and to ensure an adequate surface of coaptation.

Because the posterior aspect of the mitral annulus is not contiguous with the fibrous skeleton of the heart, pathologic annular dilation may result from chronic regurgitation associated with atrial and ventricular enlargement. Regardless of the leaflet and chordal techniques used, an annuloplasty ring or band often is necessary to restore the normal circumference and shape of the mitral valve to match the available leaflet tissue. The appropriate ring size for the amount of leaflet tissue is determined by the surface area of the anterior leaflet; a standard-length band has been used by some groups with excellent results.[39] Absence of an annuloplasty at the time of mitral valve repair is one of the strongest predictors of repair failure, resulting in recurrent moderate or severe mitral regurgitation.[40]

SURGICAL MORBIDITY AND MORTALITY OF MITRAL VALVE REPAIR

Mitral valve repair is associated with an operative mortality rate of 3% or less.[41-45] This figure is close to 1% in high-volume centers.[46] The most common cause of death is heart failure. Predictors of death include advanced age; poor NYHA functional class; atrial fibrillation; low ejection fraction; high left ventricular end-systolic dimensions; and other comorbidities such as diabetes, obesity, renal disease, and chronic lung disease.[41,47,48] In an analysis from the Society of Thoracic Surgeons National Adult Cardiac Surgery Database, major postoperative complications of mitral valve repair before discharge include prolonged (>24 hours) ventilatory support (7.3% of patients), renal failure (2.6%), and stroke (1.4%).[48] Reoperation during initial hospitalization was reported in 6.3% of patients. Approximately 5% of patients have thromboembolism develop in the first 5 years after initial surgery.[41,49] Intraoperative conversion to mitral valve replacement occurs in 2% to 10% of cases. Other rare complications of mitral valve repair include damage to important structures around the mitral apparatus such as the left circumflex coronary artery, the bundle of His, and the aortic valve.

RECURRENT MITRAL REGURGITATION AND REOPERATION RATES

The most important late complication of mitral valve repair is recurrent mitral regurgitation. The recurrence rate is higher in patients with functional mitral regurgitation. Recent reports of recurrent moderate to severe mitral regurgitation range from 5% to 29%.[40,50] Other reports cite recurrence of moderate to severe mitral regurgitation in 1% to 2% of patients per year during mid-term follow-up.[40,51] The reoperation rate is very low in degenerative mitral valve surgery; 15-year freedom from reoperation is 95%.[21] Reoperation to treat recurrent mitral regurgitation after primary repair is required in approximately 0.5% to 1.5% of patients per year.[45,47] The most common cause of recurrent mitral regurgitation is progression of the underlying degenerative process of the original valve. Leaflet shortening or scarring, ring dehiscence, and infective endocarditis also may cause recurrent regurgitation. In patients with functional mitral regurgitation, conventional ring annuloplasty is prone to failure. Recurrent severe mitral regurgitation is reported in 25% of patients as early as 1 year after surgery.[52] Other rare complications following mitral valve repair include pannus in-growth triggered by the mitral annuloplasty ring and hemolysis that may justify the need for reoperation.

RESULTS OF MITRAL VALVE REPAIR VERSUS REPLACEMENT

Mitral valve replacement can be performed with either a mechanical valve or a bioprosthetic valve. Mechanical valves, on one hand, are associated with the risk of thromboembolism and require lifelong anticoagulation. On the other hand, bioprosthetic valves are associated with the risk of valve deterioration and failure. There is also the risk of prosthetic valve endocarditis. If the chordae tendineae are severed during mitral valve replacement, the ventricular wall is no longer anchored to the valve apparatus, and the tethering effect of the chordae is lost. As a result, left ventricular wall stress increases and left ventricular function deteriorates in the long term.[53-56]

Successful mitral valve repair is achieved in approximately 90% of all surgical cases of chronic mitral regurgitation regardless of lesions or associated leaflet dysfunction.[57] Mitral valve repair is preferable to replacement for most patients undergoing surgery for mitral regurgitation. The advantages of mitral valve repair include lower rates of thromboembolism, higher resistance to endocarditis, effective late durability (reportedly for as long as 25 years), and no need for anticoagulation in most patients.[58,59] Repair has been demonstrated to be superior in the setting of combined coronary bypass procedure, reoperation, double-valve procedure, and in the older adult population.[60-63] Mitral valve repair should be the standard of care whenever possible.

However, to date no prospective randomized trials have compared mitral valve repair with replacement. Studies reported thus far are not completely isolated from bias or heterogeneity in the cohort. Data from observational studies suggest a benefit of mitral valve repair.[64-66] A meta-analysis compared mitral valve repair with replacement for degenerative mitral valve disease and suggested lower survival rates in mitral valve replacement compared with repair.[64] Another report showed a significant 5-year survival benefit for patients who underwent mitral valve repair versus replacement, but no difference in quality of life.[65] However, in a study of patients who underwent an isolated primary operation for degenerative mitral valve disease, there was no significant difference in survival at 5, 10, or 15 years between mitral valve repair versus replacement among propensity-matched cohorts.[66]

Individual and institutional experience is crucial in determining the likelihood of the success of a mitral valve repair. High-volume centers tend to have the lowest mortality rates and the greatest proportion of patients undergoing mitral valve repair rather than replacement.[46] In contemporary practice, mitral valve replacement for degenerative disease as a primary operation should be infrequent. The most common scenario for a replacement should be an end-stage Barlow disease, typically seen in older adults with longstanding disease. If valve replacement is necessary, a chordal sparing procedure should be considered to preserve the annular-papillary continuity. Although calcified leaflet segments require resection, noncalcified segments with intact chordae can be incorporated into the annulus with sutures used to implant the prosthesis.

ADVANCEMENTS IN MITRAL VALVE REPAIR

The principles of mitral valve repair have evolved since the classic Carpentier technique, which primarily involves quandrangular leaflet resection, transposition of normal chordae to other areas of prolapsing leaflet tissue, and placement of an annuloplasty ring or band.[20] Because the mitral annulus is a dynamic, saddle-shaped structure, newer annuloplasty rings have increasingly attempted to replicate the natural shape and provide flexibility for the annulus. Optimal size and material properties of an annuloplasty ring are important because they change the geometry and dynamics of the mitral annulus after implantation and directly affect the durability of mitral valve repair. Annuloplasty rings with a disproportional reduction in the septal-lateral dimension are designed to restore leaflet coaptation in functional mitral regurgitation. Annuloplasty rings of different shapes and rigidity have been studied, as have their effects on anterior mitral leaflet and mitral annular dynamics in animal models, with the goal of improving long-term durability of the mitral valve repair.[67]

Recently, surgeons in selective centers have gained experience in minimally invasive approaches to mitral valve repair. Although minimally invasive surgery may broadly refer to avoidance of a full sternotomy, robotic approach to mitral valve repair is becoming increasingly popular, especially in patients who are young and asymptomatic. In a recent series of 261 consecutive cases of robotic mitral valve repair for posterior leaflet prolapse, no deaths were reported, although the cohort was skewed toward a low-risk group.[68] In addition, the robotic approach to mitral valve repair has been limited to degenerative posterior leaflet prolapse, which has the most extensive experience, and overall outcomes depend greatly on the experience of the surgeons. Data comparing the quality of repair and outcomes of minimally invasive approach to conventional surgery are still insufficient. There is also growing experience with minimally invasive mitral valve repair performed through a right mini-thoracotomy. In a single-center series involving 1339 patients, the 30-day mortality rate was 2.4%, the 5-year survival rate was 82.6%, and the reoperation rate was 3.7%.[69] These results are similar to those of traditional surgery. However, these minimally invasive approaches still require further evaluation with respect to widespread generalizability and cost effectiveness.

Edge-to-edge approximation of the leaflets (the Alfieri technique) has reemerged in traditional mitral valve repair.[70,71] This technique typically is used with other repair techniques and annuloplasty because recurrent mitral regurgitation and a high risk for reoperation often result when this technique is used without an annuloplasty ring. One risk of edge-to-edge repair is restriction of the the mitral orifice, which could potentially lead to mitral stenosis if thickening or stiffening of the leaflets is present.

For complex ischemic mitral valve disease, some procedures have focused on the subannular procedures to approximate the papillary muscles, pull the papillary muscles toward the annulus to release leaflet tethering, or cut secondary chordae to reduce tethering of the leaflets.[72] Most patients with mitral regurgitation undergoing coronary bypass are treated with a simple annuloplasty ring or band.

PERCUTANEOUS APPROACHES TO MITRAL REGURGITATION

A variety of new percutaneous approaches to mitral valve disease are in early clinical use or undergoing preclinical investigation. Recent reviews of this broad area have been published.[73,74] The edge-to-edge surgical technique has been modified for a percutaneous approach, such as the MitraClip (Abbott Vascular, Santa Clara, CA). This device can be applied on opposing prolapsed segments of the mitral leaflets as a practical approach for patients with a simple localized prolapsed segment such as A2, P2, or both. The pathology and mechanism of mitral regurgitation need to be thoroughly assessed to determine the suitability for repair with the device. TEE, especially RT3DTEE, is critical to guide device deployment so that an immediate assessment of the device stability and results of the repair can be made.

As in the case of deployment of clips to the leaflet edges, multiple TEE views are important to center the clips over the mitral valve orifice and align the clips with the leaflet edges. The clip is oriented perpendicular to the coaptation line, and simultaneous perpendicular planes can be obtained.[75] The clip is closed when the leaflets have fallen into the clip arms. The degree of reduction of mitral regurgitation can be immediately assessed. If the initial results are suboptimal, the clip can be repositioned, or a second clip can be deployed. The mid-term results of this percutaneous approach have shown similar improvements in clinical outcomes but superior safety compared with traditional surgery, despite lower success at reducing mitral regurgitation. Of the patients with successful procedure, 77% had less than 2+ mitral regurgitation on discharge.[76] In patients with severe symptomatic mitral regurgitation deemed to be at high surgical risk because of comorbidities, the MitraClip procedure has been shown to reduce severity of mitral regurgitation in the majority of patients, with improvement in clinical symptoms and left ventricular reverse remodeling at 1-year follow-up.[77] However, this percutaneous approach does not address the shape of the dilated or distorted annulus without an accompanying annuloplasty. For surgical experience with the edge-to-edge technique not accompanied by an annuloplasty, 30% of patients require reoperation for significant recurrent mitral regurgitation at 5 years compared with 8% of those with an annuloplasty.[70,78]

There is significant interest in placing devices in the coronary sinus to push against the posterior mitral annulus to improve coaptation of the posterior and anterior mitral valve leaflets by reducing the overall circumference and the anteroposterior diameter of the mitral annulus. However, the coronary sinus does not lie directly adjacent to the posterior mitral annulus and often is not in the same plane as the annulus.[79] Given the variability of the anatomy and position of the coronary sinus and the great cardiac vein, the dimensions of the coronary sinus from both the mitral annulus and the center of the mitral valve orifice need to be accurately determined.[80] The position of the cardiac veins in relation to the mitral annulus may predict the procedural success and also the course of the left circumflex artery, whose branches need to be assessed prior to the deployment of the device. With the left circumflex coronary artery or its branches lying between the mitral annulus and the coronary sinus, placement of the device may compromise the left circumflex artery.[81] Although cardiac computed tomography and magnetic resonance imaging can provide such information prior to the procedure, it is prudent to use RT3DTEE as a guide with regard to the anatomic landmarks during the procedure and to assess the immediate results after deployment of the devices.

RECOMMENDATIONS FOR MITRAL VALVE SURGERY

Long-term survival following mitral valve repair is similar to age-matched controls, provided the operation is performed before onset of symptoms, ventricular dysfunction, or atrial fibrillation.[59] Patients undergoing mitral valve surgery with advanced symptoms do poorly compared with less symptomatic patients, so surgery should always be recommended at the onset of symptoms in otherwise low-risk patients. Long-term survival is compromised in patients after mitral surgery if the initial ejection fraction has fallen below 60%. An ejection fraction below 60% is a trigger for surgical consideration.

The current recommendation for mitral valve repair in the treatment of severe degenerative mitral regurgitation is based on observational data. Whether early surgery should be recommended for asymptomatic patients who have severe mitral regurgitation without left ventricular dysfunction or dilation, atrial fibrillation, or pulmonary hypertension is still a subject of great debate. Some investigators have found evidence of reduced morbidity and mortality with surgery and recommend early surgery, whereas others have found similar outcomes for watchful waiting.[42,82,83] Because of the advantages of repair over replacement, the threshold for performing mitral valve repair has definitely been lowered, with the degree of reduction individualized by local institutional expertise. Patients with mitral regurgitation who have early or questionable symptoms or even those who are asymptomatic often are recommended for surgery, especially if the repair rate exceeds 90%, according to the American College of Cardiology Foundation/American Heart Association guidelines.[84,85] However, the European Society of Cardiology guidelines recommend watchful waiting with medical therapy and close follow-up.[86]

Mitral valve repair has matured and evolved beyond the first generation of techniques and devices, building on an improved knowledge of the pathophysiology and limitations of prior approaches as well as extensive experience. Newer techniques and annuloplasty rings have been designed to increase the effectiveness and durability of mitral valve repair. It is hoped that these devices will gain evidence to show improved repair outcomes and ultimately lead to wider adoption in general practice by cardiac surgeons. Percutaneous approaches to mitral valve repair are still in development. Novel percutaneous repair approaches are built on lessons learned from traditional surgical techniques and are designed to be safer, more effective, and durable. Echocardiography, particularly RT3DTEE, has significantly contributed to the improvement in the assessment of pathology and success during and after mitral valve repair from both surgical and percutaneous approaches.

CASE STUDIES

CASE 1 (Figures 7-1 to 7-6, Videos 7-1 to 7-5)

A 57-year-old man with mitral valve regurgitation showed evidence of enlargement of ventricular dimensions. He also had declining function status.

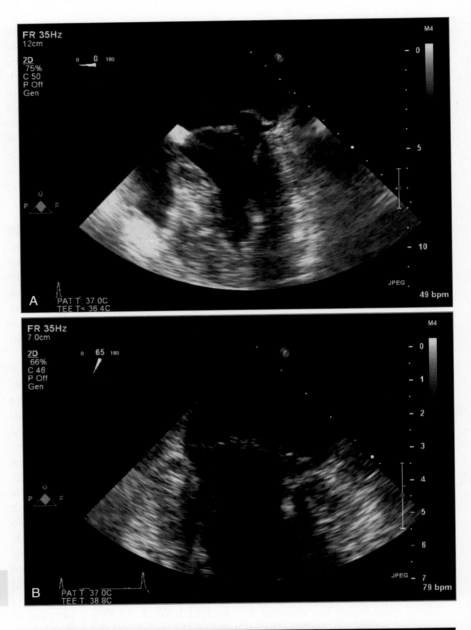

Figure 7-1 Prolapse of posterior leaflet P2, possibly anterior leaflet A2, before repair.

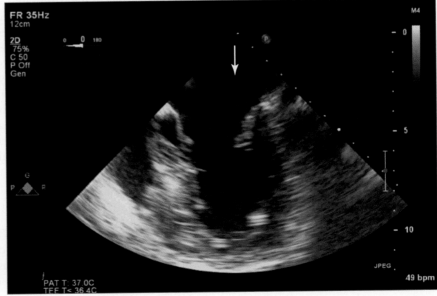

Figure 7-2 Two-dimensional transesophageal echocardiography showing posterior leaflet (likely P2) prolapse.

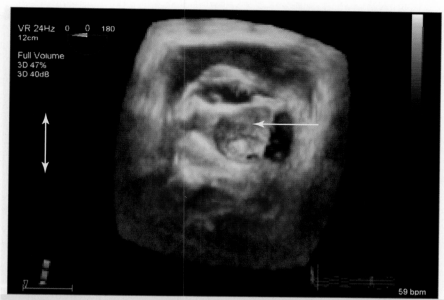

Figure 7-3 Three-dimensional prolapse of posterior leaflet P2. The prolapse of anterior leaflet A2 is much more difficult to appreciate (*arrow*).

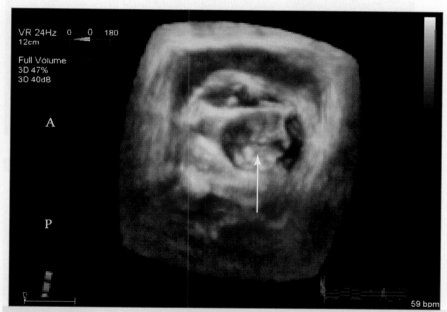

Figure 7-4 The surgeon's view of three-dimensional transesophageal echocardiography of posterior leaflet P2 prolapse (*arrow*). There is also some minor prolapse of anterior leaflet A2, directly anterior.

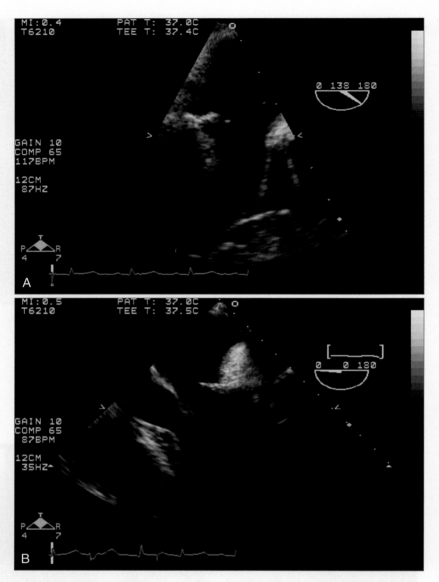

Figure 7-5   A, A long-axis, mid-esophageal transesophageal echocardiography (TEE) view shows systolic anterior motion (SAM) after mitral valve repair. **B,** A four-chamber TEE view demonstrates very mild SAM after mitral valve repair. No additional intervention was needed for the SAM.

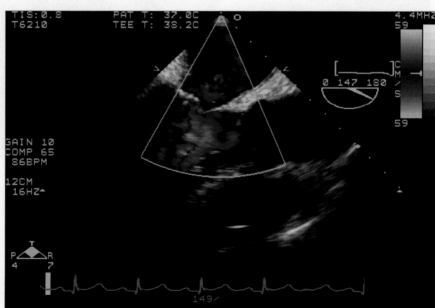

Figure 7-6   Postrepair echocardiography shows only trace regurgitation.

Intraoperative echocardiography confirmed that the pathology was predominantly in the central portion of the posterior mitral leaflet (P2), with marked hooding of the segment. There was also mild prolapse of the middle segment (A2) of the anterior leaflet. 2DE color Doppler showed a small central regurgitant jet and a bigger eccentric, anteriorly directed jet. Visual inspection confirmed that the central portion of the posterior mitral leaflet had markedly excess motion and elongated chordate. The P1 and P3 segments were well supported. The patient underwent radical mitral valve reconstruction and left atrial appendage amputation. The central portion of the posterior segment was resected by triangular resection, and the posterior leaflet was reconstituted with interrupted sutures tied on the ventricular side. A partial annular ring was placed. Immediately after repair, there was minimal and intermittent systolic anterior motion of the chordal apparatus with residual trace mitral regurgitation.

CASE 2 (Figures 7-7 to 7-14, Videos 7-6 to 7-12)

A 70-year-old man with a recent history of symptomatic mitral regurgitation had noted dyspnea with exertion. He had recently been diagnosed with atrial fibrillation, although he was unaware of it. Echocardiography showed preserved left ventricular function with severe mitral regurgitation emanating from a flail P2 segment of the posterior leaflet. The chordae tendinae to the posterior mitral leaflet were ruptured. 3DTEE confirmed that the valvular prolapse was limited to P2. The jet of the mitral regurgitation was directed anteriorly. He underwent mitral valve repair with a minimally invasive approach. Intraoperative

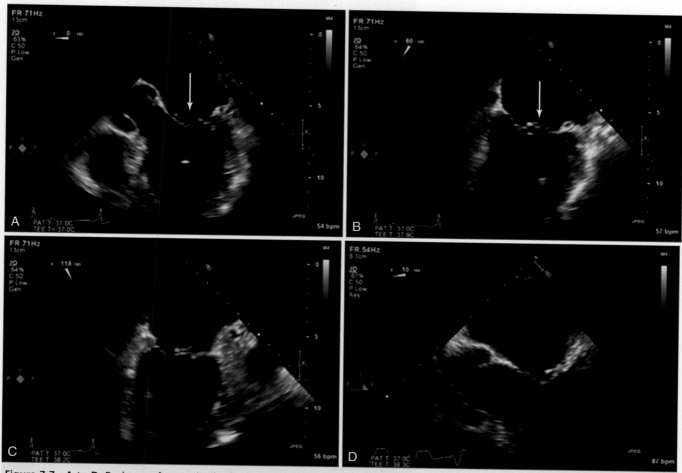

Figure 7-7 **A to D,** Prolapse of posterior leaflet P2 (*arrows*).

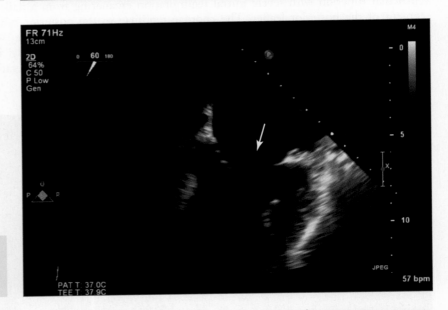

Figure 7-8 Two-dimensional transesophageal echocardiography showing posterior leaflet prolapse and flail chordae.

Figure 7-9 Two-dimensional transesophageal echocardiography showing posterior leaflet prolapse. Bicommisural view with posterior tilt shows prolapse is most likely P2 (*arrow*).

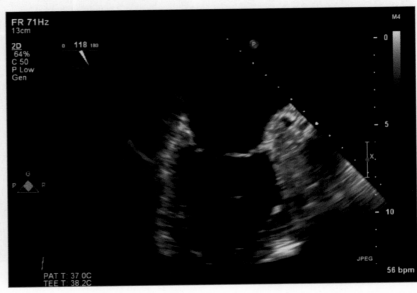

Figure 7-10 Two-dimensional transesophageal echocardiography showing direct anteroposterior view (118 degrees). This view should line up anterior leaflet A2 and posterior leaflet P2, which shows P2 prolapse with flail chordae (thin structure with movement independent of the valve leaflet).

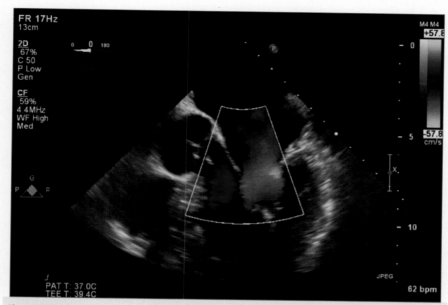

Figure 7-11 Prolapse of posterior leaflet P2 showing anteriorly directed mitral regurgitation jet.

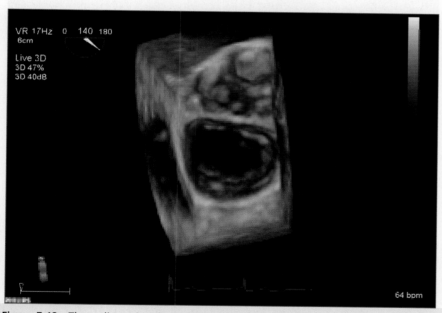

Figure 7-12 Three-dimensional transesophageal echocardiography confirms posterior leaflet P2 prolapse only, with ruptured chordae tendinae shown with motion independent of the posterior leaflet.

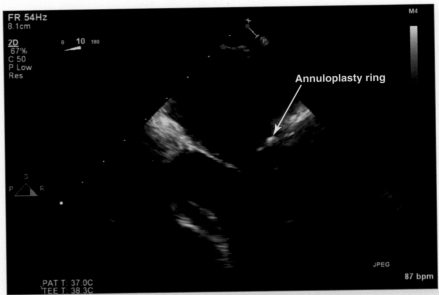

Figure 7-13 Postrepair two-dimensional transesophageal echocardiography shows excellent coaptation of the mitral leaflets, an annuloplasty ring, and no systolic anterior motion or mitral stenosis.

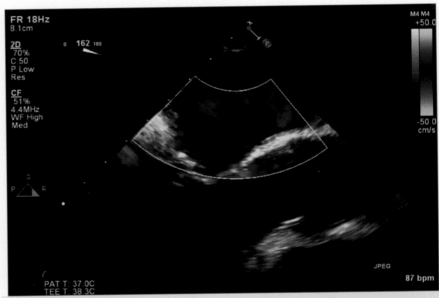

Figure 7-14 Postrepair echocardiography showing only a trace degree of mitral regurgitation.

examination of the leaflet showed obvious and pronounced rupture of multiple cords along the mid-portion of the posterior leaflet of the mitral valve, with evident thickening and prolapse. This was resected in a triangular fashion, and the posterior leaflet was reconstructed with interrupted sutures. After surgical repair, there was only trace mitral regurgitation and no evidence of mitral stenosis or systolic anterior motion.

CASE 3 (Figures 7-15 to 7-21, Videos 7-13 to 7-18)

A 79-year-old woman had mitral regurgitation and evolving congestive heart failure. Her left ventricular dimensions were enlarging, and she was referred for surgery. Echocardiographic studies showed severe prolapse of the posterior mitral

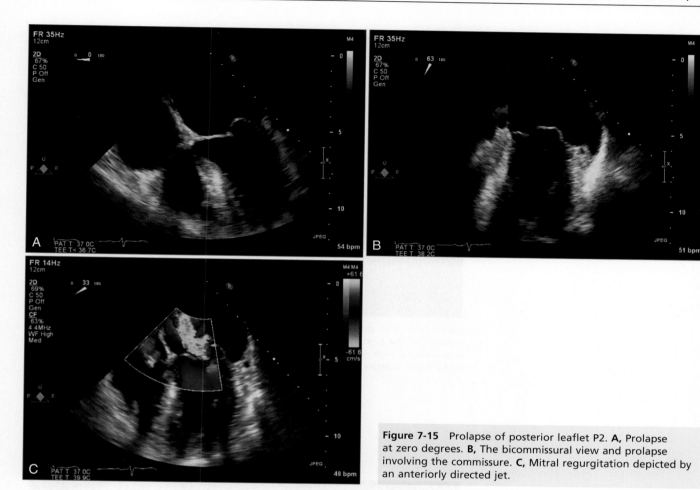

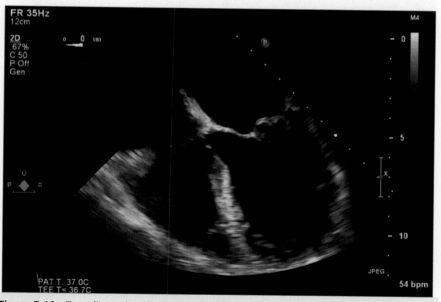

Figure 7-15   Prolapse of posterior leaflet P2. **A,** Prolapse at zero degrees. **B,** The bicommissural view and prolapse involving the commissure. **C,** Mitral regurgitation depicted by an anteriorly directed jet.

Figure 7-16   Two-dimensional transesophageal echocardiography shows classic prolapse of the posterior leaflet of the mitral valve.

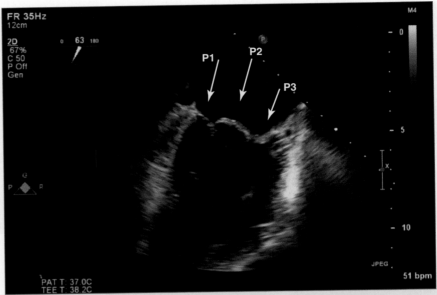

Figure 7-17   Two-dimensional transesophageal echocardiography shows classic prolapse of the posterior leaflet P2. Involvement of P3 also is suggested. The bicommisural view with posterior tilt in this case should show P2 in the middle of the mitral valve capture (*arrows*).

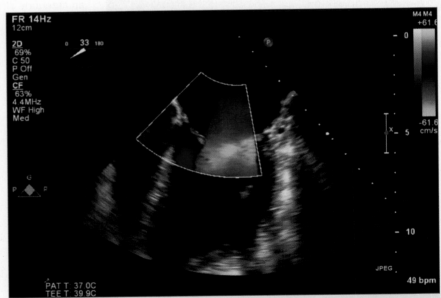

Figure 7-18   Two-dimensional transesophageal echocardiography with anteriorly directed mitral regurgitation.

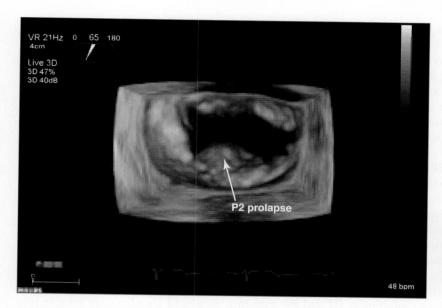

Figure 7-19 Three-dimensional transesophageal echocardiography (3DTEE) image showing extensive posterior leaflet prolapse, particularly of P2 and part of P3. In this case, 3DTEE better demonstrates that the prolapse is both P2 and P3 compared with two-dimensional TEE.

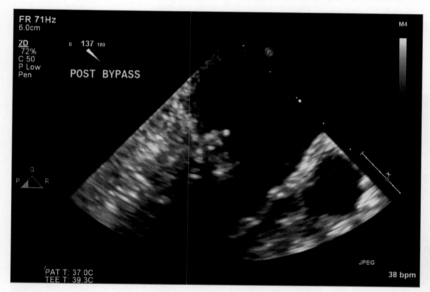

Figure 7-20 Trivial amount of systolic anterior motion and optimal coaptation of the repaired posterior leaflet with the anterior leaflet seen.

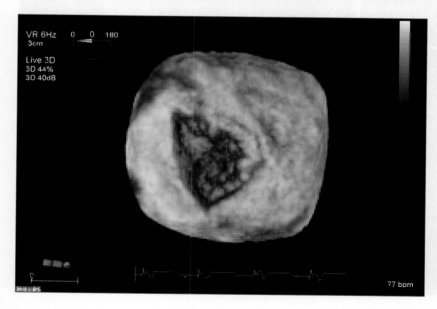

Figure 7-21 Three-dimensional transesophageal echocardiography (3DTEE) of the mitral valve after repair showing optimal coaptation of the mitral valve leaflets. Unfortunately, the quality of the 3DTEE was suboptimal.

valve leaflet, particularly P2, which was thickened and redundant. Involvement of P3 was suggested by 2DTEE and confirmed by 3DTEE. There was moderate to severe mitral regurgitation. She underwent radical mitral valve reconstruction that incorporated an annuloplasty band. A triangular resection of the central portion of P2 segment was performed, and the resection site was reconstituted with interrupted simple sutures. An annuloplasty band was sutured to the mitral annulus. Echocardiographic images after repair showed mild systolic anterior motion of the chordal apparatus and no residual mitral regurgitation.

CASE 4 (Figures 7-22 to 7-26, Videos 7-19 to 7-22)

A 68-year-old man had a history of progressive exertional dyspnea over the previous 10 months. He had a long history of heart murmur but had been asymptomatic until approximately 10 months ago. Evaluation showed severe mitral regurgitation with heavily calcified mitral annulus. The patient also had a history of transient ischemic attack with monocular blindness. Echocardiographic studies showed calcification of the posterior mitral annulus with severe prolapse of the posterior (P2 and P3) mitral leaflet. A portion of the P2 and P3 segments was flail. Intraoperatively, a large amount of calcium was noted involving the posterior annulus at P2 and P3 segments. Ruptured chordae were present into the P2 and P3 segments. Decalcification of the mitral annulus was performed first, and the mitral valve was reconstructed. Several neochordae were placed

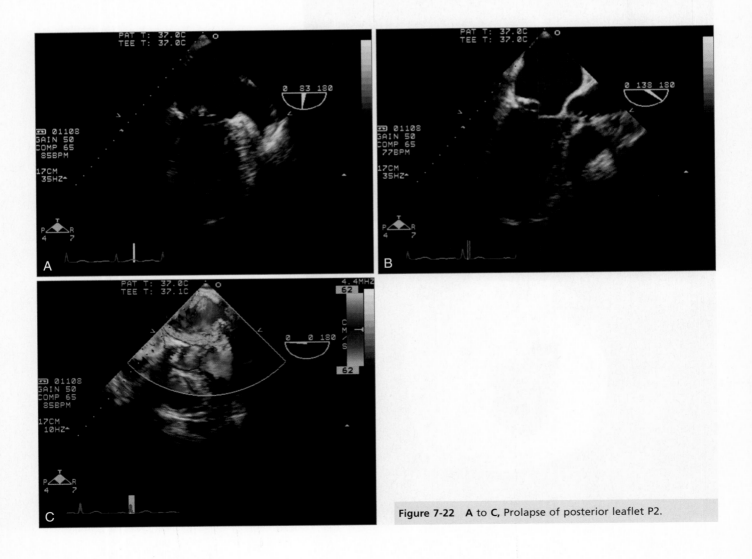

Figure 7-22 **A** to **C**, Prolapse of posterior leaflet P2.

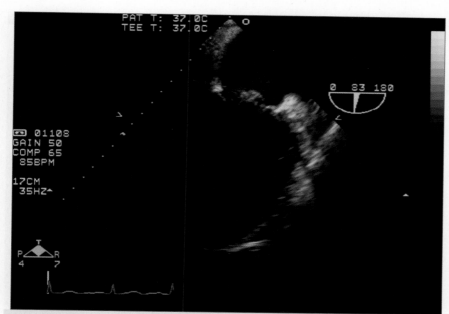

Figure 7-23 Two-dimensional transesophageal echocardiography (2DTEE) at an 83-degree view showing prolapse of posterior leaflet P2 with extensive "hooding" of the leaflet and some chordae tendinae seen in the left atrium. Whether the involvement is all P2 or also includes P3 is difficult to tell by 2DTEE.

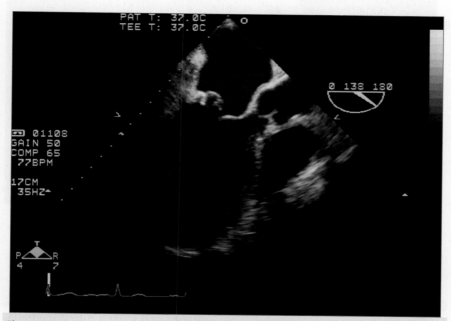

Figure 7-24 Two-dimensional transesophageal echocardiography at a 138-degree view showing posterior leaflet prolapse with extensive "hooding" of the posterior leaflet and some chordae tendinae seen in the left atrium.

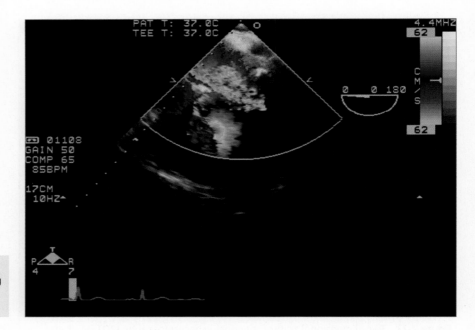

Figure 7-25 Two-dimensional transesophageal echocardiography showing extreme mitral regurgitation with a posteriorly directed jet.

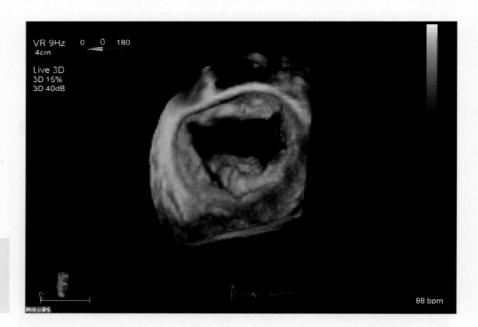

Figure 7-26 Three-dimensional transesophageal echocardiography of prolapse of posterior leaflet segments P2 and P3 with chordae tendinae visible. The extent of flail chordae is notable.

through the fibrous heads of several papillary muscle heads and brought to the ruptured chordae.

CASE 5 (Figures 7-27 to 7-34, Videos 7-23 to 7-28)

A 66-year-old man with history of hyperlipidemia and known mitral regurgitation recently had an episode of transient ischemic attack and visual loss. Serial echocardiography documented worsening mitral regurgitation from a flail posterior leaflet. Coronary angiography showed severe distal left main artery and proximal left circumflex artery lesions. TEE showed severe mitral regurgitation caused by flail posterior leaflet near the junction of the P1 and P2 segments. There were ruptured chordae tendinae to the posterior mitral leaflet at the P1-P2 junction. The jet of mitral regurgitation was directed anterolaterally. Confirmation of P1 and P2 prolapse was confirmed by 3DTEE. Coronary bypass surgery

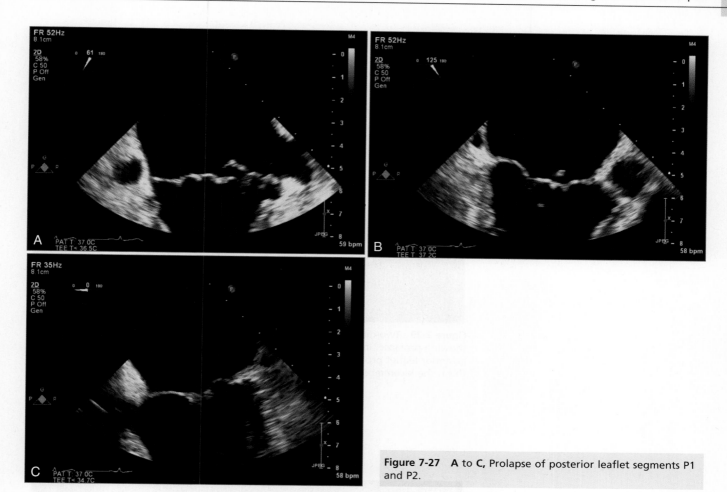

Figure 7-27   **A** to **C,** Prolapse of posterior leaflet segments P1 and P2.

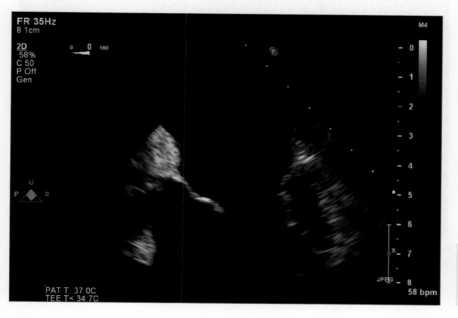

Figure 7-28   Two-dimensional transesophageal echocardiography at zero degrees. At this angle the prolapse, which is dramatic, is not seen.

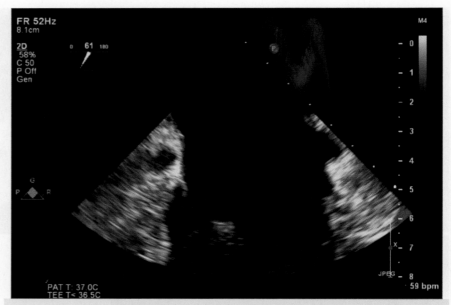

Figure 7-29 Two-dimensional transesophageal echocardiography at a 61-degree view showing prolapse. Interestingly, it is not entirely clear that what is seen here is posterior leaflet prolapse. The prolapse is suggested to involve the commissures since this is the bicommissural view.

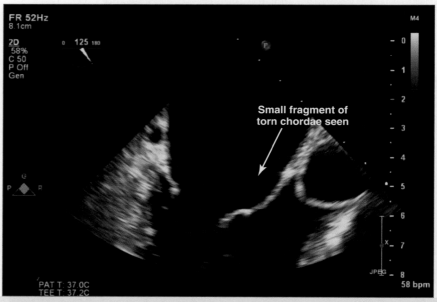

Figure 7-30 In this 125-degree view, the ruptured chordae of the posterior leaflet are visualized and there is minimal posterior leaflet prolapse.

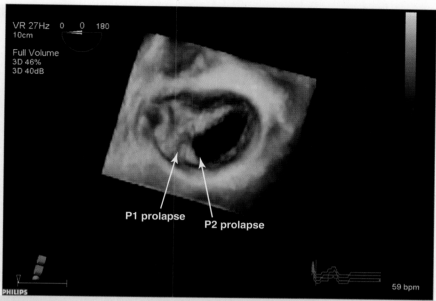

Figure 7-31   Three-dimensional transesophageal echocardiography showing prolapse of posterior leaflet segments P1 and P2.

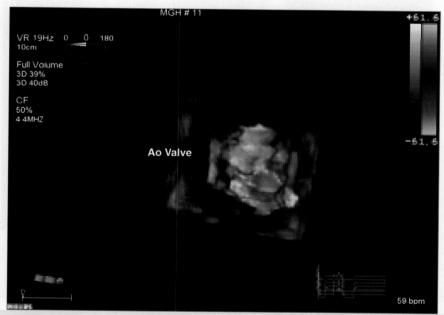

Figure 7-32   Three-dimensional transesophageal echocardiography of mitral regurgitation. The mitral regurgitation jet is anteriorly directed. Ao, aortic.

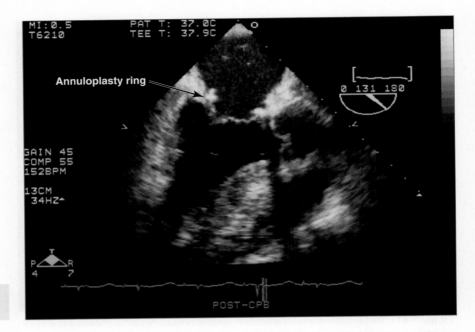

Figure 7-33 Mitral valve repair showing mitral annuloplasty ring.

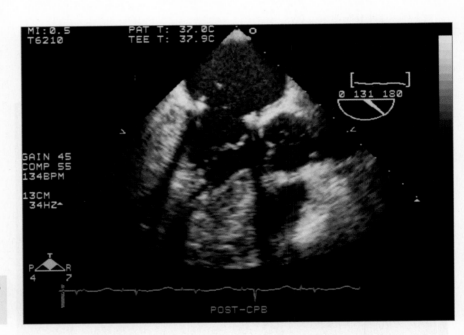

Figure 7-34 Mitral valve repair showing no prolapse and adequate coaptation of the mitral leaflets.

was performed. A portion of the flail posterior segments was resected, and the individual leaflet edges were then reapproximated with interrupted sutures.

CASE 6 (Figures 7-35 to 7-41, Videos 7-29 to 7-34)

A 65-year-old man was involved in a low-speed motor vehicle accident secondary to cardiac arrest. He was found to be in ventricular fibrillation from which he was resuscitated. He underwent a cooling protocol, and subsequent coronary angiography demonstrated no evidence of obstructive coronary artery disease. However, he had dilated cardiomyopathy with severely depressed ejection fraction and associated severe mitral regurgitation and pulmonary hypertension. TEE was performed to evaluate the etiology of his mitral regurgitation. Prolapse was

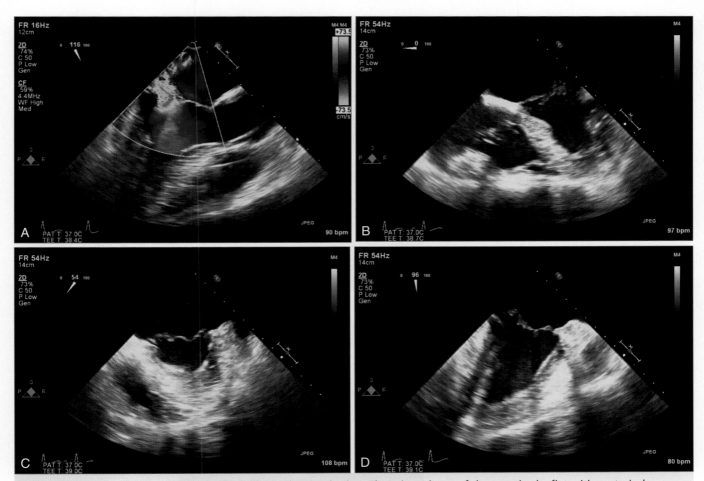

Figure 7-35 **A** to **D,** Severe posteriorly directed mitral regurgitation. There is prolapse of the anterior leaflet with posteriorly directed mitral regurgitation.

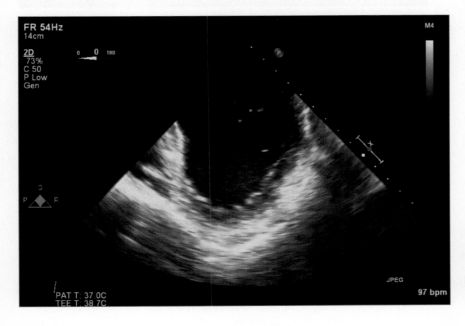

Figure 7-36 Two-dimensional transesophageal echocardiography at zero degrees showing myxomatous changes to the mitral valve. Because this is a "sweep," the anterior leaflet prolapse is seen in the initial part of the sweep on the left.

Figure 7-37 Anterior leaflet prolapse. The bicommissural view shows that the posterior leaflet is not involved.

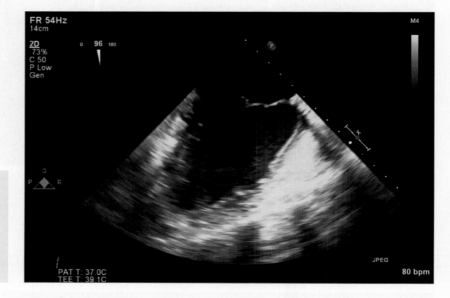

Figure 7-38 Prolapse is shown by transesophageal echocardiography at a 96-degree view, but the actual scallop involved is difficult to determine. Surprisingly, it looks most like posterior leaflet prolapse, but this is not true; the flail chordal structures are so long that they are seen posteriorly and suggest posterior leaflet prolapse.

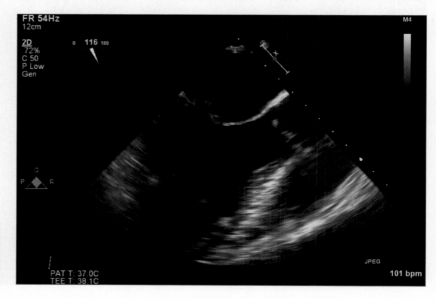

Figure 7-39 Two-dimensional transesophageal echocardiography showing anterior leaflet prolapse with ruptured chordae that are freely prolapsing into the left atrium.

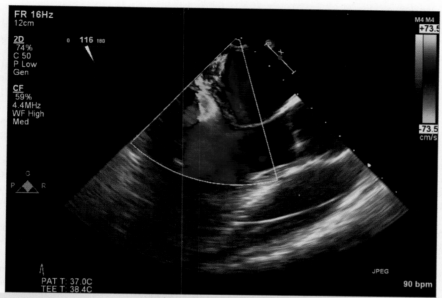

Figure 7-40 Two-dimensional transesophageal echocardiography showing severe prolapse of the anterior leaflet with severe posteriorly directed mitral regurgitation.

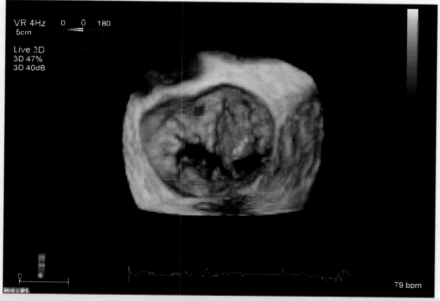

Figure 7-41 Three-dimensional transesophageal echocardiography showing prolapse of anterior leaflet segment A2 extending to A3.

present, with partial flail of the posteromedial portion of the anterior mitral leaflet, including the posteromedial portion of the A2 and all A3 segments. There were mobile echodensities on the tip of the anterior mitral leaflet suggestive of ruptured chordae tendinae. The jet of mitral regurgitation was directed posteriorly. Visual inspection of the mitral valve showed that the A2 segment was completely flail secondary to ruptured chordae. Given the acute nature of the patient's illness, the anterior mitral leaflet was resected, and he underwent mitral valve replacement with a mechanical prosthesis. This case clearly illustrates that the 3DTEE is of much more diagnostic value compared with 2DTEE.

See **expertconsult.com** *for five additional case studies with images and videos.*

References

1. Freed LA, Levy D, Levine RA, et al: Prevalence and clinical outcome of mitral-valve prolapse. *N Engl J Med* 341:1–7, 1999.
2. Adams DH, Anyanwu AC, Rahmanian PB, et al: Large annuloplasty rings facilitate mitral valve repair in Barlow's disease. *Ann Thorac Surg* 82:2096–2100, 2006.
3. Maffessanti F, Marsan NA, Tamborini G, et al: Quantitative analysis of mitral valve apparatus in mitral valve prolapse before and after annuloplasty: A three-dimensional intraoperative transesophageal study. *J Am Soc Echocardiogr* 24:405–413, 2011.
4. Disse S, Abergel E, Berrebi A, et al: Mapping of a first locus for autosomal dominant myxomatous mitral-valve prolapse to chromosome 16p11.2-p12.1. *Am J Hum Genet* 65:1242–1251, 1999.
5. Freed LA, Acierno JS, Jr, Dai D, et al: A locus for autosomal dominant mitral valve prolapse on chromosome 11p15.4. *Am J Hum Genet* 72:1551–1559, 2003.
6. Barlow JB, Pocock WA: Mitral valve prolapse, the specific billowing mitral leaflet syndrome, or an insignificant non-ejection systolic click. *Am Heart J* 97:277–285, 1979.
7. Abrams J: Mitral valve prolapse: A plea for unanimity. *Am Heart J* 92:413–415, 1976.
8. Ling LH, Enriquez-Sarano M, Seward JB, et al: Clinical outcome of mitral regurgitation due to flail leaflet. *N Engl J Med* 335:1417–1423, 1996.
9. Rosen SE, Borer JS, Hochreiter C, et al: Natural history of the asymptomatic/minimally symptomatic patient with severe mitral regurgitation secondary to mitral valve prolapse and normal right and left ventricular performance. *Am J Cardiol* 74:374–380, 1994.
10. Otsuji Y, Handschumacher MD, Liel-Cohen N, et al: Mechanism of ischemic mitral regurgitation with segmental left ventricular dysfunction: Three-dimensional echocardiographic studies in models of acute and chronic progressive regurgitation. *J Am Coll Cardiol* 37:641–648, 2001.
11. Savage EB, Ferguson TB, Jr, DiSesa VJ: Use of mitral valve repair: Analysis of contemporary United States experience reported to the Society of Thoracic Surgeons National Cardiac Database. *Ann Thorac Surg* 75:820–825, 2003.
12. Iung B, Baron G, Butchart EG, et al: A prospective survey of patients with valvular heart disease in Europe: The Euro Heart Survey on Valvular Heart Disease. *Eur Heart J* 24:1231–1243, 2003.
13. Rankin JS, Burrichter CA, Walton-Shirley MK: Trends in mitral valve surgery: A single practice experience. *J Heart Valve Dis* 18:359–366, 2009.
14. O'Gara P, Sugeng L, Lang R, et al: The role of imaging in chronic degenerative mitral regurgitation. *JACC Cardiovasc Imag* 1:221–237, 2008.
15. Foster GP, Isselbacher EM, Rose GA, et al: Accurate localization of mitral regurgitant defects using multiplane transesophageal echocardiography. *Ann Thorac Surg* 65:1025–1031, 1998.
16. Chikwe J, Adams DH, Su KN, et al: Can three-dimensional echocardiography accurately predict complexity of mitral valve repair? *Eur J Cardiothorac Surg* 41:518–524, 2012.
17. Ben Zekry S, Nagueh SF, Little SH, et al: Comparative accuracy of two- and three-dimensional transthoracic and transesophageal echocardiography in identifying mitral valve pathology in patients undergoing mitral valve repair: Initial observations. *J Am Soc Echocardiogr* 24:1079–1085, 2011.
18. Enriquez-Sarano M, Schaff HV, Orszulak TA, et al: Valve repair improves the outcome of surgery for mitral regurgitation. A multivariate analysis. *Circulation* 91:1022–1028, 1995.
19. Adams DH, Filsoufi F: Another chapter in an enlarging book: Repair degenerative mitral valves. *J Thorac Cardiovasc Surg* 125:1197–1199, 2003.

20. Filsoufi F, Carpentier A: Principles of reconstructive surgery in degenerative mitral valve disease. *Semin Thorac Cardiovasc Surg* 19:103–110, 2007.
21. Braunberger E, Deloche A, Berrebi A, et al: Very long-term results (more than 20 years) of valve repair with Carpentier's techniques in nonrheumatic mitral valve insufficiency. *Circulation* 104:I8–I11, 2001.
22. Jebara VA, Mihaileanu S, Acar C, et al: Left ventricular outflow tract obstruction after mitral valve repair: Results of the sliding leaflet technique. *Circulation* 88:II-34, 1993.
23. Maslow AD, Regan MM, Haering JM, et al: Echocardiographic predictors of left ventricular outflow tract obstruction and systolic anterior motion of the mitral valve after mitral valve reconstruction for myxomatous valve disease. *J Am Coll Cardiol* 34:2096–2104, 1999.
24. Quigley RL: Prevention of systolic anterior motion after repair of the severely myxomatous mitral valve with an anterior leaflet valvuloplasty. *Ann Thorac Surg* 80:179–182, 2005.
25. Brown ML, Abel MD, Click RL, et al: Systolic anterior motion after mitral valve repair: Is surgical intervention necessary? *J Thorac Cardiovasc Surg* 133:136–143, 2007.
26. Adams DH, Anyanwu AC, Rahmanian PB, et al: Large annuloplasty rings facilitate mitral valve repair in Barlow's disease. *Ann Thorac Surg* 82:2096–2100, 2006.
27. Mesana TG, Ibrahim M, Kulik A, et al: The "hybrid flip-over" technique for anterior leaflet prolapse repair. *Ann Thorac Surg* 83:322–323, 2007.
28. Mesana T, Ibrahim M, Hynes M: A technique for annular plication to facilitate sliding plasty after extensive mitral valve posterior leaflet resection. *Ann Thorac Surg* 79:720–722, 2005.
29. Grewal J, Mankad S, Freeman WK, et al: Real-time three-dimensional transesophageal echocardiography in the intraoperative assessment of mitral valve disease. *J Am Soc Echocardiogr* 22:34–41, 2009.
30. Chikwe J, Adams DH, Su KN, et al: Can three-dimensional echocardiography accurately predict complexity of mitral valve repair? *Eur J Cardiothorac Surg* 41:518–524, 2012.
31. Adams DH, Anyanwu AC, Sugeng L, Lang RM: Degenerative mitral valve regurgitation: Surgical echocardiography. *Curr Cardiol Rep* 10:226–232, 2008.
32. Yosefy C, Hung J, Chua S, et al: Direct measurement of vena contracta area by real-time 3-dimensional echocardiography for assessing severity of mitral regurgitation. *Am J Cardiol* 104:978–983, 2009.
33. Manda J, Kesanolla SK, Hsuing MC, et al: Comparison of real time two-dimensional with live/real time three-dimensional transesophageal echocardiography in the evaluation of mitral valve prolapse and chordae rupture. *Echocardiography* 25:1131–1137, 2008.
34. Chen X, Sun D, Yang J: Preoperative assessment of mitral valve prolapse and chordae rupture using real time three-dimensional transesophageal echocardiography. *Echocardiography* 28:1003–1010, 2011.
35. David TE: Artificial chordae. *Semin Thorac Cardiovasc Surg* 16:161–168, 2004.
36. Seeburger J, Kuntze T, Mohr FW: Gore-tex chordoplasty in degenerative mitral valve repair. *Semin Thorac Cardiovasc Surg* 19:111–115, 2007.
37. Falk V, Seeburger J, Czesla M, et al: How does the use of polytetrafluoroethylene neochordae for posterior mitral valve prolapse (loop technique) compare with leaflet resection? A prospective randomized trial. *J Thorac Cardiovasc Surg* 136:1205, 2008.
38. Carpentier AF, Pellerin M, Fuzellier JF, Relland JY: Extensive calcification of the mitral valve annulus: Pathology and surgical management. *J Thorac Cardiovasc Surg* 111:718–729, 1996.

39. Brown ML, Schaff HV, Li Z, et al: Results of mitral valve annuloplasty with a standard-sized posterior band: Is measuring important? *J Thorac Cardiovasc Surg* 138:886–891, 2009.

40. Flameng W, Herijgers P, Bogaerts K: Recurrence of mitral valve regurgitation after mitral valve repair in degenerative valve disease. *Circulation* 107:1609–1613, 2003.

41. Gillinov AM, Cosgrove DM, Blackstone EH, et al: Durability of mitral valve repair for degenerative disease. *J Thorac Cardiovasc Surg* 116:734–743, 1998.

42. Rosenhek R, Rader F, Klaar U, et al: Outcome of watching waiting in asymptomatic severe mitral regurgitation. *Circulation* 113:2238–2244, 2006.

43. Mohty D, Orszulak TA, Schaff HV, et al: Very long-term survival and durability of mitral valve repair for mitral valve prolapse. *Circulation* 104:I1–I7, 2001.

44. Akins CW, Hilgenberg AD, Buckley MJ, et al: Mitral valve reconstruction versus replacement for degenerative or ischemic mitral regurgitation. *Ann Thorac Surg* 58:668–675, 1994.

45. Lee EM, Shapiro LM, Wells FC: Superiority of mitral valve repair in surgery for degenerative mitral regurgitation. *Eur Heart J* 18:655–663, 1997.

46. Gammie JS, O'Brien SM, Griffith BP, et al: Influence of hospital procedural volume on care process and mortality for patients undergoing elective surgery for mitral regurgitation. *Circulation* 115:881–887, 2007.

47. Suri RM, Schaff HV, Dearani JA, et al: Survival advantage and improved durability of mitral repair for leaflet prolapse subsets in the current era. *Ann Thorac Surg* 82:819–826, 2006.

48. O'Brien SM, Shahian DM, Filardo G, et al: The Society of Thoracic Surgeons 2008 cardiac surgery risk models: Part 2—isolated valve surgery. *Ann Thorac Surg* 88:S23–S42, 2009.

49. Duran CG, Pomar JL, Revuelta JM, et al: Conservative operation for mitral insufficiency: Critical analysis supported by postoperative hemodynamic studies of 72 patients. *J Thorac Cardiovasc Surg* 79:326–337, 1980.

50. Suri RM, Schaff HV, Dearani JA, et al: Recurrent mitral regurgitation after repair: Should the mitral valve be re-repaired? *J Thorac Cardiovasc Surg* 132:1390–1397, 2006.

51. David TE: Outcomes of mitral valve repair for mitral regurgitation due to degenerative disease. *Semin Thorac Cardiovasc Surg* 19:116–120, 2007.

52. McGee EC, Gillinov AM, Blackstone EH, et al: Recurrent mitral regurgitation after annuloplasty for functional ischemic mitral regurgitation. *J Thorac Cardiovasc Surg* 128:916–924, 2004.

53. Yacoub M, Halim M, Radley-Smith R, et al: Surgical treatment of mitral regurgitation caused by floppy valves: Repair versus replacement. *Circulation* 64:II210–II216, 1981.

54. David TE, Uden DE, Strauss HAD: The importance of the mitral apparatus in left ventricular function after correction of mitral regurgitation. *Circulation* 68:II76–II82, 1983.

55. Goldman ME, Mora F, Guarino T, et al: Mitral valvuloplasty is superior to valve replacement for preservation of left ventricular function: an intraoperative two-dimensional echocardiographic study. *J Am Coll Cardiol* 10:568–575, 1987.

56. Pitarys CJ, II, Forman MB, Panayiotou H, Hansen DE: Long-term effects of excision of the mitral apparatus on global and regional ventricular function in humans. *J Am Coll Cardiol* 15:557–563, 1990.

57. Gillinov AM, Cosgrove DM: Mitral valve repair for degenerative disease. *J Heart Valve Dis* 11:S15–S20, 2002.

58. Ling LH, Enriquez-Saraoo M, Seward JB, et al: Clinical outcome of mitral regurgitation due to flail leaflet. *N Engl J Med* 335:1417–1423, 1996.

59. Mohty D, Orszulak TA, Schaff HV, et al: Very long-term survival and durability of mitral valve repair for mitral valve prolapse. *Circulation* 104:I1–I17, 2001.

60. Gillinov AM, Cosgrove DM, Lytle BW, et al: Reoperation for failure of mitral valve repair. *J Thorac Cardiovasc Surg* 113:467–473, 1997.

61. Gillinov AM, Faber C, Houghtaling PL, et al: Repair versus replacement for degenerative mitral valve disease with coexisting ischemic heart disease. *J Thorac Cardiovasc Surg* 125:1350–1362, 2003.

62. Gillinov AM, Blackstone EH, Cosgrove DM, III, et al: Mitral valve repair with aortic valve replacement is superior to double valve replacement. *J Thorac Cardiovasc Surg* 125:1372–1387, 2003.

63. Lee EM, Porter JN, Shapiro LM, Wells FC: Mitral valve surgery in the elderly. *J Heart Valve Dis* 6:22–31, 1997.

64. Shuhaiber J, Anderson RJ: Meta-analysis of clinical outcomes following surgical mitral valve repair or replacement. *Eur J Cardiothorac Surg* 31:267–275, 2007.

65. Jokinen JJ, Hippelainen MJ, Pitkanen OA, Hartikainen JE: Mitral valve replacement versus repair: Propensity-adjusted survival and quality-of-life analysis. *Ann Thorac Surg* 84:451–458, 2007.

66. Gillinov AM, Blackstone EH, Nowicki ER, et al: Valve repair versus valve replacement for degenerative mitral valve disease. *J Thorac Cardiovasc Surg* 135:885–893, 2008.

67. Bothe W, Kvitting JP, Swanson JC, et al: Effects of different annuloplasty rings on anterior mitral leaflet dimensions. *J Thorac Cardiovasc Surg* 139:1114–1122, 2010.

68. Mihaljevic T, Jarrett CM, Gillinov AM, et al: Robotic repair of posterior mitral valve prolapse versus conventional approaches: Potential realized. *J Thorac Cardiovasc Surg* 141:72–80, 2011.

69. Seeburger J, Borger MA, Falk V, et al: Minimal invasive mitral valve repair for mitral regurgitation: Results of 1339 consecutive patients. *Eur J Cardiothoracic Surg* 34:760–765, 2008.

70. Alfieri O, Maisano F, De Bonis M, et al: The double-orifice technique in mitral valve repair: A simple solution for complex problems. *J Thorac Cardiovasc Surg* 122:674–681, 2001.

71. Bhudia SK, McCarthy PM, Smedira NG, et al: Edge-to-edge (Alfieri) mitral repair: Results in diverse clinical settings. *Ann Thorac Surg* 77:1598–1606, 2004.

72. Levine RA, Schwammenthal E: Ischemic mitral regurgitation on the threshold of a solution: From paradoxes to unifying concepts. *Circulation* 112:745–758, 2005.

73. Mack MJ: New techniques for percutaneous repair of the mitral valve. *Heart Fail Rev* 11:259–268, 2006.

74. Block PC: Percutaneous transcatheter repair for mitral regurgitation. *J Interv Cardiol* 19:547–551, 2006.

75. Swaans MJ, Van den Branden BJ, Van der Heyden JA, et al: Three-dimensional transesophageal echocardiography in a patient undergoing percutaneous mitral valve repair using the edge-to-edge clip technique. *Eur J Echocardiogr* 10:982–983, 2009.

76. Feldman T, Foster E, Glower DD, et al; EVEREST II Investigators: Percutaneous repair or surgery for mitral regurgitation. *N Engl J Med* 364:1395–1406, 2011.

77. Whitlow PL, Feldman T, Pedersen WR, et al; EVEREST II Investigators: Acute and 12-month results with catheter-based mitral valve leaflet repair: The EVEREST II (Endovascular Valve Edge-to-Edge Repair) High Risk Study. *J Am Coll Cardiol* 59:130–139, 2012.

78. Maisano F, Caldarola A, Blasio A, et al: Midterm results of edge-to-edge mitral valve repair without annuloplasty. *J Thorac Cardiovasc Surg* 126:1987–1997, 2003.

79. Mack MJ: Coronary sinus in the management of functional mitral regurgitation: The mother lode or fool's gold? *Circulation* 114:363–364, 2006.

80. Tops LF, Van de Veire NR, Schuijf JD, et al: Noninvasive evaluation of coronary sinus anatomy and its relation to the mitral valve

annulus: Implications for percutaneous mitral annuloplasty. *Circulation* 115:1426–1432, 2007.

81. Maselli D, Guarracino F, Chiaramonti F, et al: Percutaneous mitral annuloplasty: An anatomic study of human coronary sinus and its relation with mitral valve annulus and coronary arteries. *Circulation* 114:377–380, 2006.

82. Kang DH, Kim JH, Rim JH, et al: Comparison of early surgery versus conventional treatment in asymptomatic severe mitral regurgitation. *Circulation* 119:797–804, 2009.

83. Enriquez-Sarano M, Avierinos JF, Messika-Zeitoun D, et al: Quantitative determinants of the outcome of asymptomatic mitral regurgitation. *N Engl J Med* 352:873–883, 2005.

84. American College of Cardiology; American Heart Association Task Force on Practice Guidelines: ACC/AHA 2006 guidelines for the management of patients with valvular heart disease: A report of the American College of Cardiology/American Heart Association Task Force on Practice Guidelines (writing committee to revise the 1998 guidelines for the management of patients with valvular heart disease) developed in collaboration with the Society of Cardiovascular Anesthesiologists endorsed by the Society for Cardiovascular Angiography and Interventions and the Society of Thoracic Surgeons. *J Am Coll Cardiol* 48:e1–e148, 2007.

85. Bonow RO, Carabello BA, Chatterjee K, et al: 2008 focused update incorporated into the ACC/AHA 2006 guidelines for the management of patients with valvular heart disease: A report of the American College of Cardiology/American Heart Association Task Force on Practice Guidelines (writing committee to revise the 1998 guidelines for the management of patients with valvular heart disease). *J Am Coll Cardiol* 52:e1–e142, 2008.

86. Vahanian A, Baumgartner H, Bax J, et al: Guidelines on the management of valvular heart disease: The Task Force on the Management of Valvular Heart Disease of the European Society of Cardiology. *Eur Heart J* 28:230–268, 2007.

CHAPTER 8

Prosthetic Heart Valves

G. Burkhard Mackensen, Renata G. Ferreira, and Edward A. Gill

INTRODUCTION

Although echocardiography is the imaging modality of choice for cardiac heart valves, it still has significant limitations when imaging prosthetic cardiac valves. These limitations are significant with bioprosthetic valves and are particularly problematic with mechanical valves. The classic limitation is the inability to evaluate mitral regurgitation (MR) from the apical window in patients with mechanical prosthetic valves because of reverberation artifacts and acoustic shadowing. Many of these limitations, particularly while imaging the mitral valve (MV), are overcome by transesophageal imaging; direct imaging from the left atrial side of the valve eliminates these shadowing artifacts, which reside on the ventricular aspect of the valve (**Figure 8-1; Video 8-1**). Sparse data exist regarding the use of real-time three-dimensional transthoracic echocardiography (RT3DTTE) with prosthetic valves, although in a small series of four patients with endocarditis, vegetations and/or dehiscence not recognized by two-dimensional (2D) TTE were seen.[1] Evaluation of prosthetic valves by RT3D transesophageal echocardiography (TEE) has been extensively reviewed.[2,3] In one study, RT3DTEE has been shown to be particularly accurate for diagnosing all types of prosthetic valve pathology compared with direct surgical inspection.[4] However, MV visualization, particularly valve leaflet visualization, was far superior to that of aortic or tricuspid valves. Also in this study, most of the valves were free of disease and, in fact, had recently been placed. Despite being a study of 87 patients, fewer than 40 had prosthetic valves, and the number who had metallic prosthetic valves is not clear from the report.

A notable advantage of RT3DTEE compared with 2DTEE for all mechanical valves in the mitral position is the ability to visualize the entire valve in one full-volume or 3D zoom capture compared with visualization of only a single thin slice by 2D (**Figures 8-1 to 8-6; Videos 8-1 to 8-6**). Besides live 3D imaging, RT3DTEE has the ability to acquire a 3D volume that can then be cropped and rotated to reveal pathology such as leaflet immobility, thrombi or vegetations, dehiscence, or, with the addition of 3D color, even small perivalvular leaks (see Figure 8-4 and Video 8-4). Details of the valve, such as the sewing ring, the individual stitches, the struts, and the entire leaflet motion are well visualized by RT3DTEE (see Figure 8-6 and Video 8-6). Again, such visualization is much less frequently seen in valves in either the aortic or tricuspid position.

ABNORMAL PATHOLOGY WITH MECHANICAL VALVES

Visualization of masses or the pannus on mechanical valves by RT3DTEE has not been rigorously studied because such problems are relatively uncommon. Only case reports exist of pannus formation on bileaflet mechanical valves in the mitral position evaluated by RT3DTEE, but in one published case, the pannus was identified by RT3DTEE and not seen at all by 2DTEE.[5] Thrombus formation can be more precisely evaluated by RT3DTEE than by 2DTEE; in fact, this has confirmed our observation of the ability of RT3DTEE to

143

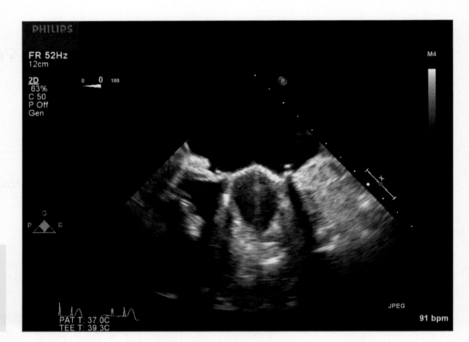

Figure 8-1   Two-dimensional mid-esophageal image of a mechanical double-tilting-disk mitral valve prosthesis captured in the closed position during systole. The image clearly illustrates the characteristic V pattern produced by the occluding disks.

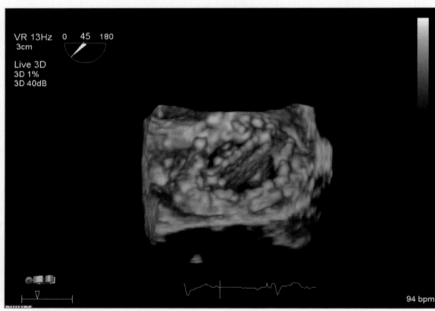

Figure 8-2   En face view of a mechanical double-tilting-disk mitral valve prosthesis captured in the open position during diastole. The image clearly illustrates the sewing ring and the two disks.

appreciate that thrombi are larger and more numerous than thrombi detected by 2DTEE.[6,7]

Periprosthetic Regurgitation

RT3DTEE is invaluable for guidance of procedures to close periprosthetic regurgitation with Amplatzer (St. Jude Medical, St. Paul, MN) vascular plugs, particularly involving the MV. This intervention and others are covered in another chapter. However, diagnosis and characterization of periprosthetic regurgitation have been evaluated somewhat systematically, and RT3DTEE has been shown to be significantly superior to 2DTEE for the determination of extent and location of periprosthetic regurgitation. In one series of 13 patients, only 2 had aortic prostheses, making statements regarding the use of RT3DTEE for aortic prosthetic regurgitation somewhat anecdotal.[8] Nevertheless, in 1 of the 2 cases, no defect was found on 2DTEE, and a substantial area of regurgitation was seen with the use of RT3DTEE.

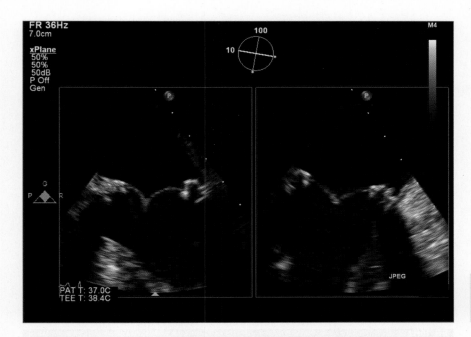

Figure 8-3 Two-dimensional echocardiographic image of a stented bioprosthetic valve in the mitral position.

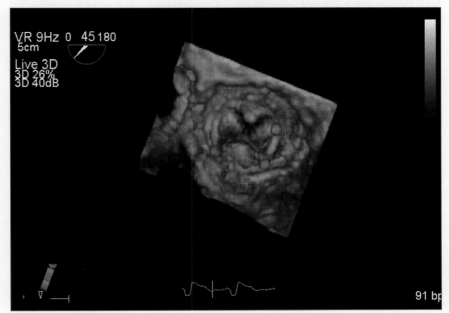

Figure 8-4 Ventricular aspect of a stented bioprosthetic valve in the mitral position imaged with three-dimensional transesophageal echocardiography.

Mitral Prosthetic Dehiscence

RT3DTEE provides additional information in patients with a postoperative MV dehiscence and therefore may help plan an optimal corrective intervention. Kronzon and colleagues,[9] in a series of 18 patients with dehisced MVs, 10 after replacement and 8 after repair, used RT3DTEE for echocardiographic evaluation. In all cases, the position of the valve dehiscence was more extensively characterized by RT3DTEE than with 2DTEE, and the position of dehiscence was confirmed to be correct in 10 of the patients by surgical findings. The presence of valve dehiscence was correctly diagnosed by 2DTEE in 17 of the 18 patients, but the type of valve ring or the position of the valve dehiscence could not be characterized in any case. Ten of the patients had posterior dehiscence, and four had lateral dehiscence. These positions were believed to be the most prominent because (1) the posterior annulus is the most difficult portion of the valve ring to reach surgically and (2) surgeons attempt to avoid the circumflex coronary artery.[9]

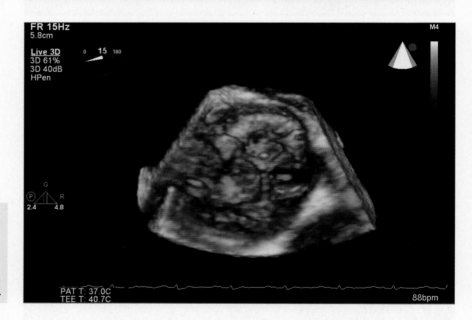

Figure 8-5   Two-dimensional mid-esophageal short-axis view of a 23-mm bioprosthetic aortic valve (PERIMOUNT Magna, Edwards Lifesciences, Irvine, CA) in the closed position. The image depicts the three stents at the commissural points.

Figure 8-6   Three-dimensional mid-esophageal en face view of a 23-mm bioprosthetic aortic valve (PERIMOUNT Magna, Edwards Lifesciences, Irvine, CA) in the closed position. The image depicts the three stents at the commissural points as well as the closure line of the three leaflets.

GUIDANCE OF PERCUTANEOUS VALVE PLACEMENT

TEE is the standard for guiding percutaneous transcatheter aortic valve implantation. Data regarding the use of RT3DTEE for this particular procedure are limited, although it is routinely performed.[10] Several potential advantages exist for RT3DTEE in this setting. The third dimension allows (1) more accurate assessment of the aortic annulus, the left ventricular outflow tract, and the aortic root size and shape; (2) measurement of the distance between the annulus and the left main coronary artery ostium; and 3) seating of the percutaneous valve while viewing the aortic valve en face and visualizing the valve leaflets and the tissue surrounding the prosthetic annulus.[11] This en face view is critically important for placement of the prosthetic valve to avoid postprocedure perivavluar regurgitation. RT3DTEE and biplane imaging also assist with the perioperative monitoring of all procedural aspects, including advancements of guidewires into the aortic valve and the placement of pigtail catheters in the sinus of Valsalva and the left ventricle, as well as balloon valvuloplasty or valve deployment. Ultimately, 2DTEE and RT3DTEE should be used as complementary imaging modalities to assess the satisfactory positioning and function of the implanted valve.

Reports of small series of transcatheter mitral valve-in-valve implantations have appeared in the literature. RT3DTEE has also been routinely used for this purpose.[12] Although this procedure is currently not available in the United States, RT3DTEE will be a mainstay for deployment of mitral valve-in-valve devices when they do become available.

Guidance of Percutaneous Valve Repair

3D echocardiography has been used for guidance during percutaneous mitral valvuloplasty and has been shown to be a suitable technique for monitoring its efficacy and complications.[13] RT3DTEE may become the gold standard in describing the morphology of commissures as a good predictor of outcome after percutaneous balloon mitral valvuloplasty.[14] Balloon valvuloplasty in patients with rheumatic MV stenosis was the first percutaneous procedure used in the management of patients with MV disease. RT3DTEE not only guides the transseptal approach, it also improves the spatial orientation of the catheter system in reference to the MV and permits immediate inspection of the MV after the valvuloplasty.[15]

Percutaneous approaches to the management of MR continue to be developed. A large number of percutaneous devices to manage mitral dysfunction have been directed at reduction of the annulus (e.g., Viacor [Viacor, Inc., Wilmington, MA], Monarch coronary sinus retracting stent [Edwards Lifesciences, Irvine, CA]), stabilization of the valve leaflet motion (e.g., MitraClip, Evalve [Abbott Vascular, Abbott Park, IL]), or reduction of leaflet restriction (Coapys [Myocor, Maple Grove, MN], subvalvular stabilization, cutting secondary chords). Recent evidence supports the utility of the simple edge-to-edge technique (MitraClip) in those not amenable to conventional surgical repairs. Based on the initial performance of edge-to-edge repair by catheter-based technology, percutaneous edge-to-edge repair was performed in the randomized, phase II Pivotal Study of a Percutaneous Mitral Valve Repair System (EVEREST II). The results of that trial suggest that percutaneous repair with the MitraClip system can be accomplished with low rates of morbidity and mortality and with acute MR reduction to less than 2+ in the majority of selected patients. This technology may soon become a less invasive alternative to surgical mitral valve repair in the future.[16,17]

TEE not only confirms the diagnosis of MR and describes MV morphology before a percutaneous MV procedure but also has been shown to be critically important in guiding the edge-to-edge repair. In brief, with the patient under general anesthesia—and with the aid of RT3DTEE, biplane viewing, and fluoroscopy—a guidewire, followed by an introducer, is advanced into the right atrium via the right femoral vein. After transseptal puncture (high posterior approach as confirmed by TEE) a 24-Fr guiding catheter is advanced into the left atrium. From this perspective, the externally controlled MitraClip delivery system is steered over the mitral orifice with continued TEE guidance. Within the left atrium, the mitral clip is oriented perpendicular to the long axis of the MV leaflet edges at the origin of the mitral regurgitation jet. In our experience, this step benefits most from the added third dimension. The clip is then advanced into the left ventricle with placement of the clip arms below the mitral leaflets. Grasping of the mitral leaflets is then performed by retraction of the clip delivery system. After confirmation of appropriate leaflet insertion into the clip and adequate reduction in MR severity by TEE, the clip is deployed. After deployment, the severity of the MR is again reassessed by both 2DTEE and 3DTEE with and without color flow Doppler.

Most of the potential complications of this percutaneous approach to MR can be monitored and diagnosed with TEE. The complications include (1) potential of aortic root puncture during atrial septal perforation (right atrium to aortic fistula), (2) right or left atrial puncture by the deployment device (cardiac tamponade), (3) increased MR during device deployment, (4) development of mitral stenosis, (5) creation of a large atrial septal defect, (6) device embolization, and (7) unsuccessful repair.

SUMMARY

In general terms, 2D and 3D imaging should be seen as complementary modalities. RT3D, especially RT3DTEE, significantly adds to the evaluation of both biologic and mechanical prostheses, especially in the MV position. The capabilities of real-time 3D acquisition—online rendering and cropping—permit accurate identification of the precise location and pathology associated with a prosthetic valve, guide corrective intervention, and will potentially help transition this modality into standard of care. One caveat exists, however; RT3DTEE is subject to the same physical laws of 2D ultrasound and is therefore prone to the same ultrasound artifacts.

CASE STUDIES

CASE 1 (Figures 8-7 and 8-8; Videos 8-7 and 8-8)

Bioprosthetic valve in the mitral position: The patient was admitted after a fall. TTE showed increased gradient across the MV. TEE and RT3DTEE showed two of the three leaflets of the valve to be immobile.

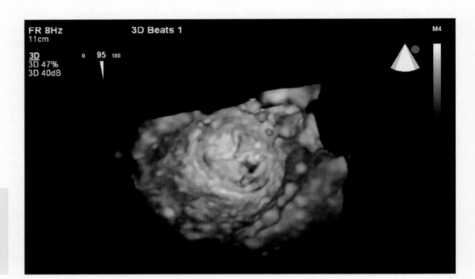

Figure 8-7 Three-dimensional transesophageal echocardiography of a bioprosthetic valve in the mitral position viewed from the left ventricular side. Note that two of the three leaflets are immobile (see Video 8-7).

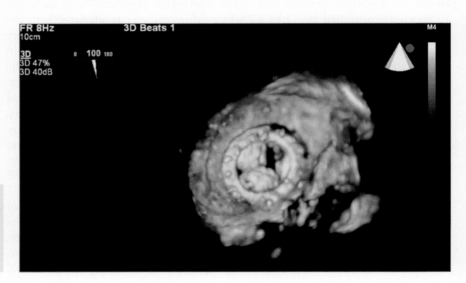

Figure 8-8 Three-dimensional transesophageal echocardiography of a bioprosthetic valve in the mitral position viewed from the left atrial side. Note that two of the three leaflets are immobile (see Video 8-8).

CASE 2 (Figures 8-9 to 8-13; Videos 8-9 to 8-12)

Prosthetic valve periprosthetic regurgitation: A bioprosthetic valve in the tricuspid position was placed because of endocarditis. After surgery, TEE was repeated because of suspicion of recurrent endocarditis. However, no vegetations or abscess cavities were appreciated, but periprosthetic regurgitation was found. This seemed to be an incidental finding because the patient had no clinical symptoms that could be the sequelae of the regurgitation.

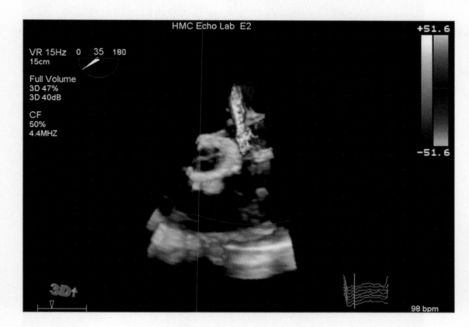

Figure 8-9 Three-dimensional transesophageal echocardiography image showing periprosthetic regurgitation. This is a bioprosthetic valve in the tricuspid position, and the regurgitant jet is seen just adjacent to the sewing ring.

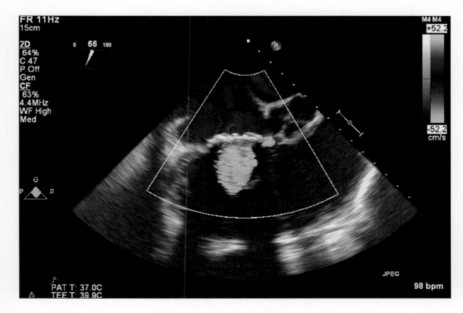

Figure 8-10 Two-dimensional transesophageal echocardiography of periprosthetic regurgitation adjacent to the sewing ring of a bioprosthetic valve in the tricuspid position (see Video 8-9).

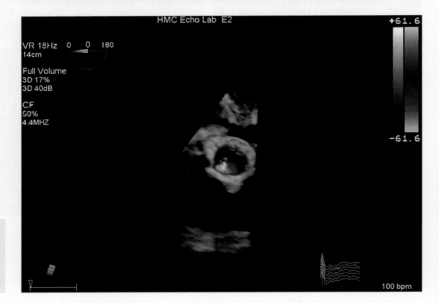

Figure 8-11 Three-dimensional transesophageal echocardiography image of periprosthetic regurgitation adjacent to the sewing ring of a bioprosthetic valve in the tricuspid position (see Video 8-10).

Figure 8-12 Three-dimensional transesophageal echocardiography image of periprosthetic regurgitation adjacent to the sewing ring of a bioprosthetic valve in the tricuspid position (see Video 8-11).

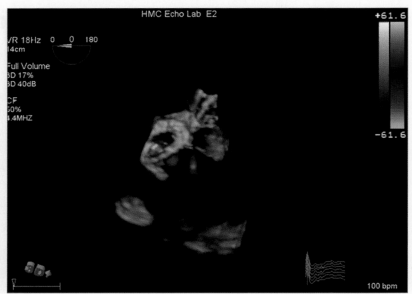

Figure 8-13 Swivel view of the periprosthetic regurgitation adjacent to bioprosthetic valve in the tricuspid position (see Video 8-12).

CASE 3 (Figures 8-14 to 8-21; Videos 8-13 to 8-16)

Left ventricular outflow tract mass: A bioprosthetic valve was present in the aortic position. TTE suggested a vegetation on the aortic valve. By TEE, a mass was seen prolapsing into the left ventricular outflow tract and was confirmed by RT3DTEE. Although endocarditis could not be excluded by TEE, it was believed to possibly represent primary valve failure. Subsequent cultures did not grow any organisms. Because of aortic regurgitation, the valve was subsequently replaced with another bioprosthetic valve.

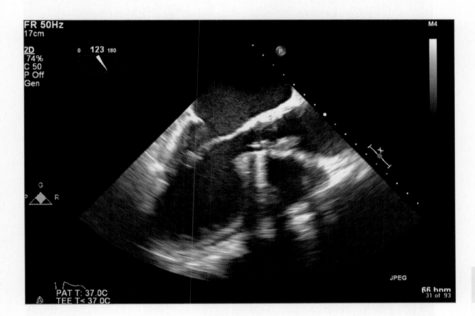

Figure 8-14 Mass seen in the left ventricular outflow tract (see Video 8-13).

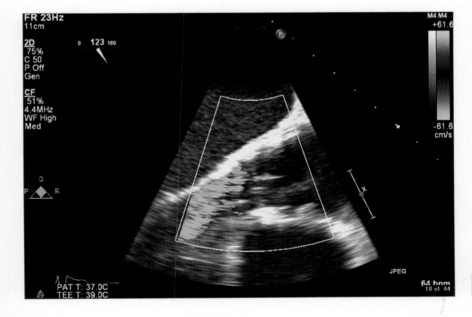

Figure 8-15 Severe aortic regurgitation.

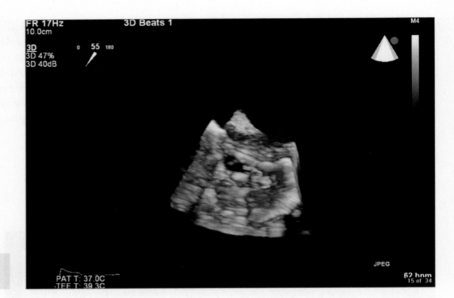

Figure 8-16 A mass in the left ventricular outflow tract (see Video 8-14).

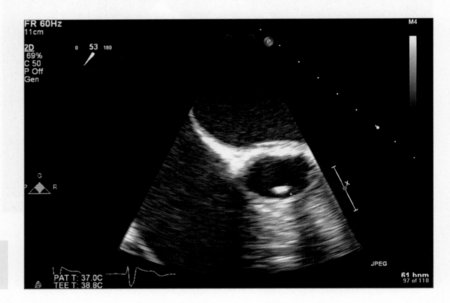

Figure 8-17 Two-dimensional transesophageal echocardiography of a mass in the left ventricular outflow tract (see Video 8-15).

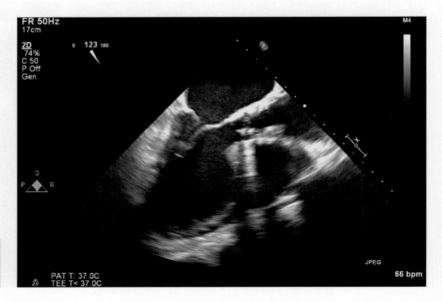

Figure 8-18 Two-dimensional transesophageal echocardiography image of a mass prolapsing into the left ventricular outflow tract.

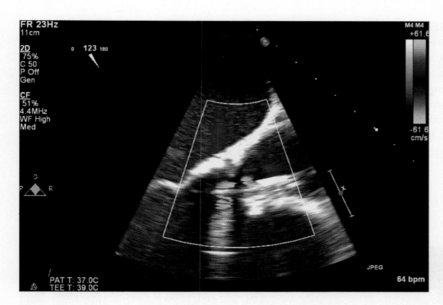

Figure 8-19 Two-dimensional transesophageal echocardiography showing severe aortic regurgitation (see Video 8-16).

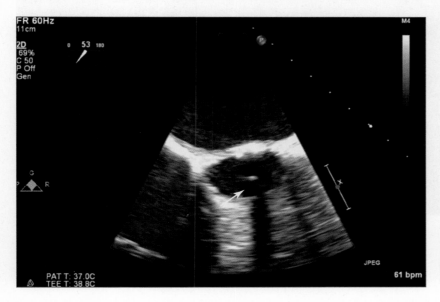

Figure 8-20 Two-dimensional transesophageal echocardiography short-axis view of the aortic valve showing a mass in the left ventricular outflow tract.

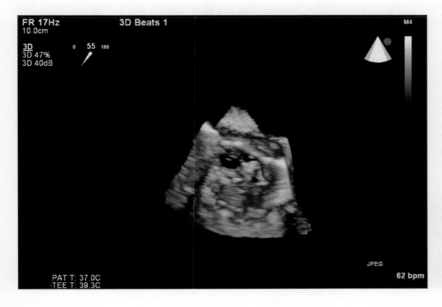

Figure 8-21 Three-dimensional transesophageal echocardiography (3DTEE) of the mass in the left ventricular outflow tract (LVOT). In this case, the mass is appreciated in its entirety with 3DTEE and is a higher percentage of the LVOT compared with two-dimensional TEE.

CASE 4 (Figures 8-22 and 8-23; Videos 8-17 and 8-18)

Thrombosis of St. Jude mitral valve: The patient had voluntarily stopped her oral anticoagulation (warfarin) for her prosthetic St. Jude MV. She was subsequently admitted for cerebrovascular accident and found to have a thrombus, thought to be embolic, in the left middle cerebral artery. TEE was performed and showed a thrombus in the left atrial appendage and a thrombus on the prosthetic MV. Visualization of the thrombus was more optimal with RT3DTEE than with 2DTEE. The size of the thrombus was measured by offline techniques; the diameter was noted to be larger with the use of RT3DTEE than with 2DTEE.

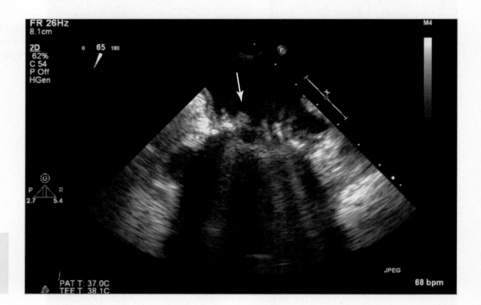

Figure 8-22 Two-dimensional transesophageal echocardiography image showing a thrombus associated with the bileaflet mitral valve (see Video 8-17).

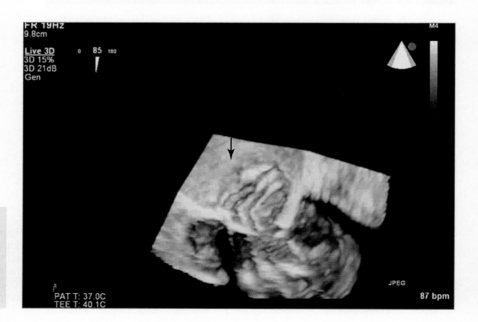

Figure 8-23 Three-dimensional transesophageal echocardiography (TEE) image in the same patient in Figure 8-22. In this case, both the length and width of the thrombus are appreciated to be greater than was demonstrated by two-dimensional TEE (see Video 8-18).

CASE 5 (Figures 8-24 to 8-30; Videos 8-19 to 8-22)

Vegetation on a prosthetic aortic valve: TEE was performed on this patient, who had blood cultures positive for *Candida tropicalis*. A vegetation was seen on the prosthetic St. Jude aortic valve.

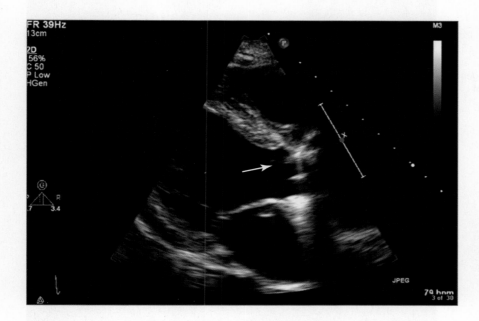

Figure 8-24 Two-dimensional transthoracic echocardiography image of a mass, presumed to be a vegetation, seen in the left ventricular outflow tract in a patient with a bileaflet mechanical valve in the aortic position. Blood cultures were positive for *Candida tropicalis*.

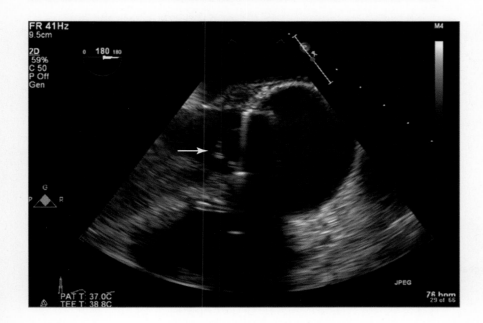

Figure 8-25 Two-dimensional transesophageal echocardiography image showing a mass in the left ventricular outflow tract consistent with a vegetation. The patient's blood cultures were positive for *Candida tropicalis*.

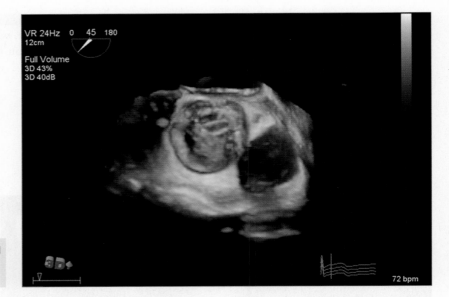

Figure 8-26 Three-dimensional transesophageal echocardiography image on the aortic side of the valve, where no mass is seen.

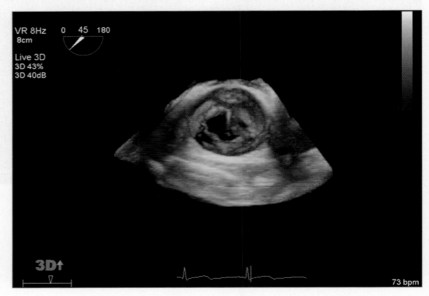

Figure 8-27 Three-dimensional transesophageal echocardiography image on the aortic side of the valve, where no mass is seen.

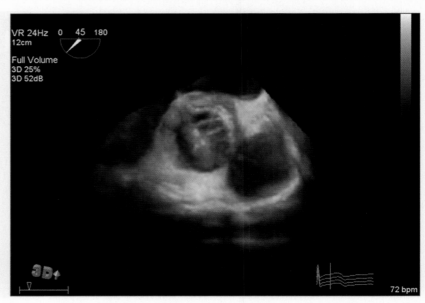

Figure 8-28 Three-dimensional transesophageal echocardiography on the aortic side of the valve, where no mass is seen.

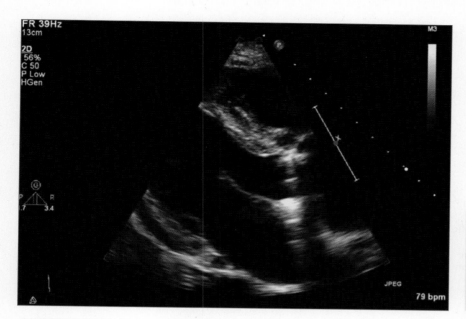

Figure 8-29 Two-dimensional transthoracic echocardiogram of a mass, presumed to be a vegetation, seen in the left ventricular outflow tract in this patient with a bileaflet mechanical valve in the aortic position. Blood cultures were positive for *Candida tropicalis*.

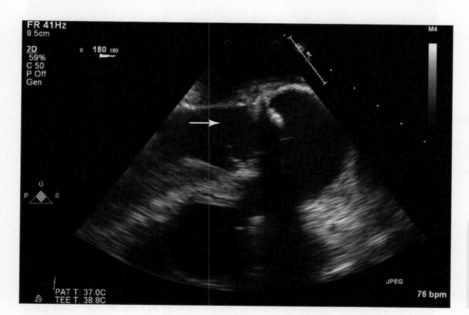

Figure 8-30 Two-dimensional transesophageal echocardiography image showing a mass in the left ventricular outflow tract consistent with a vegetation. The patient's blood cultures were positive for *Candida tropicalis*.

CASE 6 (Figures 8-31 to 8-35; Videos 8-23 to 8-26)

Fungal endocarditis of a bioprosthetic valve in the mitral position: Six months after implantation of a porcine bioprosthetic valve in the mitral position and coronary artery bypass grafting, this 74-year-old female patient was admitted with fever, symptoms of acute heart failure, and multiple episodes of syncope. TEE revealed near-complete stenosis of her stented bioprosthesis due to massive fungal endocarditis (*Exserohilum* spp.).

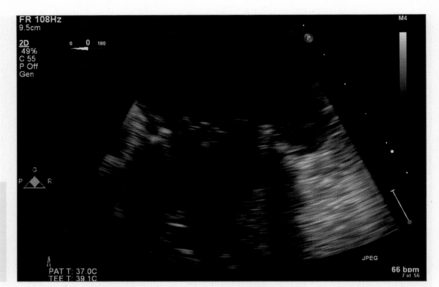

Figure 8-31 Two-dimensional mid-esophageal zoomed transesophageal echocardiography image of a completely overgrown bioprosthetic valve in the mitral position. Massive fungal endocarditis has resulted in severe mitral valve stenosis with an effective orifice area of 0.3 cm^2 (see Video 8-23).

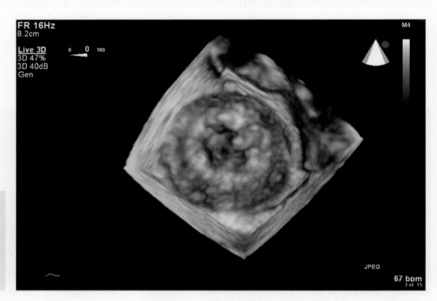

Figure 8-32 Three-dimensional transesophageal echocardiography en face view of the completely overgrown bioprosthetic valve in the mitral position shown in Figure 8-31. Note the severely stenosed mitral valve bioprosthesis with an effective orifice area of 0.3 cm^2 (see Video 8-24).

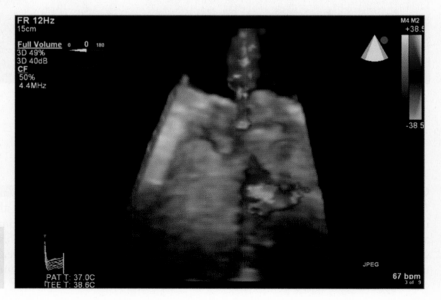

Figure 8-33 Three-dimensional transesophageal echocardiography color image of overgrown prosthetic valve indicates the extremely limited mitral valve orifice (see Video 8-25).

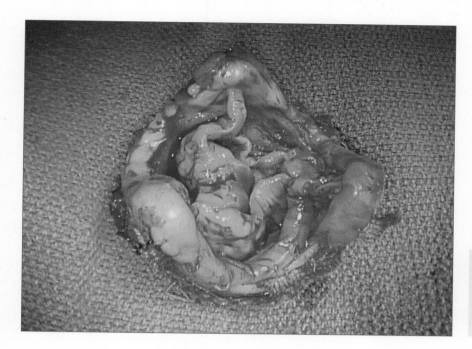

Figure 8-34   The completely overgrown bioprosthetic valve shown in Figure 8-31 as it was excised from the mitral position. Note that the fungal process has resulted in a near-complete obliteration of the bioprosthesis.

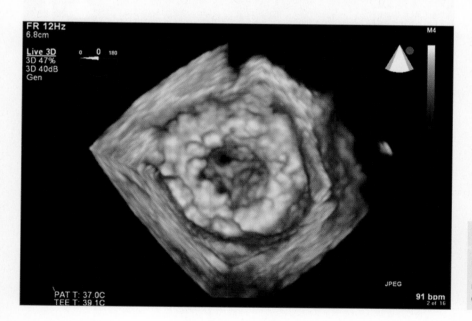

Figure 8-35   Postoperative three-dimensional (3D) en face image in the patient shown in Figure 8-31 obtained with live 3D acquisition demonstrating the replaced bioprosthesis in the mitral position (see Video 8-26).

CASE 7 (Figures 8-36 and 8-37; Videos 8-27 to 8-29)

Thrombosis of a mechanical bileaflet tilting-disk valve with a stuck anterior disk in the mitral position: This young patient had neglected to take warfarin as prescribed and was admitted to the hospital in acute renal failure with symptoms of heart failure.

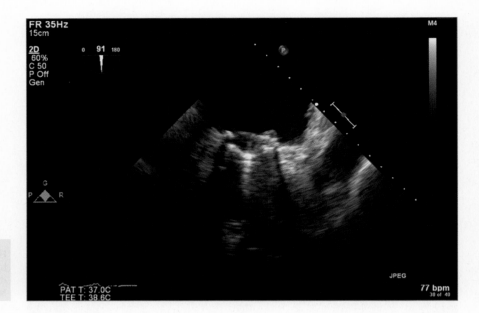

Figure 8-36 Mid-esophageal two-chamber view of the thrombosed mitral valve prosthesis with a stuck anterior leaflet (see Video 8-27).

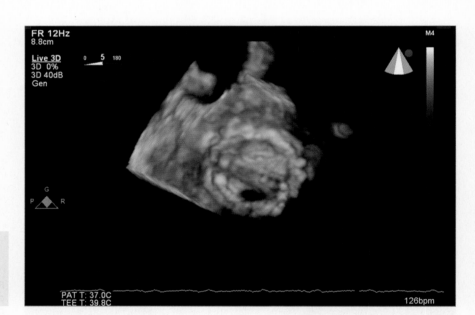

Figure 8-37 Three-dimensional transesophageal echocardiography en face view of the thrombosed mitral valve prosthesis with a stuck anterior leaflet (see Video 8-28).

CASE 8 (Figures 8-38 to 8-42; Videos 8-30 to 8-34)

A 64-year-old man who underwent coronary artery bypass grafting and St. Jude mitral valve replacement in 1998: The patient developed *Streptococcus constellatus* endocarditis and underwent repeat MV replacement in January 2008 with a CarboMedics (Sorin Group, Milan, Italy) mechanical valve. After that surgery, the patient never regained his previous state of health and had progressive loss of strength as well as increasing shortness of breath at rest and with mild activity. He was ultimately found to have persistent anemia; blood cultures were positive for methicillin-resistant *Staphylococcus epidermidis* on four occasions, and he was placed on appropriate antibiotics. TTE showed severe MR and a rocking MV prosthesis. Intraoperative TEE confirmed anterior dehiscence of the mechanical bileaflet tilting-disk valve in the mitral position along with rocking motion. The extent and location of the dehiscence are easily appreciated on the RT3DTEE en face view, but the mid-esophageal, two-chamber view with the multiplane angle at 90 degrees does not reveal the dehiscence.

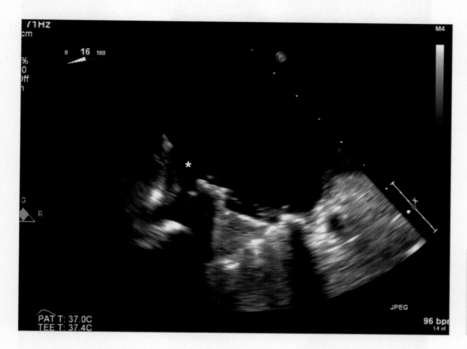

Figure 8-38 Zoomed two-dimensional transesophageal echocardiography image of an anteriorly dehisced bileaflet tilting-disk prosthesis in the mitral position. The *asterisk* indicates the dehiscence (see video 8-30).

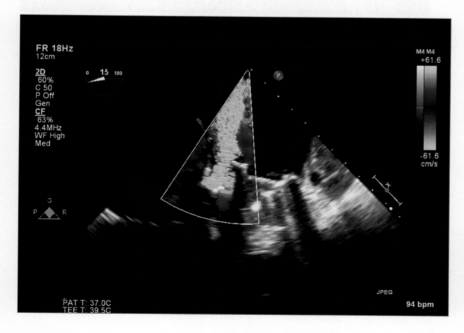

Figure 8-39 Zoomed two-dimensional transesophageal echocardiography image demonstrating the significant regurgitant jet anterior of the dehisced bileaflet tilting-disk prosthesis in the mitral position (see Video 8-31).

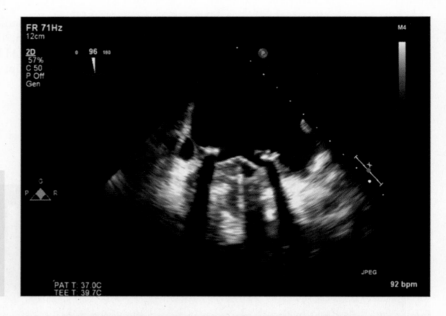

Figure 8-40 Two-dimensional transesophageal echocardiography two-chamber view of the same dehisced tilting-disk prosthesis in the mitral position shown in Figure 8-39. Note that the dehiscence is not necessarily being detected at this orientation of the multiplane angle (i.e., 96 degrees). However, the moving image demonstrates the rocking motion of the mechanical valve (see Video 8-32).

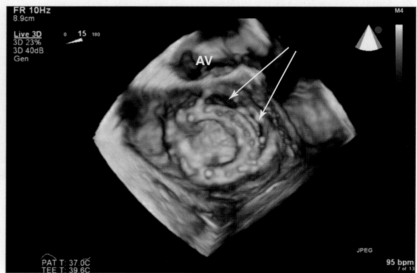

Figure 8-41 Zoomed real-time three-dimensional transesophageal echocardiography en face image of the anteriorly dehisced tilting-disk prosthesis shown in Figure 8-39. Note that the dehiscence extends at the entire anterior aspect of the valve (*arrows*) (see Video 8-33). *AV,* aortic valve.

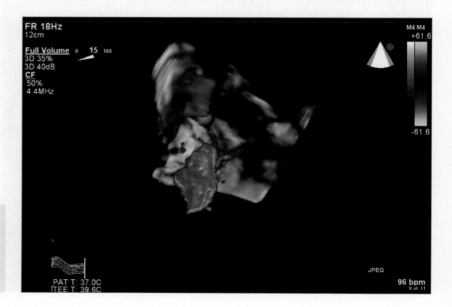

Figure 8-42 Three-dimensional color transesophageal echocardiographic image illustrates the enormous extent of the dehiscence of the mechanical valve shown in Figure 8-39 from the anterior aspect of the mitral valve annulus (see Video 8-34).

References

1. Kort S: Real-time 3-dimensional echocardiography for prosthetic valve endocarditis: Initial experience. *J Am Soc Echocardiogr* 19:130–139, 2006.

2. Tsang W, Weinert L, Kronzon I, Lang RM: Three-dimensional echocardiography in the assessment of prosthetic valves. *Rev Esp Cardiol* 64:1–7, 2011.

3. Chapman CB, Rahko PS: Three-dimensional echocardiography and mitral valve disease. *Curr Cardiol Rep* 12:243–249, 2010.

4. Sugeng L, Shernan SK, Weinert L, et al: Real-time three-dimensional transesophageal echocardiography in valve disease: Comparison with surgical findings and evaluation of prosthetic valves. *J Am Soc Echocardiogr* 21:1347–1354, 2008.

5. Ozkan M, Gunduz S, Yildiz M, Duran NE: Diagnosis of the prosthetic heart valve pannus formation with real-time three-dimensional transoesophageal echocardiography. *Eur J Echocardiogr* 11:E17, 2010.

6. Faletra FF, Moschovitis G, Auricchio A: Visualisation of thrombus formation on prosthetic valve by real-time three-dimensional transoesophageal echocardiography. *Heart* 95:482, 2009.

7. Paul B, Minocha A: Thrombosis of a bileaflet prosthetic mitral valve: A real-time three-dimensional transesophageal echocardiography perspective. *Int J Cardiovasc Imag* 26:367–368, 2010.

8. Singh P, Manda J, Hsiung MC, et al: Live/real time three-dimensional transesophageal echocardiographic evaluation of mitral and aortic valve prosthetic paravalvular regurgitation. *Echocardiography* 26:980–987, 2009.

9. Kronzon I, Sugeng L, Perk G, et al: Real-time 3-dimensional transesophageal echocardiography in the evaluation of post-operative mitral annuloplasty ring and prosthetic valve dehiscence. *J Am Coll Cardiol* 53:1543–1547, 2009.

10. Marcos-Alberca P, Zamorano JL, Sanchez T, et al: Intraoperative monitoring with transesophageal real-time three-dimensional echocardiography during transapical prosthetic aortic valve implantation. *Rev Esp Cardiol* 63:352–356, 2010.

11. Zamorano JL, Badano LP, Bruce C, et al: EAE/ASE recommendations for the use of echocardiography in new transcatheter interventions for valvular heart disease. *J Am Soc Echocardiogr* 24:937–965, 2011.

12. Cheung AW, Gurvitch R, Ye J, et al: Transcatheter transapical mitral valve-in-valve implantations for a failed bioprosthesis: a case series. *J Thorac Cardiovasc Surg* 141:711–715, 2011.

13. Dobarro D, Gomez-Rubin MC, Lopez-Fernandez T, et al: Real time three-dimensional transesophageal echocardiography for guiding percutaneous mitral valvuloplasty. *Echocardiography* 26:746–748, 2009.

14. Fatkin D, Roy P, Morgan JJ, Feneley MP: Percutaneous balloon mitral valvotomy with the Inoue single-balloon catheter: Commissural morphology as a determinant of outcome. *J Am Coll Cardiol* 21:390–397, 1993.

15. Perk G, Lang RM, Garcia-Fernandez MA, et al: Use of real time three-dimensional transesophageal echocardiography in intracardiac catheter based interventions. *J Am Soc Echocardiogr* 22:865–882, 2009.

16. Feldman T, Kar S, Rinaldi M, et al: Percutaneous mitral repair with the MitraClip system: Safety and midterm durability in the initial EVEREST (Endovascular Valve Edge-to-Edge REpair Study) cohort. *J Am Coll Cardiol* 54:686–694, 2009.

17. Mauri L, Garg P, Massaro JM, et al: The EVEREST II Trial: Design and rationale for a randomized study of the evalve mitraclip system compared with mitral valve surgery for mitral regurgitation. *Am Heart J* 160:23–29, 2010.

Tricuspid Valve

Alicia A. Bourne and Edward A. Gill

INTRODUCTION

The tricuspid valve is the largest of the four heart valves and ranges from 4 to 6 cm^2 in area. The tricuspid valve has anterior, septal, and posterior leaflets. The anterior leaflet usually is the largest, with a width of 2.2 cm. The septal and posterior leaflets are notably smaller and measure roughly 1.5 and 2.0 cm, respectively, based on autopsy series.[1] Our experience shows that the posterior leaflet often is the smallest. In many cases, the posterior leaflet is not only the smallest, it is also quite rudimentary. Disease processes of the tricuspid valve are relatively uncommon. The tricuspid valve can frequently be incompetent because of factors separate from the valve itself. Specific examples of such incompetence include right ventricular annular dilation, tricuspid annular dilation, or both as well as pulmonary hypertension. In the presence of pathology that directly involves the valve, such as bacterial endocarditis or tricuspid valve prolapse, identification of specific leaflet involvement often is critical for addressing surgical management, particularly to determine whether tricuspid valve replacement would be indicated compared with tricuspid annuloplasty.[2]

ADVANTAGES OF REAL-TIME THREE-DIMENSIONAL ECHOCARDIOGRAPHY

Real-time three-dimensional echocardiography (RT3DE) has a major advantage for imaging the tricuspid valve because of its ability to display the valve en face, which results in the visualization of all three tricuspid leaflets simultaneously; this rarely is possible with standard two-dimensional (2D) imaging. Furthermore, even on the rare occasion when imaging of the tricuspid valve en face is possible, it is possible from only one view. RT3DE allows several approaches to en face imaging of the tricuspid valve by the transthoracic approach, including RV inflow, the parasternal short-axis, apical four-chamber, and subcostal views. Dilation of the right ventricle provides a particularly satisfactory window for the visualization of the tricuspid valve with RT3DE.

Tricuspid Valve Pathology

Tricuspid stenosis is a rare pathology virtually always caused by rheumatic heart disease, especially in adults. Congenital tricuspid atresia is seen in complex congenital heart disease but is not covered in this chapter. There have now been several reports of tricuspid stenosis caused by pacemaker leads.[3] An example of tricuspid stenosis is shown in **Figure 9-1** (**Video 9-1**).

Flail tricuspid valve leaflet has become a fairly frequently detected problem, especially in tertiary centers with transplantation programs, where the tricuspid valve frequently is damaged in the process of right ventricular biopsy. Rheumatic tricuspid valve disease rarely results in the tethering of the valve leaflets so profoundly as to prevent coaptation.[4-6] This problem is a frequent outcome in carcinoid triscupid valve disease (**Figure 9-2**; **Video 9-2**). Tricuspid regurgitation is a not-infrequent complication of right ventricular pacemakers, with the wire causing the regurgitation by perforating a leaflet or by pinning one of the leaflets open. Tricuspid regurgitation is common and even normal when it is mild. Tricuspid

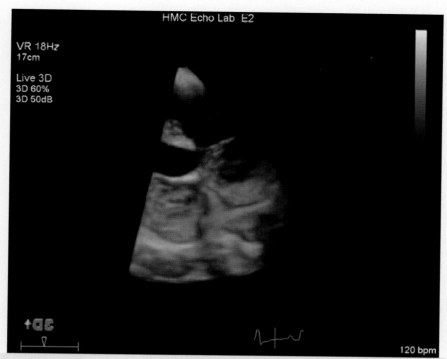

Figure 9-1 Tricuspid stenosis by three-dimensional echocardiography (see Video 9-1).

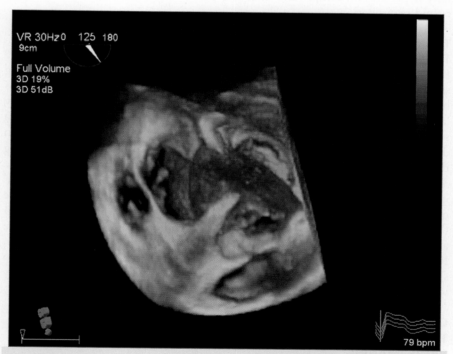

Figure 9-2 Example of a tricuspid valve by real-time three-dimensional transesophageal echocardiography. In this patient with an intracardiac mass, the tricuspid valve is on the left, with a pacer wire extruding through it into the right atrium. Despite the pacer wire helping identify the tricuspid valve, the tricuspid valve leaflets are not as well imaged as the mitral and aortic valves (see Video 9-2).

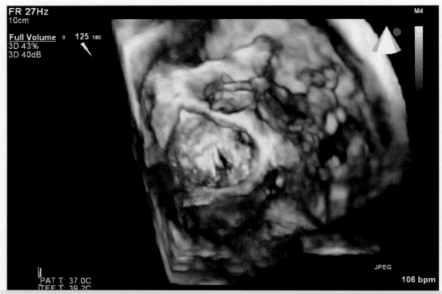

Figure 9-3 Vegetations on both the tricuspid and mitral valves in a patient with infectious endocarditis (see Video 9-3).

regurgitation frequently is seen as a result of primary or secondary pulmonary hypertension. Although any left heart abnormality can cause secondary pulmonary hypertension, mitral valve disease is particularly common, resulting in tricuspid regurgitation.

TRANSTHORACIC VERSUS TRANSESOPHAGEAL REAL-TIME THREE-DIMENSIONAL ECHOCARDIOGRAPHY

In marked contrast to the aortic valve, and particularly the mitral valve, obtaining satisfactory images from the transesophageal approach in the tricuspid valve has been found to be more challenging. 2D images of the tricuspid valve are of only fair quality by transesophageal echocardiography (TEE), and 3D images have a similar problem; although the images may be diagnostic, there is significant echo dropout of the tricuspid leaflets. However, this can be overcome by optimizing the 2DTEE images for the best possible tricuspid imaging before moving to the 3D mode: 3D zoom, live 3D, or 3D full volume. Figure 9-2 shows a 3DTEE image of the pacemaker wire traversing through the tricuspid valve. An example of a tricuspid valve vegetation imaged by RT3DTEE is shown in **Figure 9-3** (**Video 9-3**). In this case, the patient has a vegetation on both the mitral valve and the tricuspid valve. Both Figures 9-1 and 9-2 illustrate a constant in RT3DTEE imaging. Even in cases in which the image has been optimized to show the tricuspid valve, the left-sided valves typically are more optimally visualized.

CLINICAL VIGNETTES DESCRIBING USE OF REAL-TIME THREE-DIMENSIONAL ECHOCARDIOGRAPHY FOR TRICUSPID VALVE IMAGING

The following figures illustrate how RT3DE can provide impressive images of the tricuspid valve en face, with all three leaflets images simultaneously.

- Figure 9-4 (**Video 9-4**) shows an example of simultaneous visualization of the tricuspid, aortic, and mitral valves.
- Figure 9-5 (**Video 9-5**) is from a patient with severely elevated pulmonary artery (PA) systolic pressure (estimated at 75 mm Hg) by tricuspid regurgitation jet. Recurrent pulmonary emboli were the cause.

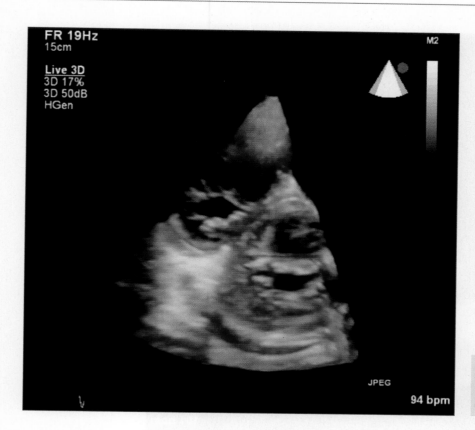

Figure 9-4 Simultaneous visualization of the tricuspid, aortic, and mitral valves by real-time three-dimensional transthoracic echocardiography (see Video 9-4).

- **Figure 9-6 (Video 9-6)** is from a patient with systemic lupus erythematosus, dyspnea, and secondary pulmonary hypertension. The right ventricle was severely dilated. PA systolic pressure was estimated at 55 mm Hg. There was severe tricuspid regurgitation from lack of coaptation of the tricuspid valve.
- **Figure 9-7 (Video 9-7)** is an RT3D transthoracic echocardiography (TTE) image from a patient with infectious endocarditis and a vegetation on the tricuspid valve. The patient had a history of intravenous drug use, cardiac murmur, chest pain, fever, and elevated white blood cell count.
- **Figure 9-8 (Video 9-8)** shows a flail tricuspid valve caused by trauma. The patient had sustained trauma to the chest in a horseback riding accident. There was severe tricuspid regurgitation. The right ventricle was moderately dilated with normal function. RT3DTTE showed the flail leaflet.
- **Figure 9-9 (Video 9-9)** shows a patient with severe congestive heart failure and a dilated left ventricle with an ejection fraction of 15%. The right ventricle was moderately dilated. Severe tricuspid regurgitation was caused by the inability of the leaflets to coapt. PA systolic pressure was estimated at 42 mm Hg.
- **Figure 9-10 (Video 9-10)** shows a patient with mitral stenosis and secondary pulmonary hypertension. There was moderate to severe right ventricular dilation, with moderately reduced systolic function. Right ventricular systolic pressure by tricuspid regurgitation jet was 51 mm Hg.
- **Figure 9-11 (Video 9-11)** is from a patient with septic shock, normal left and right ventricular function, and a mildly enlarged right ventricle. PA systolic pressure was only moderately elevated at 50 mm Hg. There was prominent pleural effusion, which may have helped obtain the image of the right heart.

Text continued on page 172

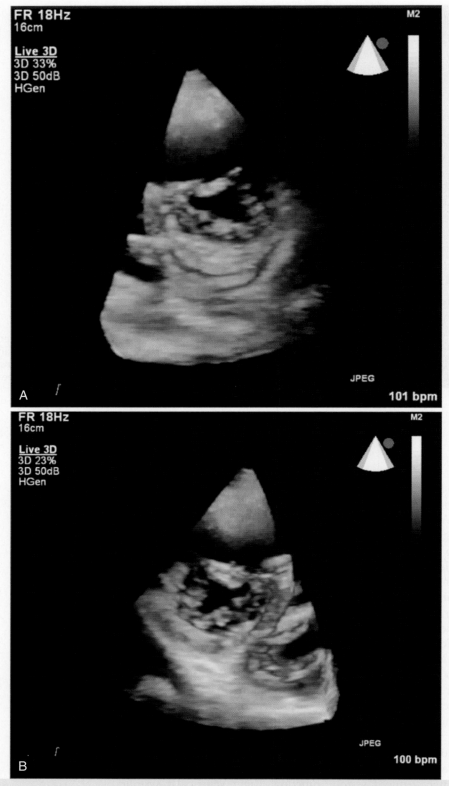

Figure 9-5 A 46-year-old patient with chronic pulmonary embolism. Shown is a severely dilated right ventricle with severely decreased function. **A,** Tricuspid valve from the right atrial side. **B,** Tricuspid valve from the right ventricular side (see Video 9-5).

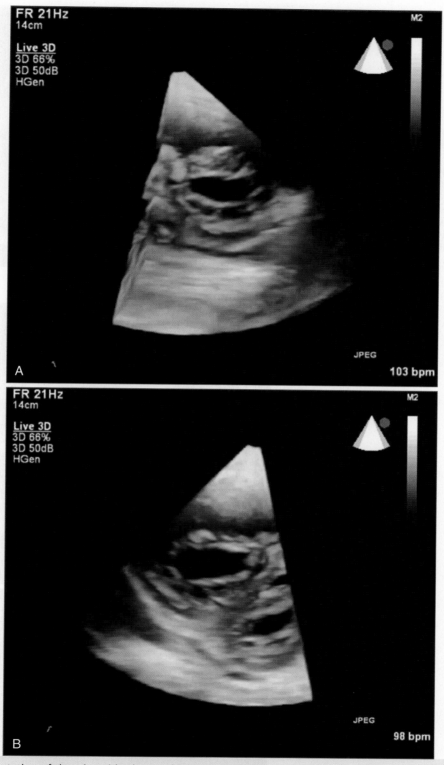

Figure 9-6   Lack of coaptation of the tricuspid valve resulting in severe tricuspid regurgitation. Real-time three-dimensional transthoracic echocardiography image of a patient with pulmonary hypertension secondary to systemic lupus erythematosus. The right ventricle was severely dilated. **A,** Tricuspid valve from the right atrial side. **B,** Tricuspid valve from the right ventricular side (see Video 9-6).

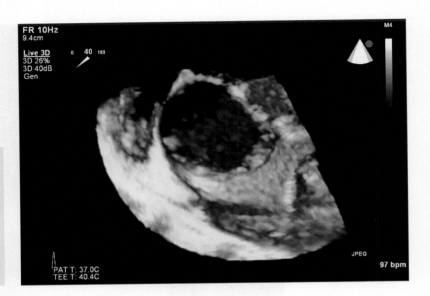

Figure 9-7 Tricuspid valve vegetation. Real-time three-dimensional transesophageal echocardiography image of a patient with an infectious vegetation on the tricuspid valve. The patient essentially had a flail tricuspid valve with the vegetation present predominantly on the anterior leaflet of the tricuspid valve. Severe tricuspid regurgitation was present. The *arrows* indicate that there is a vegetation with at least two components (see Video 9-7).

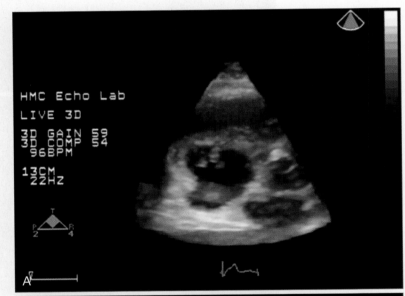

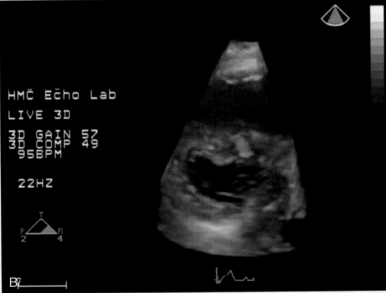

Figure 9-8 Flail tricuspid valve due to trauma. **A,** Rotating image from real-time three-dimensional transthoracic echocardiography in the parasternal short-axis view showing flail tricuspid leaflet, most likely the anterior leaflet. **B,** The flail leaflet from the right ventricular side (see Video 9-8).

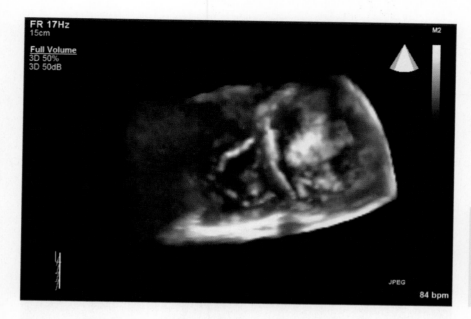

Figure 9-9 A 36-year-old patient with severe biventricular failure. The right ventricle was severely dilated, resulting in poor tricuspid valve coaptation and severe tricuspid regurgitation. The tricuspid valve is viewed from the apex, with leaflets as shown (see Video 9-9).

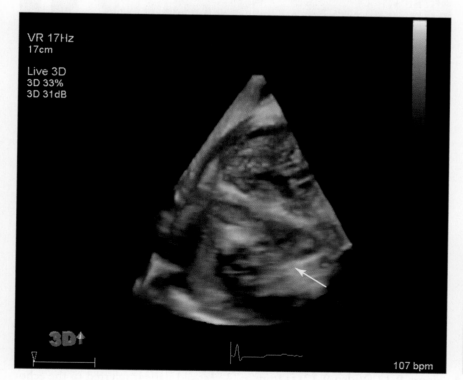

Figure 9-10 Mitral stenosis causing right ventricular dilation. Subcostal view, full-volume real-time three-dimensional transthoracic echocardiography showing prominent right ventricular dilation and a striking view of the tricuspid valve and the individual leaflets. The mitral valve is not as well visualized (*arrow*) but is associated with prominent calcification (see Video 9-10).

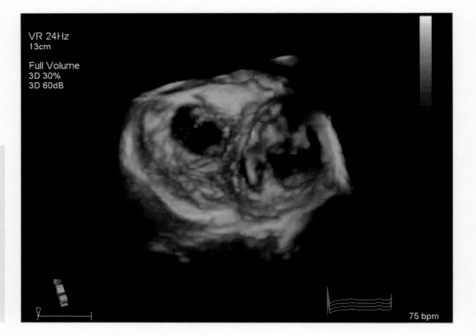

Figure 9-11 Sepsis and large pleural effusion. Real-time three-dimensional transthoracic echocardiography low parasternal, long-axis view for acquisition with subsequent cropping. This patient had no underlying valvular disease and had normal left ventricular systolic function. The right ventricle was mildly dilated, and there was moderate pulmonary hypertension, likely related to the underlying sepsis. The volume set has been cropped to show both the tricuspid and the mitral valves from the apical view (see Video 9-11).

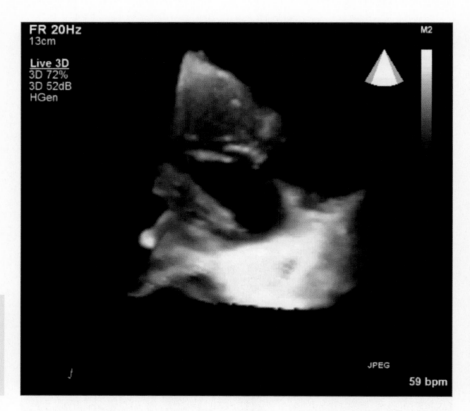

Figure 9-12 A patient with a normal heart was referred for echocardiography for evaluation of cardiac murmur. This parasternal short-axis view by real-time three-dimensional transesophageal echocardiography shows an en face view of the tricuspid valve (see Video 9-12).

- **Figure 9-12 (Video 9-12)** is from a 22-year-old patient referred to the echocardiography laboratory for evaluation of cardiac murmur. Because of very good imaging windows, the en face view of the tricuspid valve was obtained.
- **Figure 9-13 (Video 9-13)** is from a 95-year-old patient referred for echocardiography because of atrial fibrillation. The patient had severe tricuspid regurgitation with hepatic vein reversal. His right ventricle was moderately dilated but did have normal systolic function. Right ventricular systolic pressure was severely elevated and nearly systemic at 90 mm Hg, as estimated by the

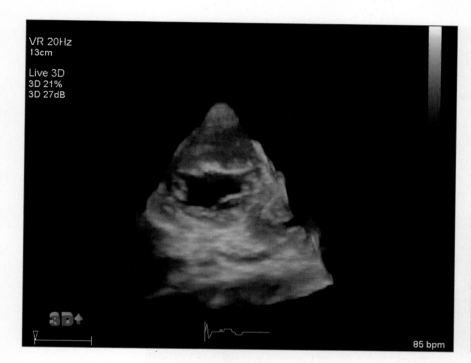

Figure 9-13 Real-time three-dimensional transesophageal echocardiography parasternal short-axis views of the tricuspid valve of a 95-year-old patient referred for echocardiography because of atrial fibrillation. The patient had severe tricuspid regurgitation with hepatic vein reversal, and the right ventricle was moderately dilated but did have normal systolic function (see Video 9-13).

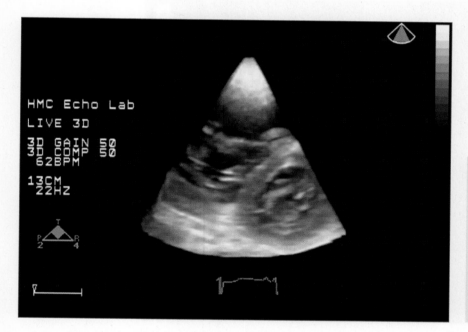

Figure 9-14 Severe right ventricular dysfunction in a 45-year-old patient. Real-time three-dimensional transthoracic echocardiography parasternal short-axis view of the tricuspid valve showing optimal imaging of the three leaflets. Imaging was particularly optimal in this patient because of severe right ventricular dilation with moderately reduced systolic function. Pulmonary artery pressure also was elevated at 76 mm Hg. Note the septal flattening (see Video 9-14).

tricuspid regurgitation jet. Four years after this echocardiogram, the patient was believed to still be alive at age 99 years.

■ **Figure 9-14 (Video 9-14)** shows a patient with severe right ventricular volume and pressure overload. The dilated, hypocontractile right ventricle provides a substrate for optimal image acquisition of the tricuspid valve.

■ **Figure 9-15 (Video 9-15)** shows images from a 51-year-old patient with severe pulmonary hypertension, systemic-level PA systolic pressure of 100 mm Hg, and chronic pulmonary emboli. The en face imaging of the tricuspid valve is excellent. From the right ventricular side, the individual leaflets can, in this case, be more clearly identified than from the right atrial side.

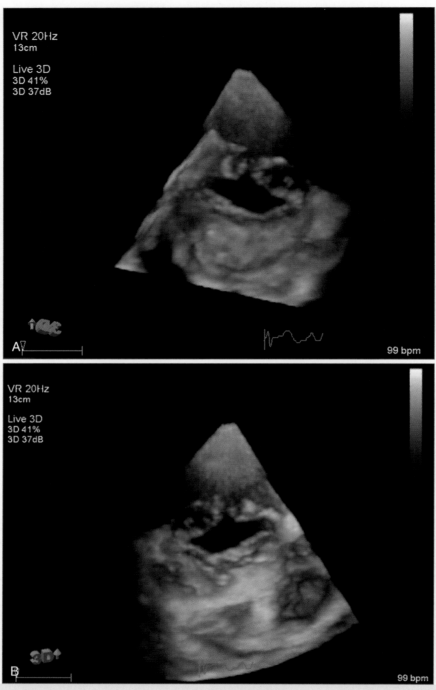

Figure 9-15 Parasternal short-axis real-time three-dimensional transthoracic echocardiography of a 51-year-old patient with systemic-level pulmonary hypertension, chronic pulmonary emboli, and right ventricular dysfunction. **A,** Right atrial side of the tricuspid valve. **B,** Right ventricular side of the tricuspid valve (see Video 9-15).

■ **Figure 9-16 (Video 9-16)** shows primary pulmonary hypertension that has resulted in severe right ventricular dilation and severe right ventricular dysfunction. The marked right ventricular dilation has allowed particularly clear imaging of the tricuspid valve from the right ventricular side. The anterior leaflet is particularly prominent. The septal leaflet appears to have been stretched by the D-shaped interventricular septum.

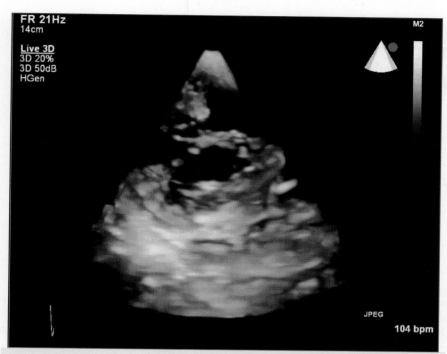

Figure 9-16 Primary pulmonary hypertension with severe right ventricular enlargement and severe right ventricular dysfunction. The right ventricle is severely dilated, which accommodated imaging of the tricuspid valve. In this case, the anterior leaflet of the tricuspid valve is notably large and well visualized (see Video 9-16).

SUMMARY

Whenever severe tricuspid regurgitation is identified, consideration must be given to either tricuspid valve repair or replacement. 3DE can provide incremental information regarding the cause of tricuspid regurgitation.

References

1. Silver MD, Lam JHC, Ranganathan N, Wigle ED: Morphology of the human tricuspid valve. *Circulation* 23:333–348, 1971.
2. Raman SV, Sparks EA, Boudoulas H, Wooley CF: Tricuspid valve disease: Tricuspid valve complex perspective. *Curr Prob Cardiol* 27(3):103–142, 2002.
3. Uijings R, Kluin J, Salomonsz R, et al: Pacemaker lead–induced severe tricuspid valve stenosis. *Circ Heart Failure* 3:465–467, 2010.
4. Faletra F, La Marchesina U, Bragato R, De Chiara F: Three-dimensional transthoracic echocardiography images of tricuspid stenosis. *Heart* 91:499, 2005.
5. Anwar AM, Geleijnse M: Evaluation of rheumatic tricuspid stenosis using real-time three-dimensional echocardiography. *Heart* 93:363, 2007.
6. Sultan FAT, Moustafa SE, Tajik J, et al: Rheumatic tricuspid valve disease: An evidence-based systematic overview. *J Heart Valve Dis* 19:374, 2010.

CHAPTER 10

Pulmonary Valve in Health and Disease

Edward A. Gill

The pulmonary valve is the smallest valve in the body and, in keeping with its size, plays a relatively uncommon role in adult cardiology. Despite the limited involvement of the pulmonary valve in adult cardiac disorders, it is important to review the clinical situations for which pulmonary valve pathology is present. Pulmonic stenosis rarely is identified in adulthood and is a problem much more frequently identified and treated in pediatric patients. Mild to moderate pulmonary regurgitation is, of course, common and normal in adults.

The most common cause of significant pulmonary regurgitation (defined as more than moderate pulmonary regurgitation) in adults is pulmonary hypertension from any cause, with or without dilation of the pulmonary valve ring. Like the tricuspid valve, the pulmonary valve typically becomes incompetent when exposed to high pressure. Less common causes of pulmonary valve regurgitation include infectious endocarditis, carcinoid syndrome, and tumor infiltration of the valve (e.g., papillary fibroelastoma).[1-5] Pulmonary hypertension can be primary or secondary; the most common secondary cause is left-sided heart failure. Pulmonary artery dilation also can ultimately result in valve ring dilation. Causes of pulmonary artery dilation include connective tissue diseases such as Marfan syndrome, Ehler-Danlos syndrome, systemic lupus erythematosus, and scleroderma. Idiopathic dilation of the pulmonary artery is a clinically described phenomenon. This entity typically is seen in older women and can result in severe pulmonary regurgitation. In the patient population at Harborview Medical Center, infective endocarditis with destruction of the valve is a not-infrequent cause of pulmonary regurgitation. The fact that we have identified several cases of pulmonary valve endocarditis in recent years is notable because the overall incidence of pulmonary valve endocarditis is quite low—estimated to be as low as 2% at autopsy series and clearly less common than tricuspid valve endocarditis.[6] Indeed, between 1960 and 1999, only 36 cases of pulmonic valve endocarditis were reported in structurally normal hearts.[7] Transesophageal echocardiography (TEE) undoubtedly has improved the diagnostic yield of pulmonic valve endocarditis compared with transthoracic echocardiography (TTE), but the true incidence remains uncertain.[8,9] Congenital absence of the pulmonary valve can be seen in association with tetralogy of Fallot or accompanying a congenital ventricular septal defect (VSD) and less commonly with atrial septal defect (ASD), coarctation of the aorta, or tricuspid atresia.[10] In practice, the valve leaflets are rudimentary and dysplastic rather than completely absent.[11] Isolated dysplastic pulmonary valve is rare and much less common than when seen in association with the previously named defects.

Three-dimensional echocardiography (3DE) of the pulmonary valve is very difficult to perform by TTE in adults, just as imaging the pulmonary valve by two-dimensional echocardiography (2DE) typically is challenging.[12] The limitation typically is ultrasound penetration due to interference from lung tissue. A clear rule of thumb regarding 3DE imaging is that if the 2DE image is poor, the 3DE image is likely to be poor or worse. **Figures 10-1** and **10-2** show a TTE image in the parasternal short-axis view with the pulmonic valve

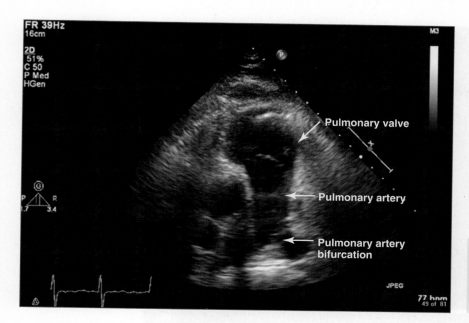

Figure 10-1 Two-dimensional transthoracic echocardiography image of a normal pulmonary valve, pulmonary artery, and pulmonary artery bifurcation (see Video 10-1).

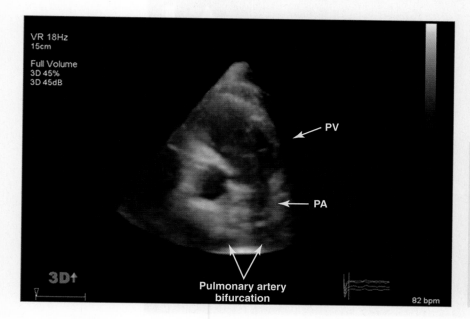

Figure 10-2 Three-dimensional (3D) image obtained from the transthoracic parasternal short-axis view of the pulmonary valve (*PV*), pulmonary artery (*PA*), and pulmonary artery bifurcation. Most notably for the pulmonary valve, the 3D image loses some of the distinguishing characteristics of the various structures compared with the two-dimensional view. The benefit of depth in this case is offset by the limited ultrasound penetration allowed by transthoracic imaging (see Video 10-2).

adjacent to the aortic valve in 2D (**Video 10-1**) and 3D (**Video 10-2**). The pulmonic valve is seen in the longitudinal view, and typically only one, or at best two, of the valve leaflets is identified. Not infrequently, the subcostal view can come in handy for viewing the pulmonary valve with surface imaging. **Figure 10-3** and **Video 10-3** show subcostal views of the pulmonary valve by 2DE and 3DE.

CASE 1

The first case is an example of detection of a pulmonary embolus using TTE. In this case, there is a saddle embolus. **Figure 10-4** and **Video 10-4** show 2D views in the parasternal long-axis and apical four-chamber view of a patient who presented with dyspnea and hypotension. The right ventricle is dilated and markedly hypocontractile. McConnell's sign is present, with severe right ventricular dysfunction that spares the apex. **Figures 10-5** and **10-6** and **Videos 10-5** and **10-6** show examples of an embolus at the bifurcation of the pulmonary artery, hence

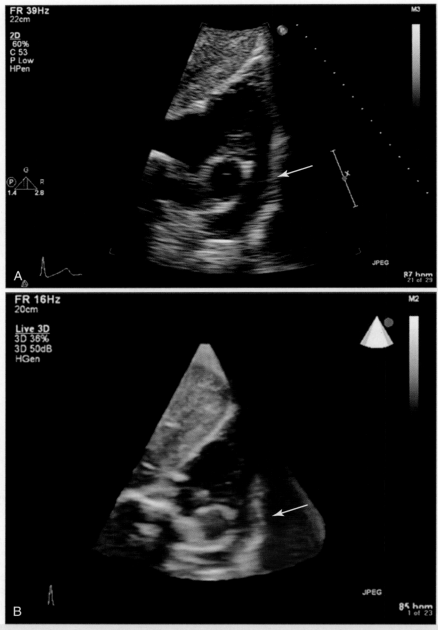

Figure 10-3 Two-dimensional (**A**) and three-dimensional (**B**) transthoracic echocardiography images by the subcostal view showing the pulmonary valve (*arrow*), pulmonary artery, and pulmonary artery bifurcation (see Video 10-3).

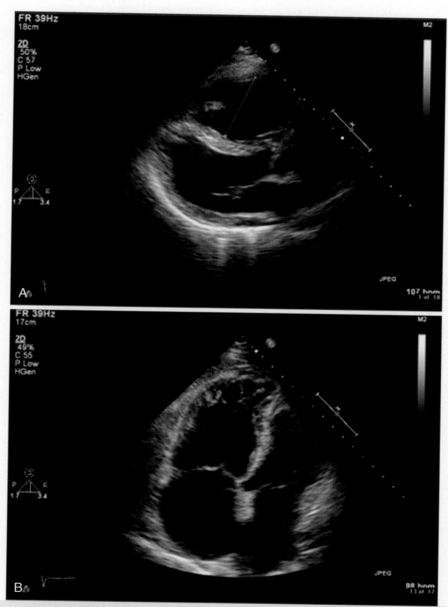

Figure 10-4   Two-dimensional transthoracic echocardiography parasternal long-axis view (**A**) and apical four-chamber view (**B**) of a patient with a saddle pulmonary embolus. Note right ventricular dilation in both views (see Video 10-4).

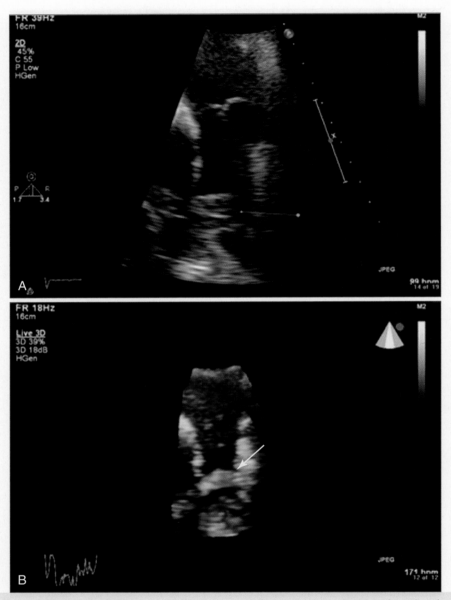

Figure 10-5   Two-dimensional (**A**) and three-dimensional (**B**) parasternal short-axis views showing thrombus (*arrow*) at the bifurcation of the pulmonary artery (*line*) (see Video 10-5).

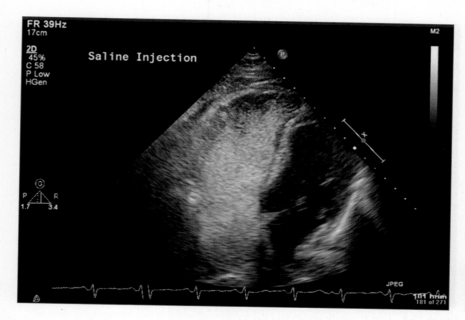

Figure 10-6 Saline contrast study showing a dilated right ventricle (see Videos 10-6 and 10-7).

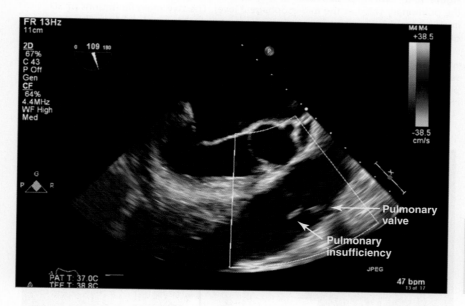

Figure 10-7 Two-dimensional transthoracic echocardiography mid-esophageal view of the pulmonary valve with a mild pulmonary regurgitation color Doppler jet (see Video 10-8).

a "saddle embolus." The right ventricular dilation and severe systolic dysfunction are emphasized even more with injection of saline contrast into the right ventricle (see Figure 10-6; **Video 10-7**).

TEE imaging is required to identify more detailed pathology of the valve. However, even standard TEE views do not easily image the pulmonary valve. The most consistent TEE view of the pulmonary valve is attained while simultaneously imaging the aortic valve in the short-axis view, typically at 50 to 90 degrees. The pulmonary valve appears in the longitudinal view and can be interrogated for regurgitation (**Figures 10-7** and **10-8**; **Videos 10-8** to **10-10**). Inconsistently, the pulmonary valve is seen almost by accident while imaging in the deep gastric view (**Figures 10-9** to **10-11**; **Videos 10-11** and **10-12**).

The position of the TEE probe for obtaining the deep gastric view is shown in Figure 10-9. The steps for obtaining the deep gastric view are as follows:

1. The TEE probe is advanced past the gastric view (typically 40 cm from the incisors) to an approximate depth of 55 cm. Throughout this manipulation, the probe angle is at zero degrees.

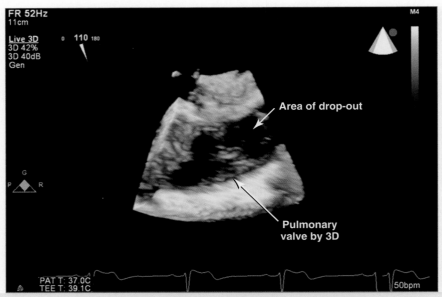

Figure 10-8   Live three-dimensional (3D) transesophageal echocardiography view of the pulmonary valve at the mid-esophageal level. The two main limitations of 3D imaging are shown in this image. First, there are notable echolucent, or "black areas," of echo dropout, which are a compromise of gain and compress settings that allow visualization of the pulmonary valve. Increasing gain would eliminate the dropout but would add additional echoes covering the pulmonary valve, making it invisible. The second limitation is difficulty viewing structures that are very thin, in this case the pulmonary valve itself. A thicker abnormal pulmonary valve with classic sclerotic changes would be more visible (see Videos 10-9 and 10-10).

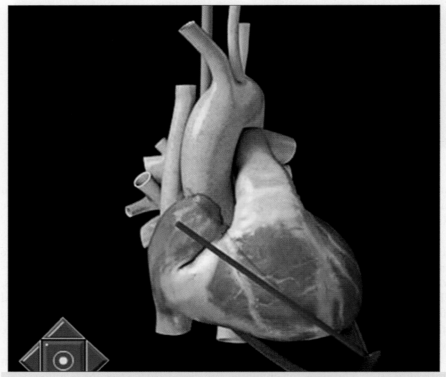

Figure 10-9   Simulation of the ideal position of the transesophageal echocardiography (TEE) probe for obtaining the deep gastric view of the pulmonary valve. This position initially is ideal for the aortic valve. Pulling the probe out slightly results in visualization of the pulmonary valve.

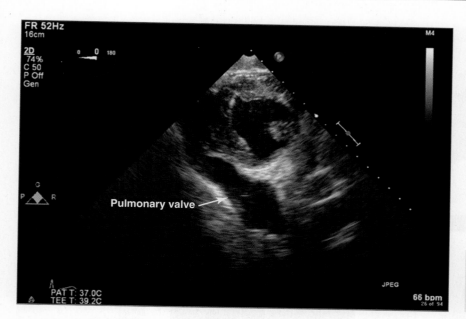

FR 52Hz
16cm

2D
74%
C 50
P Off
Gen

Pulmonary valve

PAT T: 37.0C
TEE T: 39.2C

JPEG
66 bpm

Figure 10-10 Two-dimensional transesophageal echocardiography view of the pulmonary valve from the deep gastric view (see Video 10-11).

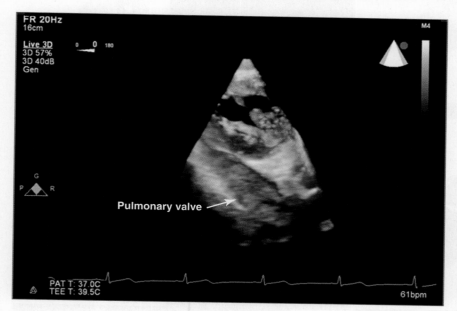

FR 20Hz
16cm

Live 3D
3D 57%
3D 40dB
Gen

Pulmonary valve

PAT T: 37.0C
TEE T: 39.5C

61bpm

Figure 10-11 Three-dimensional transesophageal echocardiography deep gastric view of the pulmonary valve. Because of its very thin leaflets, the pulmonary valve remains difficult to see (see Video 10-12).

2. The aortic valve is brought into view by the combination of flexion of the probe using clockwise manipulation of the anterior/posterior control wheel and counterclockwise manipulation of the medial/lateral wheel. This movement has the combined effect of improving contact with the stomach with anteflexion and lateral movement of the probe, aligning with the aortic valve (see Figures 10-10 and 10-11 and Videos 10-11 and 10-12).

3. By pulling the TEE probe back toward the incisors 3 to 5 cm, the pulmonary valve is brought into view.

For the most optimal views of the pulmonary valve in either 2DE or 3DE, the high esophageal view is ideal when present because of the proximity of the aorta, specifically the aortic arch. At the level of the aortic arch, the aorta provides a perfect sonographic window to see through and image the right ventricular outflow tract, the pulmonary valve, and the proximal pulmonary artery and its bifurcation (**Figure 10-12**). The only problem with this view is that it is present in only 50% to 60% of patients. Experience suggests that the view is best seen in patients with right-sided pathology, particularly dilation of the pulmonary

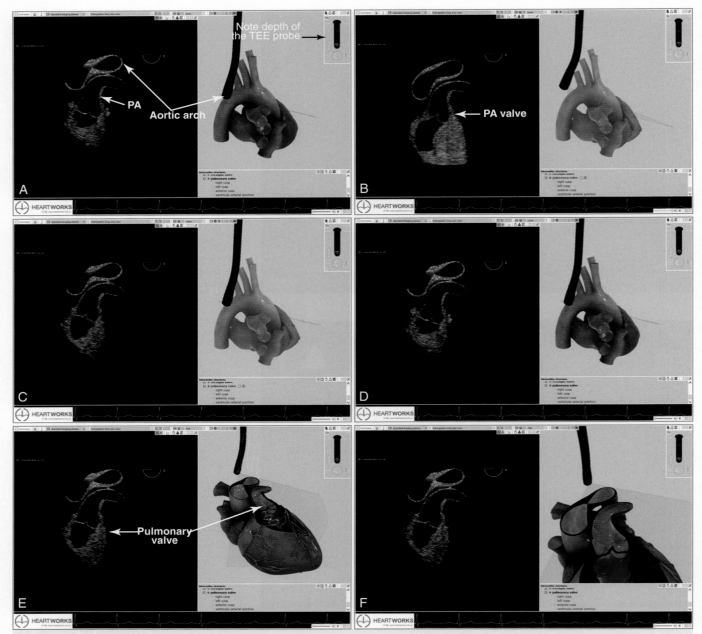

Figure 10-12   **A,** Placement of the transesophageal echocardiography (TEE) probe for acquisition of the high esophageal view is shown by TEE simulation. **B,** A similar illustration obtained by TEE simulation with emphasis on the pulmonary valve. The TEE probe is slightly retroflexed relative to the image in **A**. **C,** TEE probe position for obtaining the high esophageal view. **D,** Setup to show a cutaway of the pulmonary valve. **E,** Similar depth of the TEE probe, with similar 2D image on the left. At right, the pulmonary artery aortic arch has been partially cut away to show the pulmonary valve cusps. **F,** The position of the TEE probe has not substantially changed. A zoomed view of the aortic arch and pulmonary valve is shown.

artery. **Figures 10-13** to **10-16** and **Videos 10-13** to **10-25** show several examples of 2D and 3D TEE imaging of the pulmonary artery and valve through the high esophageal window. Figures 10-14 and 10-15 and Videos 10-19 and 10-20 show a case of pulmonary valve endocarditis, again viewed through this window.

The high esophageal view (see Figure 10-12) of the pulmonary valve is obtained by using the following manipulation:

1. The initial setup requires imaging of the descending aorta with the TEE probe facing posteriorly (see Figure 10-12, *B*). The aorta is viewed in a short-axis or transverse plane. The probe angle is at zero degrees.

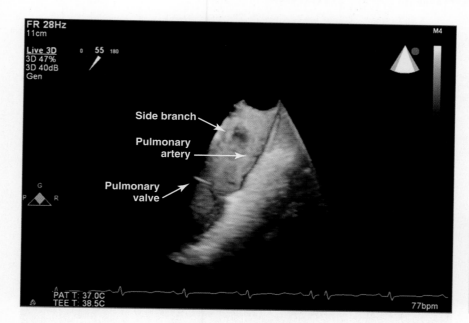

Figure 10-13 Three-dimensional transesophageal echocardiography view of the pulmonary artery, pulmonary valve, and an apparent pulmonary artery side branch. This view was obtained at the high esophageal level at the aortic arch (see Video 10-13).

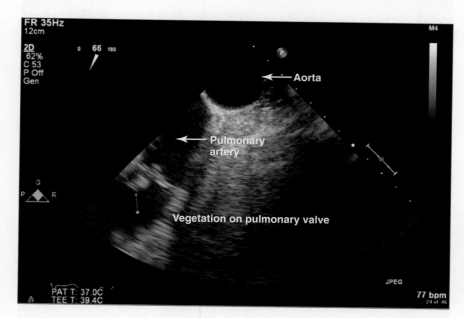

Figure 10-14 Two-dimensional transesophageal echocardiography view at the high esophageal level showing a vegetation on the pulmonary valve. The vegetation is on both the right ventricular outflow tract and pulmonary artery sides of the valve (see Video 10-19).

2. The TEE probe is then slowly retracted, moving from a depth of 30 to 35 cm to 25 to 27 cm, where the view into the aortic arch becomes prominent and is seen to "lengthen" and have a longitudinal view as opposed to the transverse view (see Figure 10-12, *C*). Depth is increased from a typical value of 4 to 6 cm for imaging the aorta to 9 to 11 cm for imaging the pulmonary artery and pulmonary valve.

3. With the aortic arch seen in its longest transverse length, the probe angle is moved from zero to 50 to 70 degrees, depending on the patient. The entire probe is rotated clockwise, or rightward, to move closer to the pulmonary artery. The medial/lateral control can help this medial movement as well (see Figure 10-12, *D*).

4. For imaging in 3D, the position obtained in Figure 10-12, *D*, can then be used to switch to live 3D. Alternatively, the 3D zoom mode can be used. The setup for optimal pulmonary artery and valve viewing, including the pulmonary artery bifurcation, is illustrated in Video 10-15.

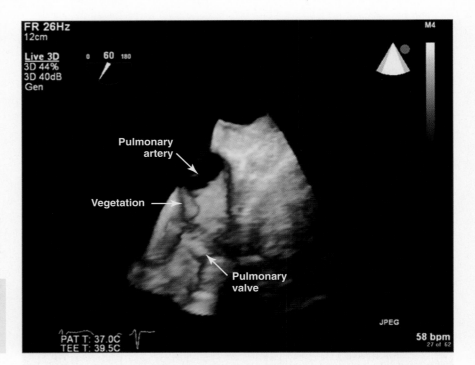

Figure 10-15 Three-dimensional view of the same vegetation seen in Figure 10-14. Note the grossly enlarged size of the vegetation compared with the two-dimensional view (see Video 10-20).

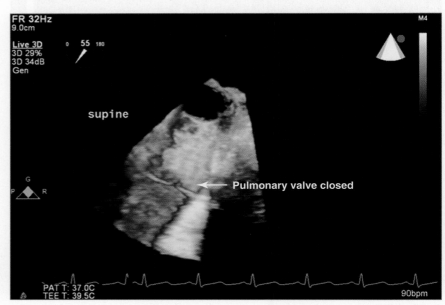

Figure 10-16 Three-dimensional transesophageal echocardiography view at the high esophageal level showing a closed pulmonary valve (see Video 10-16).

5. The operator should not be discouraged by initial failure to obtain this view because it is a high-level manipulation. Also, as mentioned, it is possible only in 50% to 60% of patients. The good news is that it tends to be more successful in patients who have pulmonary artery pathology, as demonstrated by the clinical case that follows.

The pulmonary valve is the only valve that cannot frequently be viewed en face; in fact, it would be very rare to obtain a satisfactory en face view by TTE. 3DTEE, however, occasionally can deliver an en face view of the pulmonary valve (see Video 10-9).

CLINICAL CASE

A 46-year-old man with a history of intravenous illicit drug use presented with signs and symptoms suggestive of right-sided endocarditis. Specifically, the patient reported chest pain, dyspnea, and lower extremity edema. On physical examination, a new diastolic murmur was heard over the left sternal border consistent with pulmonic valve regurgitation. Blood cultures demonstrated *Staphylococcus aureus*. The vegetation is shown by both 2DTEE and 3DTEE (see Figures 10-14 and 10-15; see Videos 10-19 and 10-20). Thus, the diagnosis of endocarditis was clearly confirmed by echocardiography.

3DE is particularly useful in congenital heart disease because like other tomographic imaging modalities such as computed tomography (CT) and magnetic resonance imaging (MRI), 3DE allows discrete visualization of adjacent structures and their important anatomic relationships. For endocarditis, 3DE frequently outperforms 2DE in assessment of vegetations from the standpoint of shape and mobility as well as size. Size in particular can be more accurately assessed by 3DE because it is a volume technique, whereas 2DE is limited to linear measurements and those of the area of the vegetation. This case of endocarditis, like many cases of right-sided endocarditis, was medically treated with a successful outcome.

CONCLUSION

Imaging the pulmonary valve with 3DE is challenging and clearly best achieved by TEE. On occasion, in thin patients, diagnostic views of the pulmonary valve are obtained by TTE, but this is an exception. The high esophageal view of the pulmonary valve can be acquired in most patients, and the striking views of the valve can be particularly useful when pathology (e.g., a vegetation) or a tumor (e.g., a papillary fibroelastoma) is present.

References

1. Hecht SR, Berger M: Right-sided endocarditis in intravenous drug users. Prognostic features in 102 episodes. *Ann Intern Med* 117:560–566, 1992.
2. Ohri SK, Schofield JB, Hodgson H: Carcinoid heart disease: Early failure of an allograft valve replacement. *Ann Thorac Surg* 58:1161, 1994.
3. Seymour J, Emanuel R, Patterson N: Acquired pulmonary stenosis. *Br Heart J* 30:776, 1968.
4. Gowda RM, Khan IA, Nair CK, et al: Cardiac papillary fibroelastoma: A comprehensive analysis of 725 cases. *Am Heart J* 146:404–410, 2003.
5. Odim J, Reehal V, Laks H, et al: Surgical pathology of cardiac tumors. Two decades at an urban institution. *Cardiovasc Pathol* 12:267–270, 2003.
6. Schroeder RA: Pulmonic valve endocarditis in a normal heart. *J Am Soc Echocardiogr* 18:197–198, 2005.
7. Ramadan FB, Beanlands DS, Burwash IG: Isolated pulmonic valve endocarditis in healthy hearts: a case report and review of the literature. *Can J Cardiol* 16:1282–1288, 2000.
8. Winslow T, Foster E, Adams JR, Schiller NB: Pulmonary valve endocarditis: improved diagnosis with biplane transesophageal echocardiography. *J Am Soc Echocardiogr* 5:206–210, 1992.
9. Shapiro SM, Young E, Ginzton LE, Bayer AS: Pulmonic valve endocarditis as an underdiagnosed disease: role of transesophageal echocardiography. *J Am Soc Echocardiogr* 5:48–51, 1992.
10. Howard S, Wan S, Freeman LJ: Congenital absence of the pulmonary valve. *Heart* 93(7):779, 2007.
11. Bharati AH, Naware A, Merchant SA: Absent pulmonary valve syndrome with tetralogy of Fallot and associated dextrocardia detected at a nearly gestational age of 26 weeks. *Ind J Radiol Imag* 18:4:352–354, 2008.
12. Kelly NF, Platts DG, Burstow DJ: Feasibility of pulmonary valve imaging using three-dimensional transthoracic echocardiography. *J Am Soc Echocardiogr* 23:1076–1080, 2010.

CHAPTER 11

Volumetric Assessment

Carly Jenkins

The rationale for the use of three-dimensional echocardiography (3DE) in a clinical setting is growing stronger. The four main areas in which the value of 3DE has been investigated include (1) the analysis of cardiac volumes and left ventricular mass, (2) ischemic heart disease, (3) congenital heart disease, and (4) valvular pathology. Although various versions of 3DE have been in use since the early 1970s, "live" or real-time 3DE (RT3DE) has only been in use since the early 2000s (**Figures 11-1** and **11-2**; **Videos 11-1** and **11-2**).[1]

3DE can display, in real time, the views and motions of deeper cardiac structures, which are unavailable by two-dimensional echocardiography (2DE), and therefore is capable of providing superior diagnostic information (**Figures 11-3** to **11-5**; **Videos 11-3** to **11-5**). This is particularly advantageous given the complex spatial relations of cardiac structures, especially in the fields of acquired valvular disease, atrial and ventricular septal defects, and left ventricular remodelling.[2-4] It can also display exact assessments of left atrial volume.[5,6] 3DE is particularly well suited for volumetric analysis of the right ventricle since it has such an irregular shape. The ability of 3DE to simulate surgical views helps facilitate vital surgical decisions such as the accurate assessments of the effect of percutaneous balloon valvuloplasty and the function of prosthetic valves and septal occluders. Finally, 3DE may help in making more accurate qualitative diagnosis and in the classification of congenital heart disease.[7]

To date, the analysis of left ventricular volumes, mass, and shape has been the most widely utilized clinical application of 3DE; this underscores the fact that 3DE has no geometric limitations with regard to the evaluation of the size and shape of the heart, particularly when it is distorted. Measurement of volumes and mass can be performed using automated and semiautomated software in which a wire frame tracks the endocardial borders.

QUALITATIVE AND QUANTITATIVE PROBLEMS WITH CLINICAL TWO-DIMENSIONAL ECHOCARDIOGRAPHY TODAY

Quantification of left ventricular volumes and ejection fraction (EF) is an important aspect of cardiac evaluation in all cardiac disorders. Indeed, assessment of left ventricular function is the most common indication for echocardiography. The serial assessment of left ventricular function frequently is used to guide therapy. However, repeated measurements are prone to variation because of poor image quality, geometric issues related to volume and mass calculations, performance measurements from off-axis cuts, and variations in ventricular loading.[8]

EF is a simple numeric value that reflects left ventricular function; however, it is strongly influenced by loading conditions and, in many cases, does not correlate with the patient's symptoms. More importantly, it has limited test-retest reliability.[9] Subjective visual or "eyeball" assessment of left ventricular EF (LVEF) often is performed in clinical practice but can be misleading because of irregular heart rhythms, when the left ventricular cavity is very large or very small, or when the heart rate is very low or very fast.[10] Motion mode (MM)

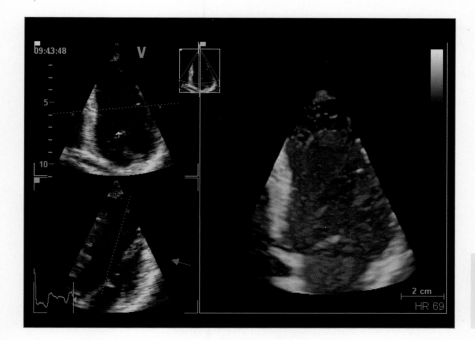

Figure 11-1 Example of a full-volume three-dimensional image with corresponding two-dimensional four- and two-chamber views (see Video 11-1). (Courtesy EchoPAC-PC, GE Vingmed.)

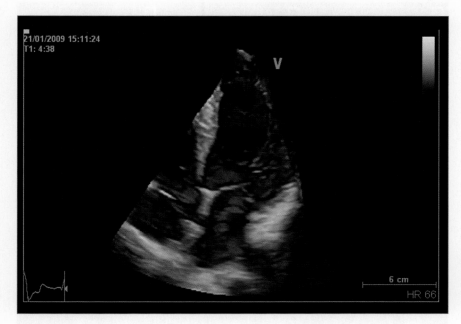

Figure 11-2 Example of a real-time three-dimensional image from the apical view (see Video 11-2). (Courtesy EchoPAC-PC, GE Vingmed.)

has been used for many decades to calculate the fractional shortening and EF from the left ventricular diameters at end diastole and end systole; however, these values have large variations because of angle dependency.[11] Studies have shown that Simpson's biplane calculation of EF can vary up to 4.1% between readers.[12,13] This variability is caused by the complex geometric assumptions and potential problems with image foreshortening presented by 2DE calculation of EF. Previous work by King et al[11] has shown the importance of cut planes on cardiac measurements. In their study, 2DE did not achieve consistent optimal positioning of standard imaging views, resulting in a high percentage (93%) of off-axis images with resultant variations in left ventricular measurements (9%).[14] Neither MM nor the Simpson's biplane technique take into account the regional variation of the whole left ventricular volume, which may occur due to myocardial infarction. Similar findings have been reported for left ventricular mass. The smallest change of mass that can be detected with 95% confidence is 59 g, which

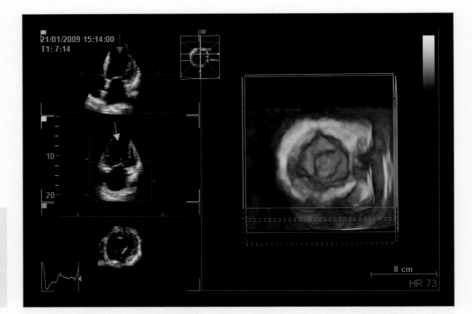

Figure 11-3 Cropped three-dimensional image, viewing from the left ventricular side through the mitral valve, with the corresponding two-dimensional images of the four-chamber, two-chamber, and short-axis views (see Video 11-3). (Courtesy EchoPAC-PC, GE Vingmed.)

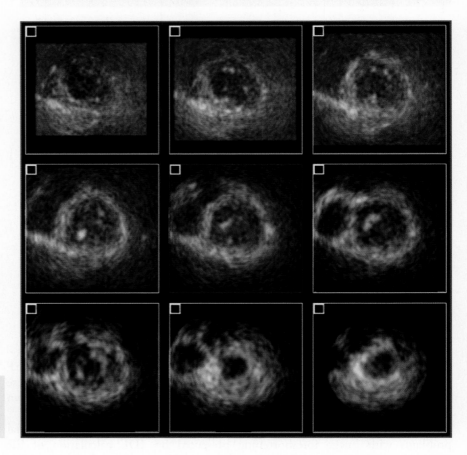

Figure 11-4 Example of nine-slice view of a full-volume three-dimensional image (see Video 11-4). (Courtesy Philips Healthcare, Andover, MA.)

compares with an average 20 to 40 g/year change in most antihypertensive therapy trials.[15]

Consequently, cardiac magnetic resonance imaging (MRI) has been proposed as a more desirable alternative for left ventricular assessment, especially in clinical trials, because of its excellent image quality and high spatial resolution.[16] Given this, cardiac MRI has become the gold standard for left ventricular volumes, EF, and left ventricular mass. However, expense, patient intolerance (e.g.,

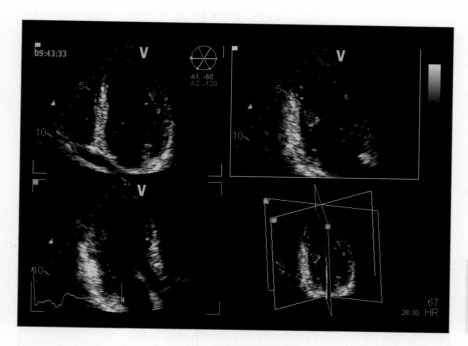

Figure 11-5 Example of a triplane image consisting of the three two-dimensional apical views cut from a full-volume three-dimensional image (see Video 11-5). (Courtesy EchoPAC-PC, GE Vingmed.)

claustrophobia, noise), a relative contraindication in patients with cardiac devices, and lack of portability have limited the use of this modality in routine clinical practice.

Despite the technical limitations of 2DE, it remains the most widely used noninvasive technique for the measurement of left ventricular size and function. These limitations may be overcome with the use of 3DE, which has less test-retest variation, better reproducibility, and better accuracy compared with 2DE.[9,17-21]

ASSESSMENT OF LEFT VENTRICULAR VOLUMES AND EJECTION FRACTION

In the past 3 decades, 3DE has developed into a clinical tool for measuring volumes, EF, and left ventricular mass. Many studies have shown that 3DE is more closely correlated to MRI with less variability than 2DE for cardiac measurements. The advancement of 3DE from a cumbersome offline tool to a real-time online process has taken it out of the research arena and into the clinical laboratory.

In the early 1990s, volumetric 3DE was developed by Duke University using a sparse matrix array transducer. This technique is based on the concept that the heart would fit into a pyramidal dataset and does not rely on the transducer movement or sequential capturing. Although the output is known as "real-time output," it actually consists of multiple 2D images displayed simultaneously.[22] Other previous 3D transducers used a modified 2D probe that had elements arranged in a single line, in which multiple windows and planes were needed to reconstruct an image. These volumetric and reconstructed volumes were found to have improved accuracy for left ventricular volumes.

These early techniques formed the basis of RT3DE. Current matrix transducers use a dense array, rather than the previous sparse array arrangement, and reportedly have more than 3000 elements.[23] RT3DE uses 256 firing elements in the form of a grid instead of a line, which enables acquisition of an online 3D volume of ultrasound data (**Figures 11-6 to 11-10; Videos 11-6 to 11-10**).

Online 3DE allows volumetric quantification using a biplane or triplane technique.[12] 3DE has the advantage of accurate delineation of the true long-axis length of the ventricle, thus increasing the accuracy of Simpson's guided biplane measurements (see Figures 11-4 and 11-5; see Videos 11-4 and 11-5). For 2DE,

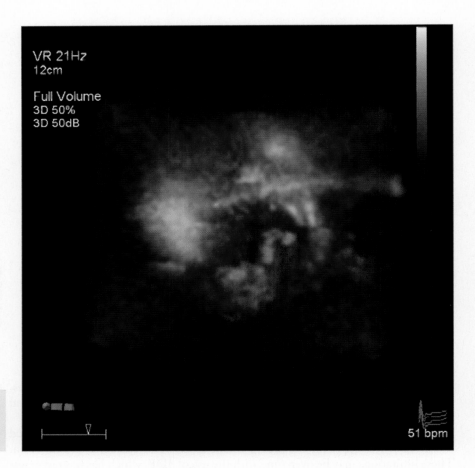

Figure 11-6 Example of normal left ventricular systolic function and wire frame over the cardiac cycle (see Video 11-6). (Courtesy TomTec, Munich, Germany.)

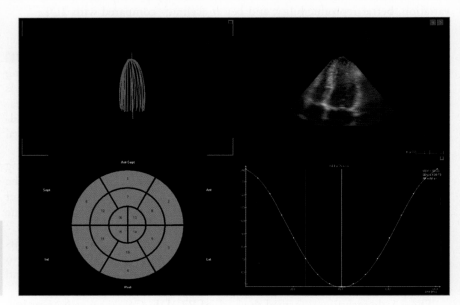

Figure 11-7 Example of endocardial border tracking of normal left ventricular systolic function and measurement of volumes (see Video 11-7). (Courtesy Philips Healthcare, Andover, MA.)

the accuracy of left ventricular volumes by Simpson's method depends on the apical four-chamber and two-chamber lengths being nearly equal. Since the geometric assumptions of the 2DE calculations depend on the accuracy of ventricular lengths, foreshortening will result in underestimation of the cross-sectional area.

Recent advancements in 3DE technology have allowed for faster assessment in full left ventricular volume measures because of the semiautomated endocardial

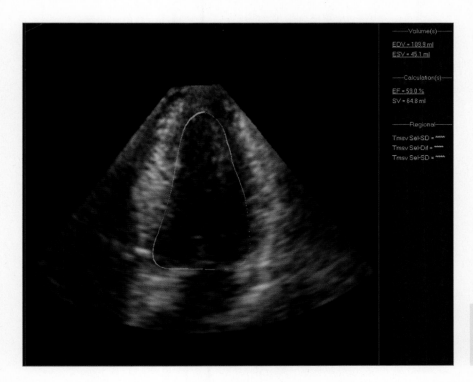

Figure 11-8 Example of poor left ventricular systolic function and the 16-segment model (see Video 11-8). (Courtesy TomTec, Munich, Germany.)

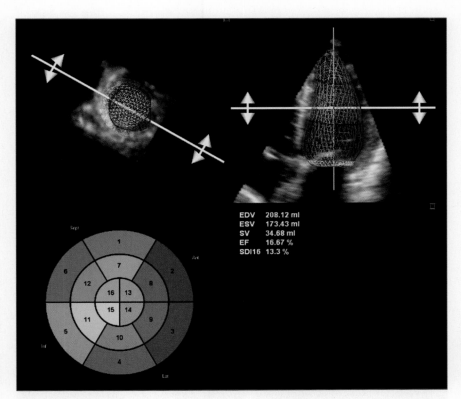

Figure 11-9 Example of poor left ventricular systolic function and a time volume curve (see Video 11-9). (Courtesy EchoPAC-PC, GE Vingmed.)

edge detection. Online measurement of left ventricular volumes is feasible and more accurate than with 2DE.[24]

Despite semiautomated measuring techniques, 3DE has been found to underestimate left ventricular volumes compared with MRI measures. The major shortcoming of 3DE relates to the image quality of the currently obtainable images (**Figure 11-11; Video 11-11**). The lower line density and frame rate

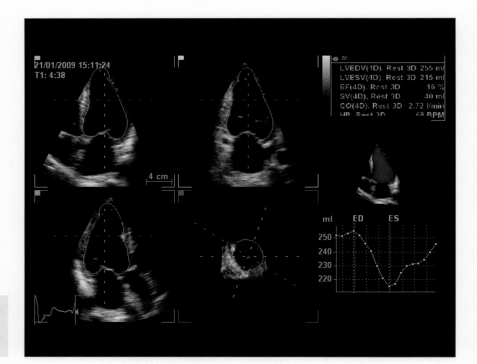

Figure 11-10 View of a three-dimensional image and the importance of cut plane. Elongation of the apex is the key to measuring volumes (see Video 11-10).

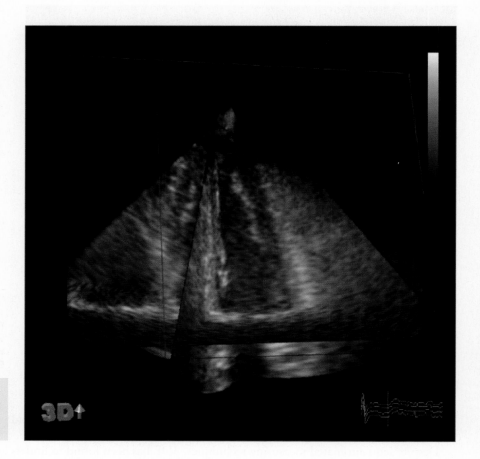

Figure 11-11 Example of a stitching artifact, one of the limitations of acquiring over four cardiac cycles (see Video 11-11). (Courtesy Philips Healthcare, Andover, MA.)

increase the difficulties in discriminating the endocardial border and are potential contributors to inaccuracies in the measurement of left ventricular volumes. In addition, even with the volume dataset, the apex can be difficult to visualize. However, more advanced software that allows the 3D volume datasets to be aligned such that the apex is optimally visualized has become available. The difficulty in endocardial border visualization often can be overcome by the use of contrast imaging, namely left ventricular opacification (LVO). Studies have demonstrated increased accuracy using LVO for both 2DE and 3DE calculation of left ventricular volumes and EF (**Figure 11-12; Videos 11-12 and 11-13**).[25]

More recently, there has been an attempt to validate a standardized protocol for measuring left ventricular volumes and EF. The first multicenter study to validate and provide information of the sources of error between MRI and 3DE found the definition of endocardial borders to be the major source of error with 3DE. In 3DE, the trabeculae are blended in with the myocardium rather than being included in the left ventricular cavity, as is the case with MRI. Another critical difference is that MRI uses short-axis slices, whereas 3DE uses long-axis slices; both use separate software for analysis. This was investigated with the use of a phantom, which found very small differences between the techniques for measured volumes (**Figures 11-13 to 11-17; Videos 11-14 to 11-25**).[21]

LEFT VENTRICULAR MASS

Previous trials have based the calculation of left ventricular mass on 2DE; the smallest change of mass that can be detected with 95% confidence is 59 g, which compares with an average 20 to 40 g/year change in most antihypertensive therapy trials. However, it recently has been shown that 2DE measurements overestimate left ventricular mass because of the large number of images that are off axis.[26] Again, similar to volumes, much of the variability in echocardiographic measurements relates to the problems posed by the use of geometric assumptions for calculations and the influence of different imaging planes from one scan to the next. Despite this, 2DE is frequently still performed in clinical practice for repeated testing. Using either the 3D guided biplane or the volumetric measurements of left ventricular mass, 3DE has been shown to be more feasible and reliable than 2DE (**Figures 11-18 to 11-20; Videos 11-26 and 11-27**).[27-29]

RIGHT VENTRICULAR FUNCTION

Echocardiography is the most widely used technique for imaging the right ventricle (RV), but assessment can be challenging because of the location of the RV behind the sternum and its crescent shape, wrapped around the left ventricle (LV) (**Figure 11-21**).[30] Endocardial tracing and calculation of volumes may be hindered by trabeculations and the presence of the moderator band within the volume. Geometric shapes are too simplistic to be applied as models for right ventricular volume calculation. Right ventricular size and function may be difficult to assess with pulmonary disease but play an important role in clinical decision making for therapy and prognosis. Previous validation studies of the RV using 3DE have used various techniques such as reconstructed 3DE, sparse array 3DE, and now RT3DE.[31-35] All have shown that this technique shows higher reproducibility than 2DE.

CLINICAL USE OF THREE-DIMENSIONAL ECHOCARDIOGRAPHY VOLUME AND EJECTION FRACTION MEASURES

The calculation of left ventricular volume and function continues to be the most commonly requested reason for echocardiography. In addition, the development of new interventions such as stem cell therapy will increase the requirement for more accurate assessment of left ventricular remodeling. The current American

Text continued on page 204

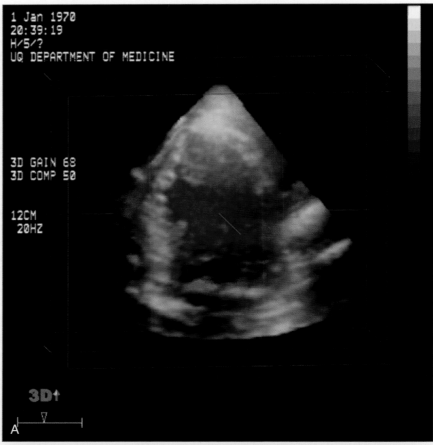

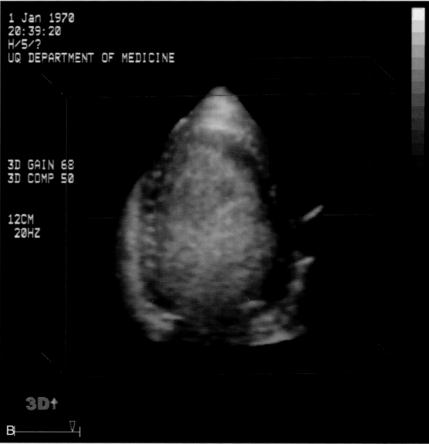

Figure 11-12 A, Example of poor three-dimensional imaging. **B,** The same patient with the use of contrast left ventricular opacification (see Videos 11-12 and 11-13).

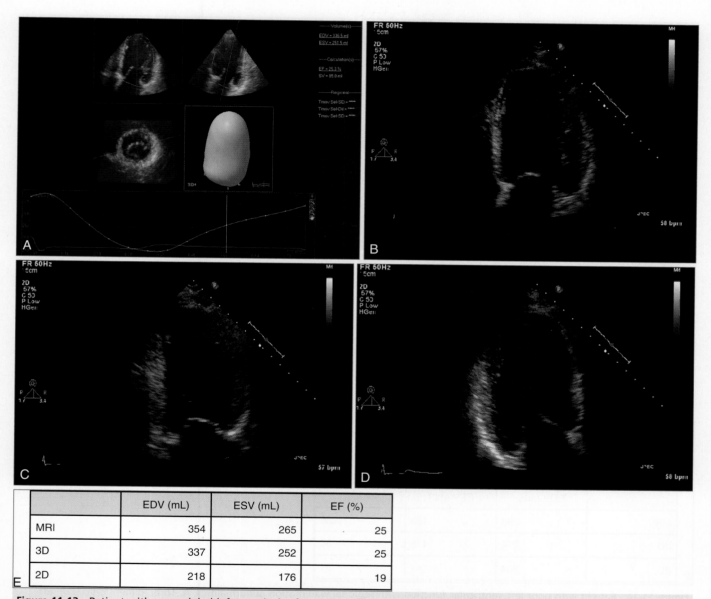

Figure 11-13 Patient with poor global left ventricular function. **A,** Three-dimensional (*3D*) left ventricular volume and ejection fraction (*EF*) measurement. **B,** Two-dimensional (*2D*) apical four-chamber view. **C,** 2D apical two-chamber view. **D,** 2D apical long-axis view. **E,** Table of measures, comparison of magnetic resonance imaging (*MRI*), 3D, and 2D results (see Videos 11-14 to 11-17). *EDV,* end-diastolic volume; *ESV,* end-systolic volume. (**A,** Courtesy Philips Healthcare, Andover, MA.)

	EDV (mL)	ESV (mL)	EF (%)
MRI	354	265	25
3D	337	252	25
2D	218	176	19

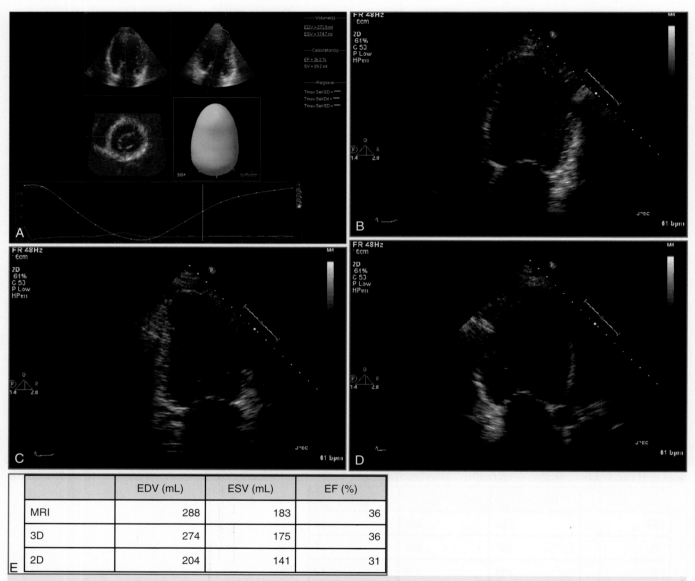

	EDV (mL)	ESV (mL)	EF (%)
MRI	288	183	36
3D	274	175	36
2D	204	141	31

Figure 11-14 Patient with poor left ventricular function with regional wall motion abnormalities. **A,** Three-dimensional (*3D*) left ventricular volume and ejection fraction (*EF*) measurement. **B,** Two-dimensional (*2D*) apical four-chamber view. **C,** 2D apical two-chamber view. **D,** 2D apical long-axis view. **E,** Table of measures, comparison of magnetic resonance imaging (*MRI*), 3D, and 2D results (see Videos 11-18 to 11-20). *EDV,* end-diastolic volume; *ESV,* end-systolic volume. (**A,** Courtesy Philips Healthcare, Andover, MA.)

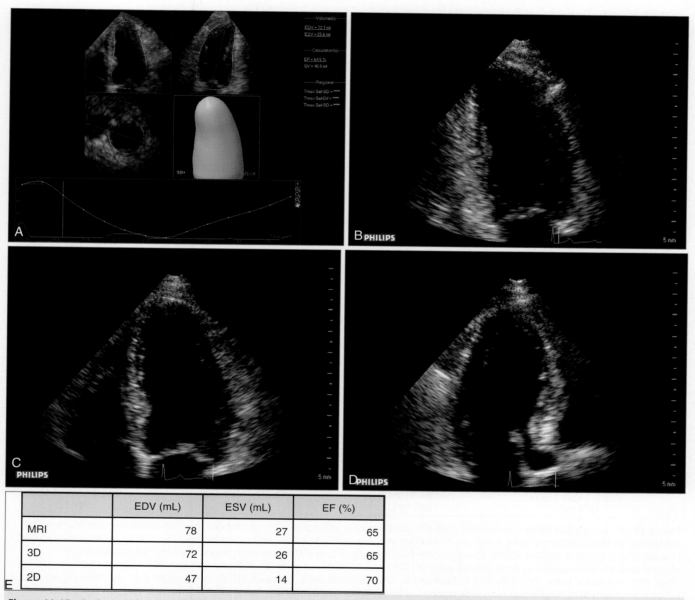

	EDV (mL)	ESV (mL)	EF (%)
MRI	78	27	65
3D	72	26	65
2D	47	14	70

Figure 11-15 Patient with normal left ventricular function. **A,** Three-dimensional (*3D*) left ventricular volume and ejection fraction (*EF*) measurement. **B,** Two-dimensional (*2D*) apical four-chamber view. **C,** 2D apical two-chamber view. **D,** 2D apical long-axis view. **E,** Table of measures, comparison of magnetic resonance imaging (*MRI*), 3D, and 2D results (see Videos 11-22 to 11-25). *EDV,* end-diastolic volume; *ESV,* end-systolic volume. (**A,** Courtesy Philips Healthcare, Andover, MA.)

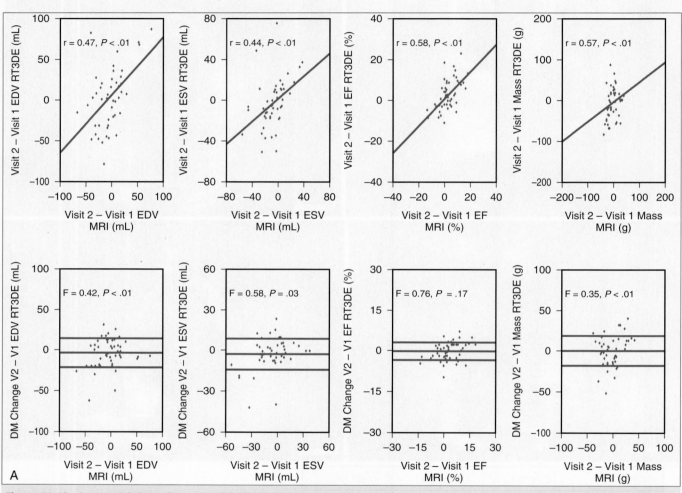

Figure 11-16 Sequential three-dimensional (*3D*) echocardiographic measurements of changes in volume and ejection fraction (*EF*) are similar to those obtained using magnetic resonance imaging (*MRI*), but two-dimensional echocardiography (*2DE*) overestimated change in end-diastolic volume (*EDV*). Changes over follow-up (*top*) and difference from mean (*DM*) change (*bottom*) with **(A)** real-time three-dimensional echocardiography (*RT3DE*) and MRI (*n* = 50) and **(B)** 2DE and MRI (*n* = 50). *ESV*, end-systolic volume; *Mass*, left ventricular mass. (From Jenkins C, Bricknell K, Chan J, Hanekom L, Marwick TH: Comparison of two- and three-dimensional echocardiography with sequential magnetic resonance imaging for evaluating left ventricular volume and ejection fraction over time in patients with healed myocardial infarction. *Am J Cardiol* 99[3]:300–306, 2007.)

Continued

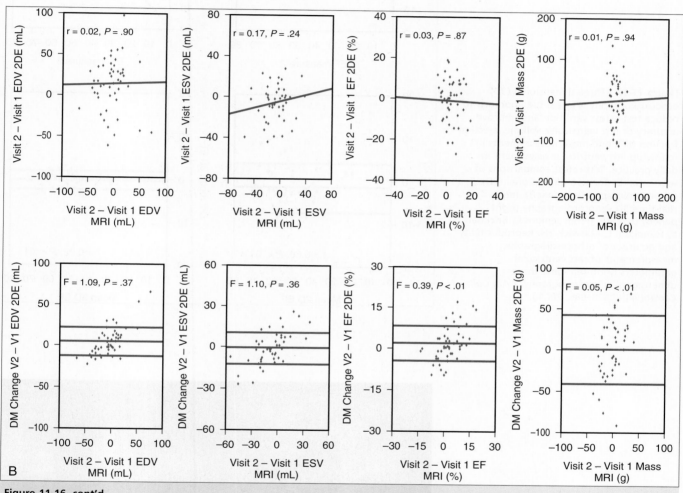

Figure 11-16, cont'd

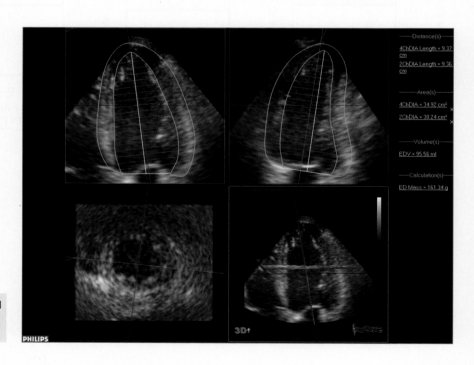

2D EJECTION FRACTION TEST-RETEST

3D EJECTION FRACTION TEST-RETEST

r = 0.66, P < .01

r = 0.92, P < .01

Figure 11-17 Three-dimensional (*3D*) echocardiography is a feasible approach to reduce test-retest variation and improve accuracy of left ventricular volume, ejection fraction (*EF*), and mass measurements in follow-up left ventricular assessment in daily practice. Test-retest comparisons of sequential EF for two-dimensional (*2D*) echocardiography (*left panels*) and real-time 3D echocardiography (*right panels*) (*n* = 50). (From Jenkins C, Bricknell K, Hanekom L, Marwick TH: Reproducibility and accuracy of echocardiographic measurements of left ventricular parameters using real-time three-dimensional echocardiography. *J Am Coll Cardiol* 44[4]:878–886, 2004.)

Figure 11-18 Example of three-dimensional biplane left ventricular mass measurement. (Courtesy Philips Healthcare, Andover, MA.)

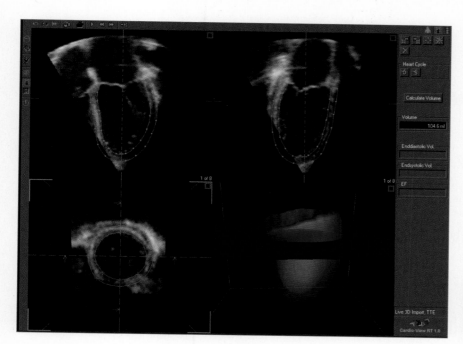

Figure 11-19 Example of three-dimensional left ventricular mass measurement (see Video 11-26). (Courtesy TomTec, Munich, Germany.)

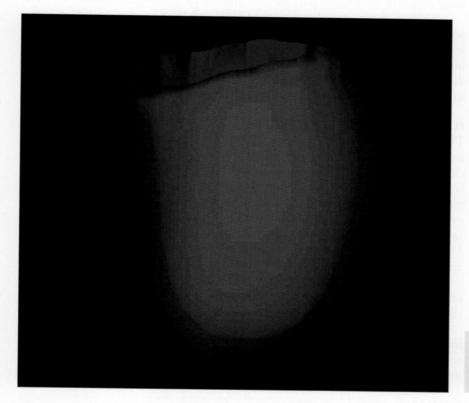

Figure 11-20 Left ventricular mass, a view of the endocardial and endocardial shell (see Video 11-27). (Courtesy TomTec, Munich, Germany.)

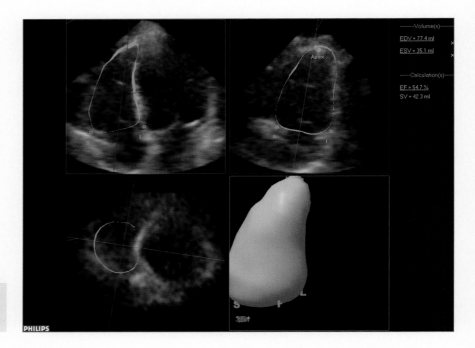

Figure 11-21 Example of right ventricular end-diastolic shape. (Courtesy Philips Healthcare, Andover, MA.)

College of Cardiology Foundation and American Heart Association guidelines for the management of heart failure recommend the use of left ventricular dimensions and 2DE EF for this purpose.[36] A number of studies have shown that 3DE has overcome many of the limitations of 2DE with less test-retest variation, better reproducibility, and better accuracy in left ventricular volume estimations. A recent study by Hare et al[37] has shown differences in the classification of patients into EF thresholds using 3DE compared with 2DE, which may affect treatment decisions, especially with regard to device therapy. Moreover, 3DE appears to be superior to 2DE for evaluating left ventricular size in long-term follow-up.

FUTURE DIRECTIONS OF VOLUME ASSESSMENT

The development of real-time acquisition of volumetric images, as opposed to reconstruction of 2DE images from multiple cycles, has made 3DE a realistic clinically applicable tool for the first time. Previous 3DE transducers have had a larger footprint and decreased image quality from lower line density and frame rates. In the past few years, there have been significant developments in 3DE transducer technology. Full volumetric assessment can now be performed in a single heartbeat, thus eliminating stitching artifact (see Figure 11-11; see Video 11-11), which occurs with multiple-beat acquisition. In addition, the actual size and footprint of RT3DE transducers have dramatically decreased such that some are virtually identical in size to those used for 3D imaging. This has resulted in greater acceptance of the 3DE technology as well as improved workflow by eliminating the need to switch transducers to perform 3D imaging.

In the future, technical improvements will see 3DE transducers with a smaller footprint, allowing wider angle acquisitions with increased spatial and temporal resolutions. More sophisticated online automated endocardial border tracking software will allow faster volume and EF assessment.

SUMMARY

3DE is clearly superior to 2DE for the sequential measurement of both left ventricular and right ventricular volumes and function, with accuracy and reproducibility similar to those obtained by MRI. It is an effective long-term imaging tool when sequential measurement of volumes is sought to guide management decisions. A recent study has shown that reduction of error in the estimation of left ventricular volumes with 3DE allows this method to make a greater incremental contribution to the prediction of adverse outcomes compared with 2DE.[38] The accurate measurement of left ventricular EF is now a critical part of the guidelines for patients to qualify for life-saving device therapies, such as cardiac resynchronization therapy and implantable cardiac defibrillators.[36] It is thus critical, given the real-life implications of these EF cutoffs for decision making, that a reproducible test with limited test-retest variation is utilized to define accurately each patient's eligibility, thus maximizing the likelihood that a patient will be given the same assessment results irrespective of where he or she is evaluated. Although 3DE is emerging as the echocardiographic method of choice for volume assessment, practice guidelines do not yet recognize this evidence (**Figures 11-22** and **11-23**; **Videos 11-28** and **11-29**). The adoption of this technique in the clinical laboratory has been slow and may be limited by inexperience. An

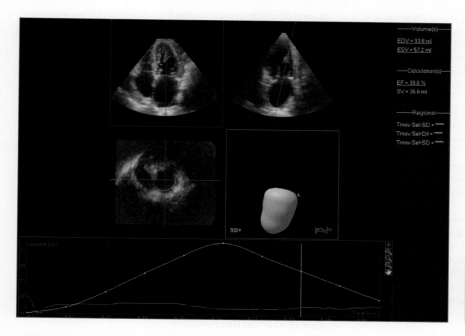

Figure 11-22 Example of left atrial volume measured in the apical view (see Video 11-28). (Courtesy Philips Healthcare, Andover, MA.)

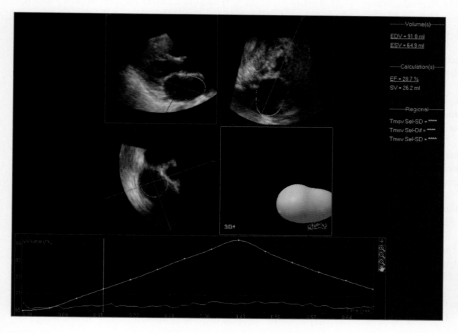

Figure 11-23 Example of left atrial volume measured in the parasternal long-axis view (see Video 11-29). (Courtesy Philips Healthcare, Andover, MA.)

interactive teaching course with rehearsal and direct mentoring appears to overcome this limitation and may improve the acceptance of this technique.[39]

3DE is now the gold standard echocardiographic measurement of choice for the accurate calculation of left ventricular volumes and EF. As more reproducible measurements are sought to guide management decisions, the demand for 3DE will grow accordingly and is likely to soon be incorporated into mainstream cardiac guidelines.

References

1. Dekker DL, Piziali RL, Dong E, Jr.: A system for ultrasonically imaging the human heart in three dimensions. *Comput Biomed Res* 7:544–553, 1974.

2. Zamorano J, Cordeiro P, Sugeng L, et al: Real-time three-dimensional echocardiography for rheumatic mitral valve stenosis evaluation: An accurate and novel approach. *J Am Coll Cardiol* 43:2091–2096, 2004.

3. van den Bosch AE, Ten Harkel DJ, McGhie JS, et al: Characterization of atrial septal defect assessed by real-time 3-dimensional echocardiography. *J Am Soc Echocardiogr* 19:815–821, 2006.

4. Kapetanakis S, Kearney MT, Siva A, et al: Real-time three-dimensional echocardiography: A novel technique to quantify global left ventricular mechanical dyssynchrony. *Circulation* 112:992–1000, 2005.

5. Artang R, Migrino RQ, Harmann L, et al: Left atrial volume measurement with automated border detection by 3-dimensional echocardiography: Comparison with magnetic resonance imaging. *Cardiovasc Ultrasound* 7:16, 2009.

6. Jenkins C, Bricknell K, Marwick TH: Use of real-time three-dimensional echocardiography to measure left atrial volume: Comparison with other echocardiographic techniques. *J Am Soc Echocardiogr* 18:991–997, 2005.

7. Seliem MA, Fedec A, Cohen MS, et al: Real-time 3-dimensional echocardiographic imaging of congenital heart disease using matrix-array technology: Freehand real-time scanning adds instant morphologic details not well delineated by conventional 2-dimensional imaging. *J Am Soc Echocardiogr* 19:121–129, 2006.

8. Mondelli JA, Di Luzio S, Nagaraj A, et al: The validation of volumetric real-time 3-dimensional echocardiography for the determination of left ventricular function. *J Am Soc Echocardiogr* 14:994–1000, 2001.

9. Jenkins C, Bricknell K, Hanekom L, Marwick TH: Reproducibility and accuracy of echocardiographic measurements of left ventricular parameters using real-time three-dimensional echocardiography. *J Am Coll Cardiol* 44:878–886, 2004.

10. Foster E, Cahalan MK: The search for intelligent quantitation in echocardiography: "Eyeball," "trackball" and beyond. *J Am Coll Cardiol* 22:848–850, 1993.

11. King DL, Harrison MR, King DL, Jr., et al: Ultrasound beam orientation during standard two-dimensional imaging: Assessment by three-dimensional echocardiography. *J Am Soc Echocardiogr* 5:569–576, 1992.

12. Otterstad JE, Froeland G, St John SM, Holme I: Accuracy and reproducibility of biplane two-dimensional echocardiographic measurements of left ventricular dimensions and function. *Eur Heart J* 18:507–513, 1997.

13. Otterstad JE: Measuring left ventricular volume and ejection fraction with the biplane Simpson's method. *Heart* 88:559–560, 2002.

14. Nijland F, Kamp O, Verhorst PM, et al: Early prediction of improvement in ejection fraction after acute myocardial infarction using low dose dobutamine echocardiography. *Heart* 88:592–596, 2002.

15. Gottdiener JS, Livengood SV, Meyer PS, Chase GA: Should echocardiography be performed to assess effects of antihypertensive therapy? Test-retest reliability of echocardiography for measurement of left ventricular mass and function. *J Am Coll Cardiol* 25:424–430, 1995.

16. Bottini PB, Carr AA, Prisant LM, et al: Magnetic resonance imaging compared to echocardiography to assess left ventricular mass in the hypertensive patient. *Am J Hypertens* 8:221–228, 1995.

17. Jacobs LD, Salgo IS, Goonewardena S, et al: Rapid online quantification of left ventricular volume from real-time three-dimensional echocardiographic data. *Eur Heart J* 27:460–468, 2006.

18. Gopal AS, Shen Z, Sapin PM, et al: Assessment of cardiac function by three-dimensional echocardiography compared with conventional noninvasive methods. *Circulation* 92:842–853, 1995.

19. Sugeng L, Mor-Avi V, Weinert L, et al: Quantitative assessment of left ventricular size and function: Side-by-side comparison of real-time three-dimensional echocardiography and computed tomography with magnetic resonance reference. *Circulation* 114:654–661, 2006.

20. Jaochim NH, Sugeng L, Corsi C, et al: Volumetric analysis of regional left ventricular function with real-time three-dimensional echocardiography: Validation by magnetic resonance and clinical utility testing. *Heart* 93:572–578, 2007.

21. Mor-Avi V, Jenkins C, Kuhl HP, et al: Real-time 3-dimensional echocardiographic quantification of left ventricular volumes: Multicenter study for validation with magnetic resonance imaging and investigation of sources of error. *JACC Cardiovasc Imag* 1:413–423, 2008.

22. von Ramm OT, Smith SW: Real time volumetric ultrasound imaging system. *J Digit Imag* 3:261–266, 1990.

23. Houck RC, Cooke JE, Gill EA: Live 3D echocardiography: A replacement for traditional 2D echocardiography? *AJR Am J Roentgenol* 187:1092–1106, 2006.

24. Jenkins C, Chan J, Hanekom L, Marwick TH: Accuracy and feasibility of online 3-dimensional echocardiography for measurement of left ventricular parameters. *J Am Soc Echocardiogr* 19:1119–1128, 2006.

25. Jenkins C, Moir S, Chan J, et al: Left ventricular volume measurement with echocardiography: A comparison of left ventricular opacification, three-dimensional echocardiography, or both with magnetic resonance imaging. *Eur Heart J* 30:98–106, 2009.

26. Abramov D, Helmke S, Rumbarger L, et al: Overestimation of left ventricular mass and misclassification of ventricular geometry in heart failure patients by two-dimensional echocardiography in comparison with three-dimensional echocardiography. *Echocardiography* 27:223–229, 2010.

27. Mor-Avi V, Sugeng L, Weinert L, et al: Fast measurement of left ventricular mass with real-time three-dimensional echocardiography: Comparison with magnetic resonance imaging. *Circulation* 110:1814–1818, 2004.

28. Kuhl HP, Hanrath P, Franke A: M-mode echocardiography overestimates left ventricular mass in patients with normal left ventricular shape: A comparative study using three-dimensional echocardiography. *Eur J Echocardiogr* 4:312–319, 2003.

29. Rodevand O, Bjornerheim R, Kolbjornsen O, et al: Left ventricular mass assessed by three-dimensional echocardiography using rotational acquisition. *Clin Cardiol* 20:957–962, 1997.

30. Ho SY, Nihoyannopoulos P: Anatomy, echocardiography, and normal right ventricular dimensions. *Heart* 92(Suppl 1):i2–i13, 2006.

31. Pini R, Giannazzo G, Di Bari M, et al: Transthoracic three-dimensional echocardiographic reconstruction of left and right ventricles: In vitro validation and comparison with magnetic resonance imaging. *Am Heart J* 133:221–229, 1997.

32. Heusch A, Koch JA, Krogmann ON, et al: Volumetric analysis of the right and left ventricle in a porcine heart model: Comparison of three-dimensional echocardiography, magnetic resonance imaging and angiocardiography. *Eur J Ultrasound* 9:245–255, 1999.

33. Shiota T, Jones M, Chikada M, et al: Real-time three-dimensional echocardiography for determining right ventricular stroke volume in an animal model of chronic right ventricular volume overload. *Circulation* 97:1897–1900, 1998.

34. Schindera ST, Mehwald PS, Sahn DJ, Kececioglu D: Accuracy of real-time three-dimensional echocardiography for quantifying right ventricular volume: Static and pulsatile flow studies in an anatomic in vitro model. *J Ultrasound Med* 21:1069–1075, 2002.

35. Jenkins C, Chan J, Bricknell K, et al: Reproducibility of right ventricular volumes and ejection fraction using real-time three-dimensional echocardiography: Comparison with cardiac MRI. *Chest* 131:1844–1851, 2007.

36. Cheitlin MD, Armstrong WF, Aurigemma GP, et al: ACC/AHA/ASE 2003 guideline update for the clinical application of echocardiography: Summary article. A report of the American College of Cardiology/American Heart Association Task Force on Practice Guidelines (ACC/AHA/ASE Committee to Update the 1997 Guidelines for the Clinical Application of Echocardiography). *J Am Soc Echocardiogr* 16:1091–1110, 2003.

37. Hare JL, Jenkins C, Nakatani S, et al: Feasibility and clinical decision-making with 3D echocardiography in routine practice. *Heart* 94:440–445, 2008.

38. Jenkins C, Stanton T, Marwick TH: What is the best predictor of outcome: Ejection fraction or global strain? *Eur Heart J* 31:1062, 2010.

39. Jenkins C, Monaghan M, Shirali G, et al: An intensive interactive course for 3D echocardiography: Is "crop till you drop" an effective learning strategy? *Eur J Echocardiogr* 9:373–380, 2008.

CHAPTER 12

Assessment of Left Ventricular Mechanical Dyssynchrony

Cliona Kenny and Mark J. Monaghan

Real-time three-dimensional echocardiography (RT3DE) has proven to be the most reliable and reproducible echocardiographic measure of left ventricular volumes, ejection fraction (EF), and mass.[1,2] The advent of the matrix array transducer and improvements in parallel processing technologies have improved the temporal and spatial resolution of the volumes acquired, and full left ventricle (LV) datasets can now be obtained in a single heartbeat on some commercial systems.[3]

Mechanical dyssynchrony, an uncoordinated pattern of left ventricular contraction, has been described in a variety of patient cohorts, including those with left ventricular systolic dysfunction and right ventricular pacing. A reliable and reproducible measure of left ventricular mechanical dyssynchrony has proved elusive, as evidenced by the Predictors of Response to CRT (PROSPECT) study, which demonstrated poor agreement between multiple two-dimensional (2D), M-mode echocardiographic, and tissue Doppler measures of dyssynchrony in patients undergoing cardiac resynchronization therapy (CRT).[4] The inability to image the entire LV simultaneously also was noted as a drawback to these measures.

Kapetanakis and colleagues[5] proposed RT3DE quantification of regional myocardial function as an accurate measure of left ventricular mechanical dyssynchrony, which might overcome the shortcomings of traditional measures of dyssynchrony. This method is based on the construction of a cast of the LV using semiautomated endocardial border recognition throughout the cardiac cycle. The cast is then segmented into 16 or 17 segments around a central axis, corresponding to American Society of Echocardiology guidelines (**Figure 12-1**; **Video 12-1**). Segmental volume or time curves are constructed, and a dyssynchrony index (SDI-16 or SDI-17) is calculated on the basis of the standard deviation of the time to minimal segmental volume as a percentage of the R-R interval (**Figure 12-2**; **Video 12-2**). Indexing to the R-R interval allows comparison of the systolic dyssynchrony index (SDI) between subjects with differing heart rates. This method has been validated against cardiac magnetic resonance imaging (MRI) and single-photon emission computed tomography for the assessment of left ventricular dyssynchrony and has been shown to correlate well with other echocardiographic measures of dyssynchrony, such as tissue Doppler.[6-8]

TIME AND VOLUME CURVES

The software for LV analysis produces plots of the absolute segmental volume against time as well as normalized volume curves. When the absolute volumes are normalized such that the greatest volume represents 100%, the difference between 100% and the average of the minimum segmental volumes represents the EF. Segmental volume curves may be viewed individually, but the pattern of segmental contraction is useful and forms the basis of the SDI. The minimum volume point is identified on each curve. In a normal ventricle, the

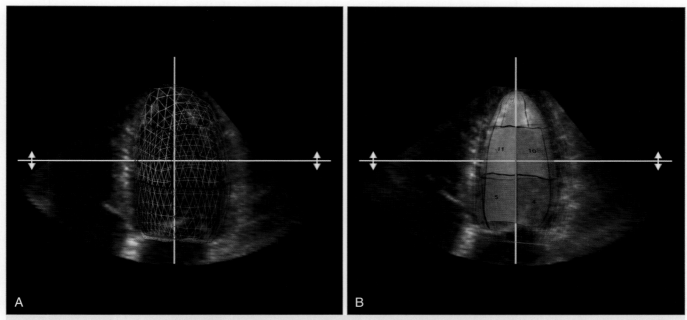

Figure 12-1 Endocardial border detection throughout the cardiac cycle produces a "cast" of the left ventricle, which is segmented according to the American Society of Echocardiography guidelines into either 16 or 17 segments (see Video 12-1).

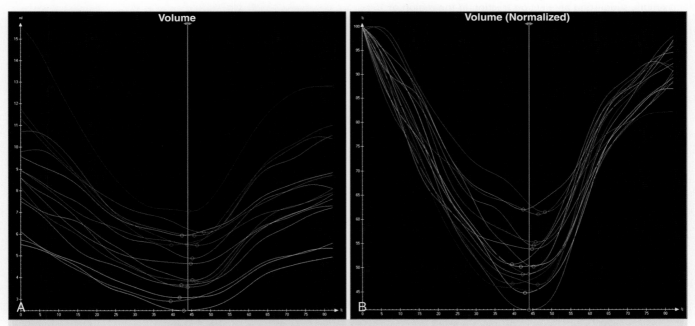

Figure 12-2 Example of time-volume (**A**) and normalized volume (**B**) curves in a patient with normal left ventricle function. The volume curves are U-shaped, and the minimum volume is within a narrow range, suggesting synchronous contraction and a low systolic dyssynchrony index. In this case, the average minimum volume is approximately 50%, suggesting an ejection fraction of roughly 50% (see Video 12-2).

spread of the minimum volume points is narrow, leading to a low standard deviation from the mean time (see Figure 12-2). The volume curves may be used to identify regional wall motion abnormalities due to differences in amplitude between segments (**Figure 12-3**). A septal flash also is readily identified using the volume curves (**Figure 12-4**).

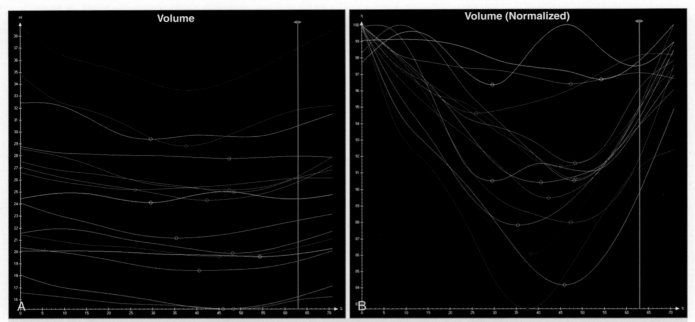

Figure 12-3 Time-volume curves in a patient with impaired left ventricular systolic function. **A,** The time-volume curves are relatively flat, with little change in absolute volume throughout the cardiac cycle, indicating severe left ventricular systolic dysfunction. **B,** The amplitude of the normalized volume curves is greater, making the minimum volume point easier to identify. The dispersion of the minimum volume points is greater compared with the patient with normal left ventricular systolic function. This indicates a high systolic dyssynchrony index and therefore significant dyssynchrony. The mean minimum volume is approximately 85% of the maximum, suggesting an ejection fraction in the region of 15%.

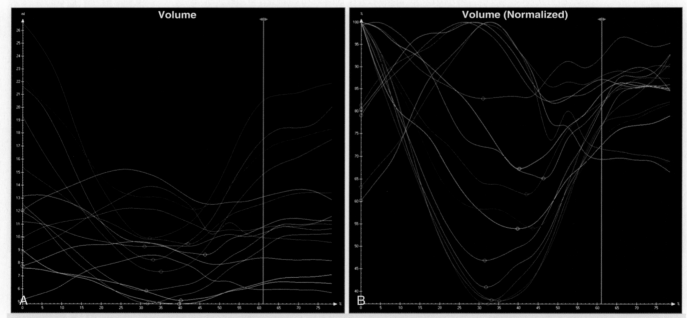

Figure 12-4 **A,** In this patient with ischemic left ventricular systolic dysfunction, the time-volume curves are relatively flat, although the U shape of some curves is preserved, suggesting regional wall motion abnormalities. **B,** When the normalized volume curves are inspected, the minimum volume of the septal and anteroseptal curves (*green and light blue curves*) occur at the beginning of systole. This is consistent with a septal flash.

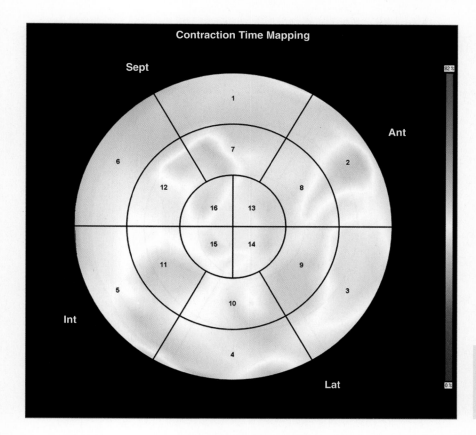

Figure 12-5   Normal static map showing homogeneous transition with a large area through white to blue (see Video 12-3). *Ant,* anterior; *Int,* interior; *Lat,* lateral; *Sept,* septal.

CONTRACTION FRONT MAPPING

Contraction front mapping analyzes temporal and spatial activation of left ventricular contraction, representing the myocardial segments that reach peak contraction every 25 ms on a color-coded polar map of the LV. As the contraction front spreads through the ventricle, the color changes from red to blue, allowing areas of late contraction to be easily identified. The normal left ventricular activation pattern is homogeneous and rapid (**Figure 12-5**; **Video 12-3**). The activation pattern in patients with left ventricular systolic dysfunction is variable, but generally a U-shaped activation pattern is noted (**Figures 12-6** and **12-7**; **Videos 12-4** and **12-5**). In our experience, the region of maximal delay most commonly appears to be the septum, leading to a predominant left-to-right color transition. No definite pattern has been established in cases of left bundle branch block, although a septal flash may be identified in some cases (**Figure 12-8**; **Video 12-6**). This tool also has been used to identify regional wall motion abnormalities at rest and during stress echocardiography.

Reproducibility of Systolic Dyssynchrony Index

Excellent reproducibility was noted in the original description of SDI.[5] The authors described test-retest variability ranging from 1% for end-diastolic volume (EDV) to 4.6% for SDI. Intraobserver variability ranged from 0.6% for EDV to 8.1% for SDI, and interobserver variability ranged from 3.5% for EDV to 6.4% for SDI. The investigators further tested the reproducibility of the technique in a two-center study involving institutions in the United Kingdom and Hong Kong.[9] To ensure that methods were comparable, a cross-site training program was devised with 20 "training" datasets. The authors reported excellent agreement at the end of the training period. Subsequently, datasets of 62 patients with reduced left ventricular systolic function who were planned for cardiac resynchronization therapy were shared between the two sites and independently analyzed.

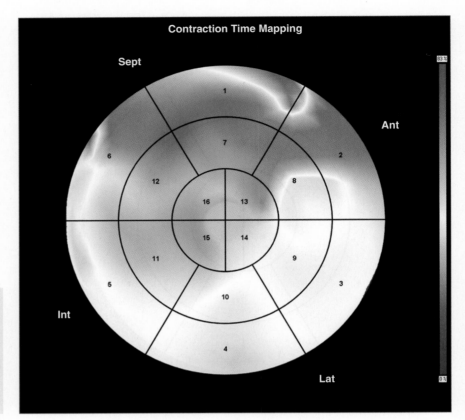

Figure 12-6 Typical static map in a dyssynchronous patient showing U-shaped earliest color transition predominantly in the basal lateral and inferolateral segments, suggesting a predominant left-to-right activation. The activation also is slower than normal; a large part of the map remains red (see Video 12-4). *Ant,* anterior; *Int,* interior; *Lat,* lateral; *Sept,* septal.

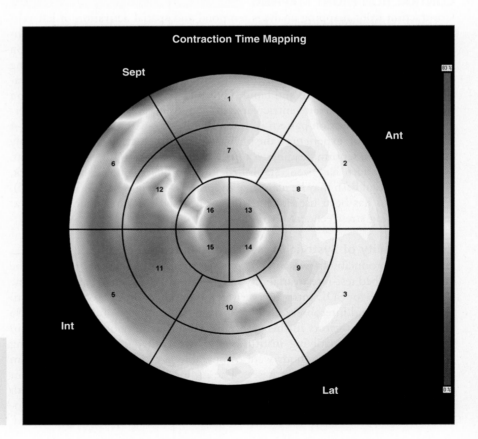

Figure 12-7 Atypical static map showing U-shaped right-to-left activation, with first color transition predominantly in the basal anteroseptal and anterior segments (see Video 12-5). *Ant,* anterior; *Int,* interior; *Lat,* lateral; *Sept,* septal.

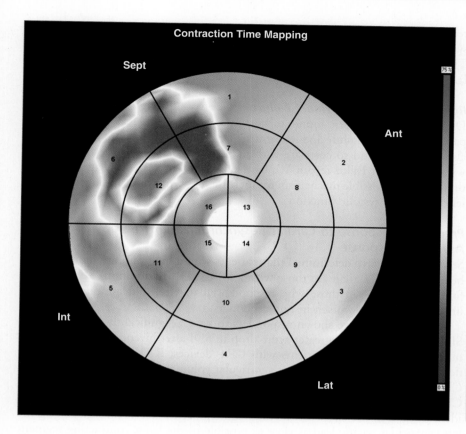

Figure 12-8   A clear septal flash is seen (*dark blue*). This is again associated with a typical predominant left-to-right transition; the next activation is seen in the basal lateral and inferolateral segments (*white*) (see Video 12-6). *Ant,* anterior; *Int,* interior; *Lat,* lateral; *Sept,* septal.

Intraclass correlation (ICC) coefficients in this study were excellent at greater than 0.8 for all parameters studied (EDV, end-systolic value [ESV], EF, and SDI). Interhospital variability was 2.9% for EDV, 1% for ESV, 7.1% for EF, and 7.6% for SDI.

Soliman and colleagues[10] elucidated reproducibility further by categorizing dataset quality in 50 randomly selected patients included in their study and noted the reproducibility of SDI to be better in patients with good-quality datasets (interobserver variability of 9% and ICC of 0.99 in patients with good-quality datasets compared with interobserver variability of 16% and ICC of 0.95 in patients with moderate-quality datasets). Overall excellent reproducibility was noted in this study (interobserver variability of 12%, intraobserver variability of 10% for SDI, and both interclass correlation coefficients >0.95).

Normal Values for Systolic Dyssynchrony Index

A number of studies have sought to establish normal values for SDI. On the basis of current evidence, the normal value of the SDI-16 appears to be approximately 3% to 4%, with a maximal value below 6% in normal individuals.[5,10-14] There appears to be a normal apex-to-base contraction gradient, which creates a peristaltic-type contraction pattern in the normal heart.[12-13] There does not appear to be a significant difference between genders, and SDI does not appear to change significantly with increasing age. A strong negative correlation between SDI-16 and EF has been shown in several studies, and SDI has been demonstrated to be independent of QRS duration.[5,7,12]

Clinical Significance of Systolic Dyssynchrony Index
Right Ventricular Pacing

Right ventricular pacing has been shown to increase the SDI and to disrupt the normal apex-to-base contraction gradient of the heart.[15] This is particularly true in patients with right ventricular apical pacing and is associated with a reduction in left ventricular ejection fraction. Baseline reduced left ventricular systolic function and high pacing burden appear to worsen this phenomenon.[16] This phenomenon suggests a potential mechanism for the worsened left ventricular systolic function observed in patients undergoing right ventricular pacing.

Role in Patients with Heart Failure

Dyssynchrony has been found to correlate with reduced exercise capacity in patients with heart failure and left ventricular systolic dysfunction. Dyssynchrony also has been found to correlate with markers of collagen synthesis in patients with tetralogy of Fallot repair. We have postulated increased collagen synthesis or fibrosis as a possible mechanism for increased dyssynchrony, leading to reduced left ventricular systolic function.

Predicting Response to Cardiac Resynchronization Therapy and Assessing Response

Several studies have determined that patients with a high SDI are more likely to benefit from CRT than are those with a lower SDI. In addition, SDI has been found to decrease in those who respond well to CRT but appears to remain unchanged or even worsen in nonresponders.

Several studies have shown responders to have a significantly higher baseline SDI and a significantly greater acute drop in SDI after biventricular (BiV) pacemaker implantation. In patients with CRT devices, RT3DE has been used to demonstrate acute changes in left ventricular volumes, EF, and SDI between the CRT-on and CRT-off modes. SDI-16 has been shown to predict response to CRT in single-center studies.[17-20] The regional volume curves generated allow identification of the latest contracting segment. There is evidence that siting the left ventricular pacing lead as close as possible to the latest contracting segment provides incremental benefit.[21] There is emerging evidence that persistently elevated SDI after CRT can identify a subpopulation of patients who will benefit from device optimization.

Technique for Left Ventricle Analysis

LV analysis may be performed with a number of software packages, all following similar principles, although the results are not directly comparable due to differences in methodology and software algorithms. Described are the steps of LV analysis using 4D LV Analysis software (TomTec, Munich, Germany).

1. The end-systolic and end-diastolic frames are identified, and the axis of the LV is identified using the apex and mitral valve annulus as landmarks (**Figure 12-9**; **Video 12-7**).
2. The endocardial border is identified at end systole and end diastole in three cut frames corresponding to the traditional 2D apical views (four-chamber, two-chamber, and long-axis views). This is performed in the same manner as Simpson's biplane view, excluding the endocardial trabeculae and papillary muscles. There is usually a tradeoff between the accuracy of estimated volumes compared with MRI and accuracy of tracking. Placing the border more subendocardially to mid-myocardially improves the correlation between 3D echocardiography and MRI volumes. However, this may be at the cost of accurate tracking, leading to a less accurate SDI. Our practice is initially to place the borders further out. However, if tracking proves inaccurate, we move the border closer to the blood-tissue interface (**Figure 12-10**; **Videos 12-8** to **12-10**).
3. These data are then used to generate a model of the LV throughout the cardiac cycle using endocardial border detection software (see Figure 12-1). The model is inspected to ensure accurate identification of the endocardial border and reliable tracking throughout the cardiac cycle. This is done in the short-axis and again in the long-axis views. This step is particularly important because

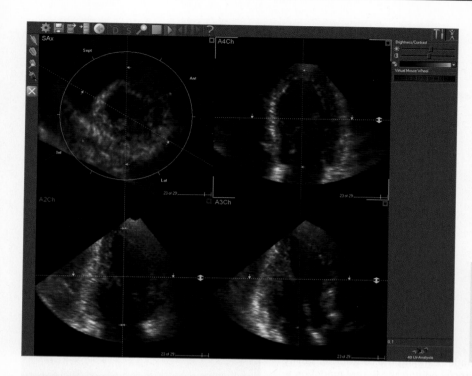

Figure 12-9 Aligning the central axis of the left ventricle. The dataset is manipulated so the axis runs from the apex to the center of the mitral valve annulus in all three cut planes. End-systolic and end-diastolic frames are identified (see Video 12-7).

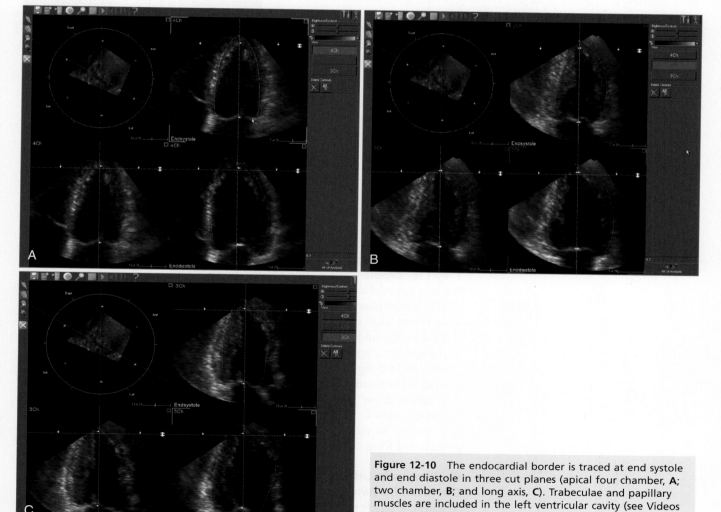

Figure 12-10 The endocardial border is traced at end systole and end diastole in three cut planes (apical four chamber, **A**; two chamber, **B**; and long axis, **C**). Trabeculae and papillary muscles are included in the left ventricular cavity (see Videos 12-8 to 12-10).

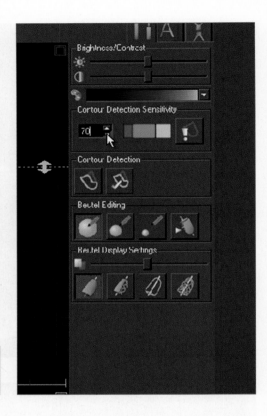

Figure 12-11 Methods to adjust tracking include changing the contour sensitivity level, adjusting the contour detection, and directly editing the Beutel model on a frame-by-frame basis.

accurate border tracking is essential for identification of the exact timing of the end-systolic subvolumes (**Video 12-11**).

4. If necessary, tracking may be adjusted in a number of ways (**Figure 12-11**). Initially, the contour detection sensitivity may be adjusted. This step makes the model more "stiff" because it increases dependence on the user-defined planes (**Video 12-12**). If tracking remains suboptimal, we return to the endocardial border identification stage and adjust the initial cut plane borders in regions where tracking is poor. It sometimes is necessary to define the border closer to the blood-tissue interface, although this does decrease the accuracy of the volume measurements (**Video 12-13**). Alternatively, the tracking may be adjusted on the Beutel model on a frame-by-frame basis. This method can increase the jerkiness of the Beutel model that is generated, again making the minimum volume more difficult to identify. This difficulty can be overcome by the "smoothing" function (**Video 12-14**).

5. Once a model that tracks satisfactorily has been achieved, ESV, EDV, EF, and SDI are calculated. At this point, we inspect the individual time-volume curves to ensure that the minimum volume has been accurately identified (**Video 12-15**). We find this easiest using the normalized time-volume curves because the greater amplitude of the curves makes the minimum volume clearer to identify (see Figures 12-2 to 12-4). If the minimum volume has been attributed to the wrong time, this is adjusted, changing the overall SDI. This process is repeated for both the 16-segment and 17-segment models. If there are outlier curves, the tracking in these segments should again be carefully inspected to ensure its accuracy. Segments that do not track well may be excluded from the final result.

Challenges in Left Ventricle Analysis
Operator Training and Experience

Assessment of left ventricular function is known for the difficulties in achieving consistent results. Formal teaching interventions have been shown to improve interobserver variability in the 2D assessment of EF, thereby ensuring good-quality results.[22] Our experience supports this conclusion in the case of 3D analysis of the LV. We have found that consistent methods among operators plays an extremely important role in achieving reproducible results because even small differences in methodology may lead to a systematic bias in results, consistent with published evidence.[23] At our institution, all operators are required to undergo a formal training program using a set of 3D datasets representing a spectrum of pathologies and dataset quality. Good agreement with the results of an expert operator is required prior to beginning clinical analysis. This method has proven to be effective for us, as evidenced by the excellent interobserver and interhospital agreement in the previously mentioned study by Kapetanakis et al.[9]

Dataset Quality

As seen in the study by Soliman and colleagues,[10] dataset quality has a large bearing on the accuracy and reproducibility of LV analysis.[10] Mor-Avi and colleagues[23] also noted poor spatial resolution as a factor accounting for discrepancies between operators. A recent study in a "real world" population by Miller and associates[24] has confirmed that image quality has a significant impact on observer variability. Our experience is significantly in keeping with this finding. Up to 15% of datasets may be rejected because of poor quality, with the proportion of unusable scans higher among patients with heart disease.[14]

The acquisition of the raw 3D dataset should be optimized for maximal volume rate and spatial resolution. This is achieved by adjusting depth and sector settings to include only the LV, the mitral valve annulus, and the aortic valve (required for spatial orientation). Acquisition is performed during sustained breath-hold to minimize translation artifacts. Optimal datasets are achieved at heart rates less than 80 beats/min. In patients with an irregular rhythm, such as atrial fibrillation or frequent ventricular ectopy, we attempt to time acquisition to obtain volumes with a regular R-R interval. Datasets that include an ectopic beat seen on the accompanying electrocardiogram can almost universally be excluded because of the presence of stitching artifact. This process frequently requires many attempts to obtain a good-quality dataset.

In all cases, we obtain multiple datasets and inspect them for dataset quality and stitching artifact at the point of acquisition. Datasets with stitching artifact are rejected. Datasets with two or more missing segments are interpreted with caution, and a comment is made regarding dataset quality when reporting the results.

Left Ventricle Analysis in Patients with Reduced Systolic Function

LV analysis is more challenging in patients with reduced LV function. This is caused by a number of factors. First, reduced LV function is associated with LV dilation resulting in larger left ventricular volumes, which are technically more challenging to acquire (**Figure 12-12; Video 12-16**). The apical echocardiographic window frequently is displaced, and the apex and anterior wall become more difficult to image. Larger volumes result in lower volume rates, a problem that can be partly overcome by four- or seven-beat acquisitions. Alternatively, the high volume rate–low scan line density acquisition option may be used, although it results in reduced spatial resolution.

Second, the increasing sphericity index as the LV dilates makes the true apex more difficult to identify and hence the central axis of the LV difficult to align (**Figure 12-13; Video 12-17**). Because the LV model is subsegmented around this axis, variation in the axis leads to alteration in subsegmental volumes and time to minimum volume.

Third, the reduction in LV function is associated with prolonged isovolumic times, which make the true end-systolic and end-diastolic frames more difficult to identify. Small absolute changes in ventricular volumes over the cardiac cycle contribute to this. As ventricular systolic function worsens and the

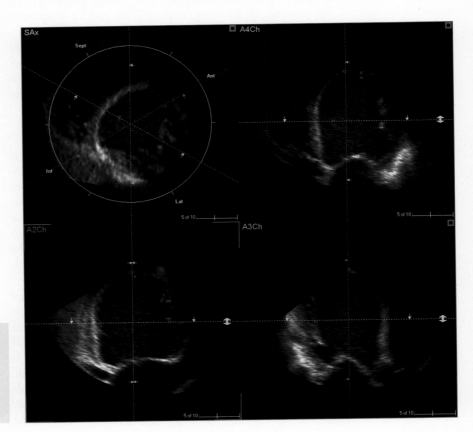

Figure 12-12 An example of poor image quality. Dilation of the left ventricle (LV) displaces the LV apex and makes the anterior wall more difficult to image. As the volume increases, it becomes difficult to include the entire LV in the dataset, although this can be partially overcome by increasing the number of cardiac cycles included in the acquisition. Another approach is to use the high volume rate–low scan line density option for acquisition, but spatial resolution will suffer, leading to reduced tracking accuracy (see Video 12-16).

Figure 12-13 Spherical left ventricle (LV). The central axis of the LV becomes difficult to align as the LV dilates and becomes spherical, making the true apex more difficult to identify. This may lead to inaccuracy in the minimum volumes (see Video 12-17).

difference between end-systolic and end-diastolic volumes decreases, small discrepancies in volume measurements result in a larger percentage error in EF (**Video 12-18**).

Fourth, the small changes in left ventricular volumes over the cardiac cycle mean that the amplitude of endocardial motion is small and therefore difficult to track. This may lead to a low signal/noise ratio, which can make the minimum volume difficult to identify. To circumvent this problem, we inspect the normalized regional volume curve rather than the lower amplitude absolute regional volume curve. We inspect each curve individually to ensure maximum curve amplitude (**Video 12-19**).

Finally, segments that do not track well may be reflected as noisy regional volume curves, making the minimum segmental volume impossible to identify. This problem may be partially overcome by ensuring optimal endocardial border tracking, by manual correction if necessary, and careful inspection of regional volume curves to ensure correct identification of the volume nadir. An outlier timing in this context may falsely increase SDI; consideration should therefore be given to excluding segments such as these.

Endocardial Border Detection

In some cases, endocardial border detection may prove difficult, particularly in patients with prominent papillary muscles or endocardial dropout over the cardiac cycle.

Future Directions

Development of new software such as speckle tracking potentially allows for more accurate endocardial border tracking. 3D speckle tracking software is now available from a number of vendors and allows assessment of left ventricular global and segmental volumes as well as novel quantification of measures of myocardial deformation. This uses several of the benefits of 3D LV analysis, overcoming 2D limitations such as foreshortening and geometric assumptions of the LV, and offers the added benefit of tracking of speckles moving in all three dimensions (**Figure 12-14**; **Videos 12-20** and **12-21**). Initial experience with this software

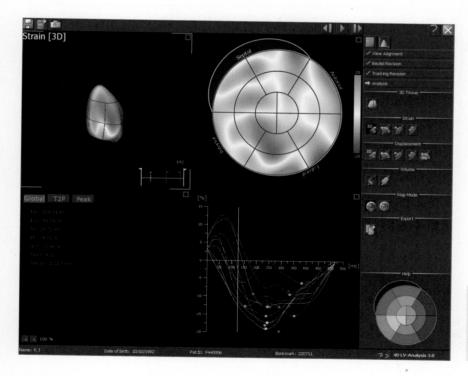

Figure 12-14   Three-dimensional strain in a patient with impaired left ventricular systolic function. The ejection fraction is 24% and global longitudinal strain is −3.5% (see Videos 12-20 and 12-21).

suggests a quicker and simpler workflow. This approach shows promise, with good reproducibility noted in one study using software from a single vendor.[25] However, it requires further validation prior to widespread use.

CASE 1: NORMAL LEFT VENTRICULAR SYNCHRONY WITH THREE-DIMENSIONAL ECHOCARDIOGRAPHY AND BROAD QRS

A 65-year-old man with longstanding dilated cardiomyopathy, attributed to a past history of viral myocarditis, presented to the CRT assessment clinic for consideration of upgrade of single-chamber defibrillator after a deterioration in heart failure symptoms. At the time of assessment, resting ECG showed sinus rhythm with left bundle branch block and QRS duration of 141 ms (**Figure 12-15**). However, 3DE did not suggest significant dyssynchrony, with an SDI-16 measured at 5.6% (**Figure 12-16; Video 12-22**). He was offered a CRT upgrade on the basis of deteriorating symptoms to New York Heart Association (NHYA) functional class III, broad QRS, and EF measured at 13%. However, the lack of 3D dyssynchrony suggested possible lack of benefit of CRT.

One month after implantation, the patient presented again with worsening heart failure symptoms. On interrogation of his device, he was found to be 93% BiV paced. LV analysis was repeated, and SDI-16 was found to be 6.3% during BiV pacing (**Figure 12-17; Video 12-23**) compared with 5.2% during intrinsic rhythm (**Figure 12-18; Video 12-24**). The pacing function of the device was switched off. The patient was referred for ventricular assist device and was placed on the waiting list for cardiac transplantation.

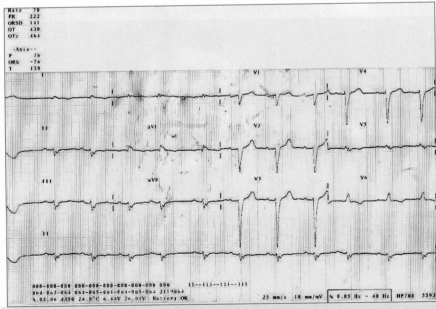

Figure 12-15   Electrocardiogram of the patient in Case 1, showing left bundle branch block with a QRS duration of 141 MS.

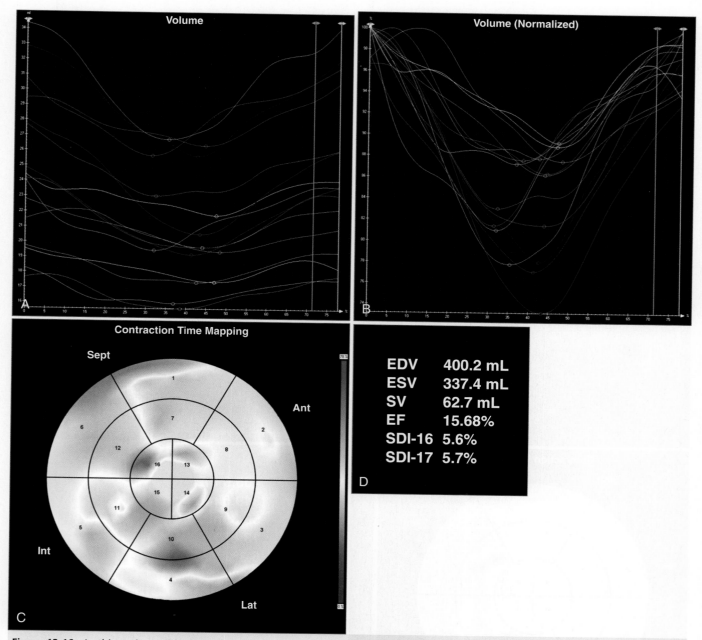

Figure 12-16   In this patient with a history of viral myocarditis, the volume curves (**A**) are of low amplitude. The normalized volume curves (**B**) show that the timing of the minimum volume is not widely dispersed, suggesting that the ventricle is not very dyssynchronous despite the electrocardiogram, which shows left bundle branch block. The static polar map (**C**) shows predominant right-to-left activation. These findings are reflected in the results (**D**), which show an intermediate systolic dyssynchrony index (*SDI*) of 5.6%, suggesting that this patient is unlikely to benefit from cardiac resynchronization therapy (see Video 12-22). *Ant,* anterior; *EDV,* end-diastolic volume; *EF,* ejection fraction; *ESV,* end-systolic volume; *Int,* interior; *Lat,* lateral; *Sept,* septal; *SV,* systolic volume.

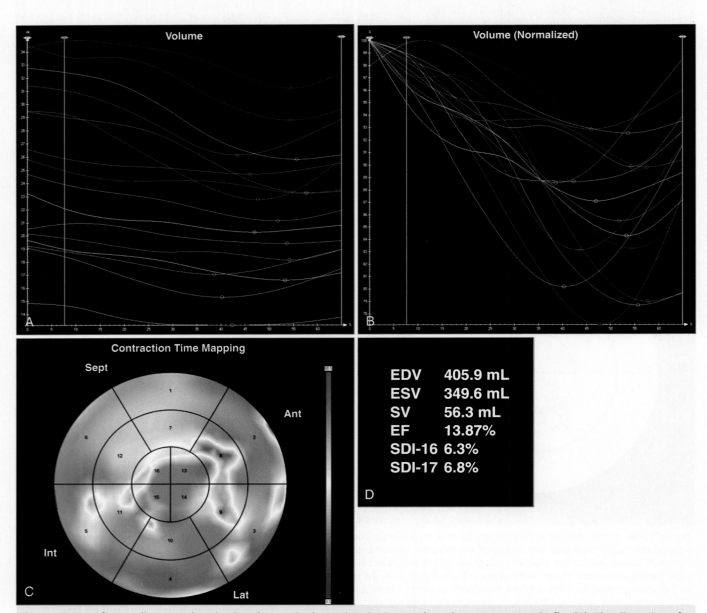

Figure 12-17   After cardiac resynchronization therapy in the patient in Case 1, the volume curves remain flat (**A**). The dispersion of the time of the minimum volume appears to have increased slightly (**B**); this is reflected in the slight increase in systolic dyssynchrony index (*SDI*) to 6.4% (**D**). The activation pattern is more homogeneous but is slower (**C**) (see Video 12-23). *Ant,* anterior; *EDV,* end-diastolic volume; *EF,* ejection fraction; *ESV,* end-systolic volume; *Int,* interior; *Lat,* lateral; *Sept,* septal; *SV,* systolic volume.

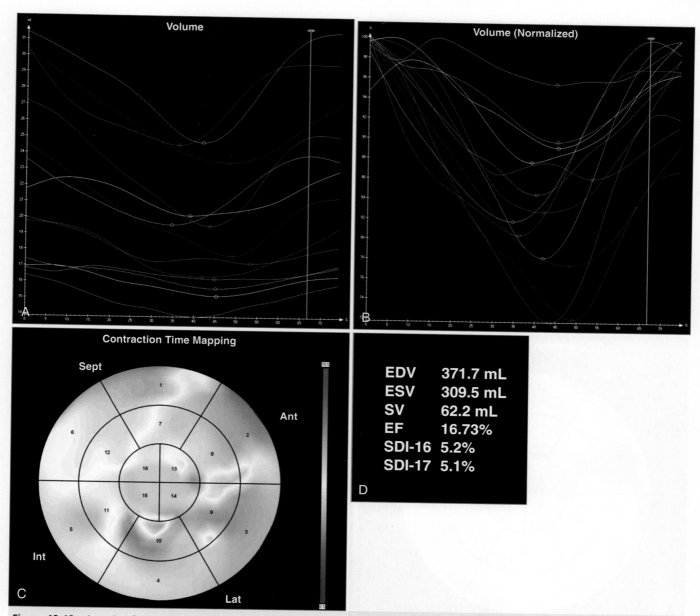

Figure 12-18 **A** to **C**, After cardiac resynchronization therapy with biventricular pacing switched off in the patient in Case 1, there is no significant change compared with biventricular pacing on. The activation pattern is once again predominantly right-to-left and occurs more rapidly. The systolic dyssynchrony index (*SDI*) is shown in **D** (see Video 12-24). *Ant,* anterior; *EDV,* end-diastolic volume; *EF,* ejection fraction; *ESV,* end-systolic volume; *Int,* interior; *Lat,* lateral; *Sept,* septal; *SV,* systolic volume.

CASE 2: ATRIAL FIBRILLATION

A 61-year-old man with a history of permanent atrial fibrillation, coronary artery disease, and previous coronary artery bypass grafting was referred for consideration of CRT. He had a history of increasing shortness of breath on exertion and paroxysmal nocturnal dyspnea. Adequate 3DE volumes were obtained for analysis and demonstrated severely reduced LV systolic function, with an EF of 13.5%, and gross dyssynchrony, with an SDI at 19.1% (**Figure 12-19**; **Video 12-25**).

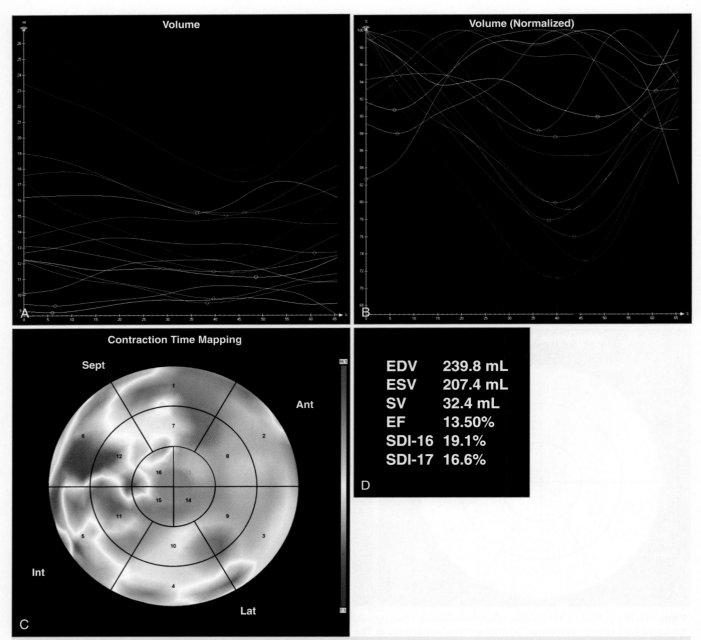

Figure 12-19 Prior to cardiac resynchronization therapy in the patient in Case 2, adequate volumes are obtained for analysis in a patient with permanent atrial fibrillation. The volumes are carefully inspected to outrule stitching artifact prior to analysis. The volume curves (**A**) are flat, consistent with reduced left ventricular systolic function (ejection fraction of 13.5%). Inspection of the normalized volume curves (**B**) facilitates identification of the minimum volume. **C,** The time of the minimum volume is broadly dispersed, with the minimum volume identified at the beginning of systole in the basal to mid-septal and basal inferior segments (*green and yellow curves*). This represents a septal flash and is clearly seen on the static contraction map, with early septal breakthrough. **D,** The systolic dyssynchrony index (*SDI*) is high at 19.1%, suggesting probable benefit from cardiac resynchronization therapy. Note that segment 13 is excluded from the analysis in this case because of poor tracking of the endocardium (see Video 12-25). *Ant,* anterior; *EDV,* end-diastolic volume; *EF,* ejection fraction; *ESV,* end-systolic volume; *Int,* interior; *Lat,* lateral; *Sept,* septal; *SV,* systolic volume.

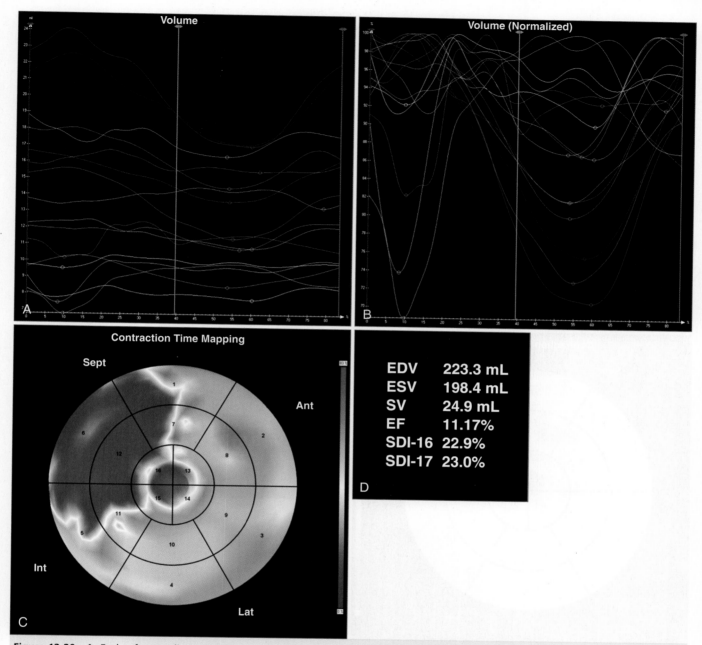

Figure 12-20   A, Early after cardiac resynchronization therapy in the patient in Case 2, there is a small increase in the amplitude of the volume curves. However, when the normalized curves are inspected (**B**), the minimum volume is seen to occur early in the septal and basal inferior segments, suggesting persistent dyssynchrony. A persistent septal flash is seen on the static contraction map (**C**), and the systolic dyssynchrony index (*SDI*) remains high (**D**). On clinical evaluation, the patient was noted to have rapidly conducted atrial fibrillation, leading to a low percentage of biventricular pacing (see Video 12-26). *Ant,* anterior; *EDV,* end-diastolic volume; *EF,* ejection fraction; *ESV,* end-systolic volume; *Int,* interior; *Lat,* lateral; *Sept,* septal; *SV,* systolic volume.

Following CRT-D implantation, he was noted to have poor ventricular rate control despite high-dose β-blocker therapy, with rates ranging from 90 to 100 beats/min. This resulted in inadequate BiV pacing therapy, at just 34% BiV pacing (**Figure 12-20; Video 12-26**). Atrioventricular node ablation was performed and resulted in 100% BiV pacing. LV analysis performed 4 days after his

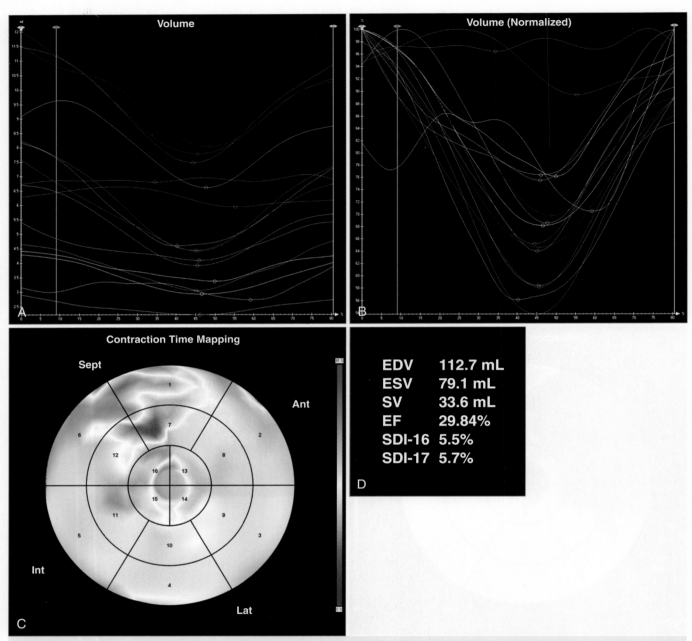

Figure 12-21   After atrioventricular node ablation, the patient in Case 2 underwent biventricular pacing 100% of the time. Repeat left ventricle analysis conducted 3 months after the procedure showed a marked increase in the amplitude of the volume curves. The segmental minimum volumes timings (**A**) are seen to occur closer together on the normalized volume graph (**B**). The early septal nadir also has disappeared. The septal flash has disappeared on the static polar map (**C**). Significant reverse remodeling has occurred. **D,** Successful resynchronization therapy is reflected in the near-normal systolic dyssynchrony index (*SDI*) of 5.5% (see Video 12-27). *Ant,* anterior; *EDV,* end-diastolic volume; *EF,* ejection fraction; *ESV,* end-systolic volume; *Int,* interior; *Lat,* lateral; *Sept,* septal; *SV,* systolic volume.

atrioventricular node ablation showed that the EF had increased, with reduction in SDI to 10.2%, suggesting significant benefit from BiV pacing. This improved further at a follow-up visit 3 months later, with improvement in EF to 30% and reduction in SDI to 5.5% (**Figure 12-21**; **Video 12-27**). Symptomatically, the patient had an excellent benefit following his two procedures.

CASE 3: SUBOPTIMAL LEAD POSITION

A 77-year-old woman with a history of idiopathic dilated cardiomyopathy, with broad QRS duration and significant dyssynchrony on 3DE assessment (SDI, 16.1%), underwent CRT-defibrillator implantation (**Figure 12-22; Video 12-28**). Over the subsequent 6 months, she noted a progressive deterioration in heart failure symptoms. Repeat 3DE analysis of the LV indicated persistent dyssynchrony (**Figure 12-23; Video 12-29**). Postimplantation chest radiograph and

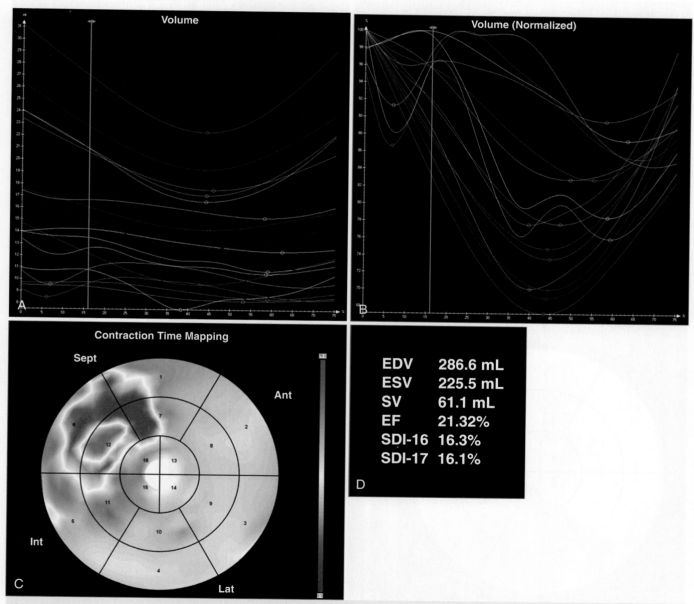

Figure 12-22 Prior to cardiac resynchronization therapy in the patient in Case 3, the volume curves are low amplitude (**A**), and there is significant dispersion of the timing of the minimum volume seen on the normalized volume curves (**B**), with early minimum volume of the septum (*green curves*). This represents a septal flash, which is seen on the static polar map (**C**), and there is significant dyssynchrony (**D**), suggesting a probable benefit from cardiac resynchronization therapy (see Video 12-28). *Ant*, anterior; *EDV*, end-diastolic volume; *EF*, ejection fraction; *ESV*, end-systolic volume; *Int*, interior; *Lat*, lateral; *Sept*, septal; *SV*, systolic volume.

coronary sinus venography films from the device were reviewed, and it was noted that the LV lead had been placed in an anteroseptal branch. An alternative posterior vein was noted for lead deployment, and the patient underwent lead repositioning (**Figure 12-24**). Following device revision, her clinical condition considerably improved, with reduced dose of diuretic and improved exercise capacity. Subsequent repeat measurement of left ventricular SDI demonstrated a significant improvement in dyssynchrony (**Figure 12-25; Video 12-30**).

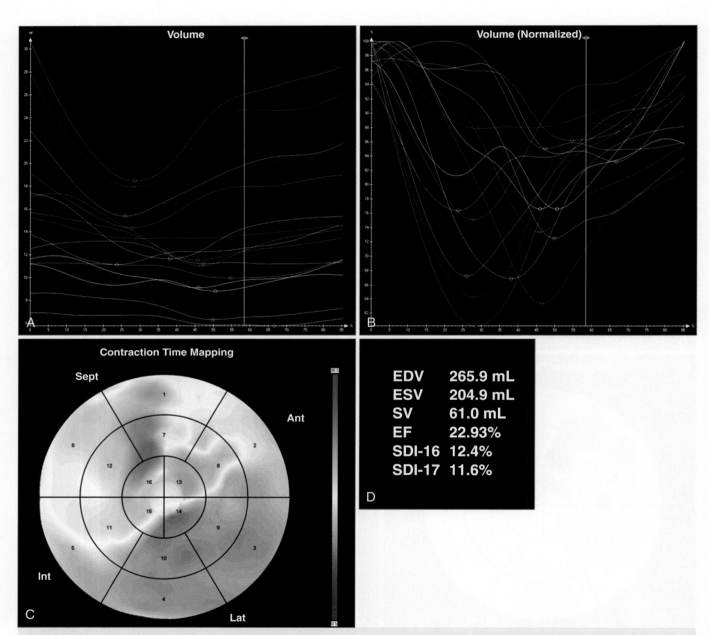

EDV	265.9 mL
ESV	204.9 mL
SV	61.0 mL
EF	22.93%
SDI-16	12.4%
SDI-17	11.6%

Figure 12-23 After cardiac resynchronization therapy in the patient in Case 3, there is no significant improvement in the volume curves (**A**), and the minimum volume timings remain broadly dispersed (**B**). The contraction pattern has changed and now is seen to spread from left to right (**C**), but the ventricle remains dyssynchronous, and ventricular function has not improved (**D**) (see Video 12-29). *Ant,* anterior; *EDV,* end-diastolic volume; *EF,* ejection fraction; *ESV,* end-systolic volume; *Int,* interior; *Lat,* lateral; *Sept,* septal; *SV,* systolic volume.

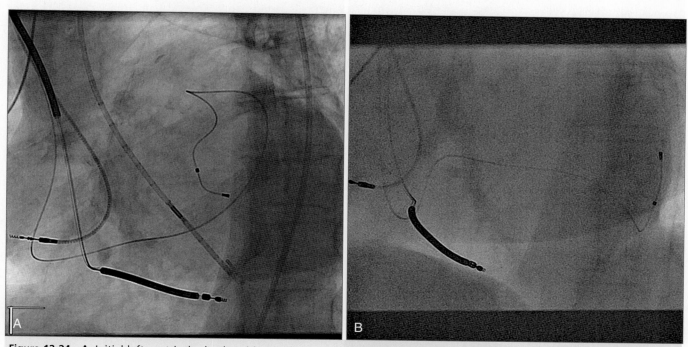

Figure 12-24 **A,** Initial left ventricular lead position in the patient in Case 3 as viewed in left anterior oblique projection. **B,** Comparable view of the left ventricular lead position after procedure to resituate the lead.

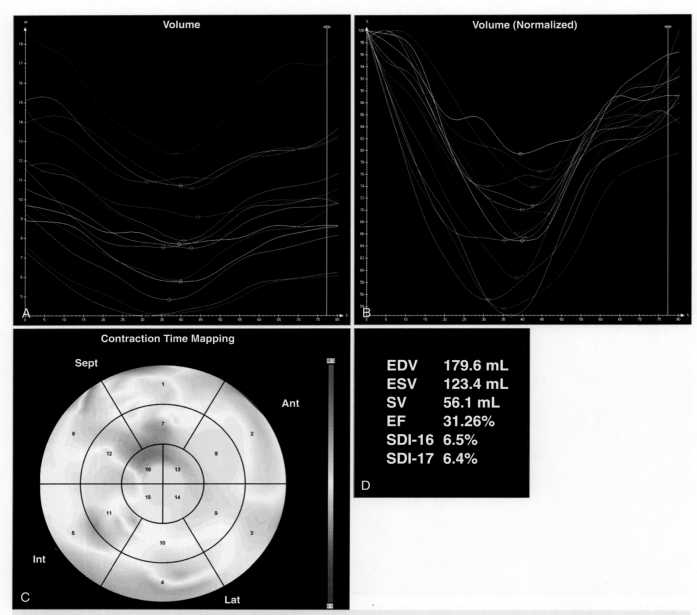

Figure 12-25   Left ventricle (LV) analysis conducted 3 months after repositioning of the left ventricular lead in the patient in Case 3. The amplitude of the volume curves has increased significantly (**A**) and the range minimum volume time is narrower (**B**), demonstrating resynchronization. A homogeneous pattern of activation is seen on the static contraction map (**C**), and there is evidence of significant reverse remodeling (**D**). This correlated with an excellent symptomatic improvement (see Video 12-30). *Ant,* anterior; *EDV,* end-diastolic volume; *EF,* ejection fraction; *ESV,* end-systolic volume; *Int,* interior; *Lat,* lateral; *Sept,* septal; *SV,* systolic volume.

CASE 4: DYSSYNCHRONY DESPITE NORMAL QRS DURATION

An 80-year-old man with a background of coronary artery disease and previous coronary artery bypass grafting was referred for consideration of implantable cardioverter-defibrillator therapy on primary prevention grounds. He had a history of exertional breathlessness and was in NYHA class III. He was known to have left ventricular systolic impairment, with an EF of approximately 30%. During his assessment, QRS duration was noted to be 96 ms, with delayed precordial R-wave progression (**Figure 12-26**); 24-hour ECG monitoring revealed four beats of ventricular tachycardia. The patient was referred for 3DE, which showed an EF of 33% and an SDI of 18.8% (**Figure 12-27; Video 12-31**). This result suggested potential benefit from CRT, although falling outside current guidelines; reimbursement therefore was subsequently denied.

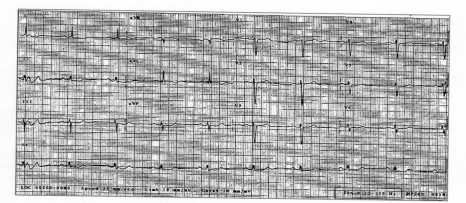

Figure 12-26 The electrocardiogram in the patient in Case 4 demonstrates sinus rhythm with normal QRS duration. Despite the narrow QRS complex, three-dimensional left ventricular analysis shows significant dyssynchrony.

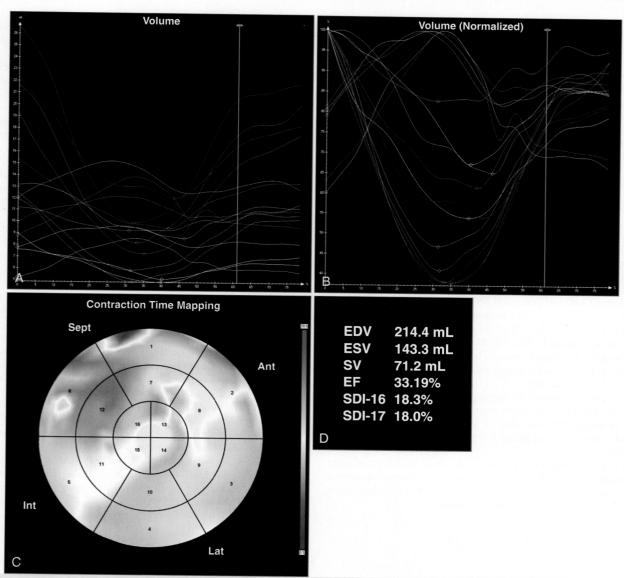

Figure 12-27 The regional volume curves demonstrate left ventricular systolic dysfunction, with regional wall motion abnormalities, in the patient in Case 4. The inferoposterior, septal, and anteroseptal volume curves are flat, with some preservation of the amplitude of the anterolateral (*red and dark blue*) curves. There is a prominent septal flash seen on the normalized volume curves (**A**), with the minimum volume of the septal and anteroseptal curves (*green and light blue curves*) detected at the beginning of systole (**B**). **C,** The static map demonstrates predominant left-to-right activation, with representation of the akinesis of the septum and anteroseptum (*remains red*), and septal flash seen in segment 1 only. **D,** There is clear dyssynchrony despite the normal QRS duration, suggesting that the patient may derive benefit from cardiac resynchronization therapy. *Ant,* anterior; *EDV,* end-diastolic volume; *EF,* ejection fraction; *ESV,* end-systolic volume; *Int,* interior; *Lat,* lateral; *Sept,* septal; *SV,* systolic volume.

References

1. Sugeng L, Mor-Avi V, Weinert L, et al: Quantitative assessment of left ventricular size and function: Side-by-side comparison of real-time three-dimensional echocardiography and computed tomography with magnetic resonance reference. *Circulation* 114:654–661, 2006.
2. Jenkins C, Bricknell K, Hanekom L, Marwick TH: Reproducibility and accuracy of echocardiographic measurements of left ventricular parameters using real-time three-dimensional echocardiography. *J Am Coll Cardiol* 44:878–886, 2004.
3. Monaghan M, Bax J, Franke A, et al: 3-dimensional echocardiographic assessment of left ventricular dyssynchrony: An alternative viewpoint. *JACC Cardiovasc Imag* 2:1334–1335, 2009.
4. Chung ES, Leon AR, Tavazzi L, et al: Results of the predictors of response to CRT (PROSPECT) trial. *Circulation* 117:2608–2616, 2008.
5. Kapetanakis S, Kearney MT, Siva A, et al: Real-time three-dimensional echocardiography: A novel technique to quantify global left ventricular mechanical dyssynchrony. *Circulation* 112:992–1000, 2005.
6. Marsan NA, Henneman MM, Chen J, et al: Real-time three-dimensional echocardiography as a novel approach to quantify left ventricular dyssynchrony: A comparison study with phase analysis of gated myocardial perfusion single photon emission computed tomography. *J Am Soc Echocardiogr* 21:801–807, 2008.
7. Takeuchi M, Jacobs A, Sugeng L, et al: Assessment of left ventricular dyssynchrony with real-time 3-dimensional echocardiography: Comparison with Doppler tissue imaging. *J Am Soc Echocardiogr* 20:1321–1329, 2007.
8. Vieira MLC, Cury AF, Naccarato G, et al: Analysis of left ventricular regional dyssynchrony: Comparison between real time 3D echocardiography and tissue Doppler imaging. *Echocardiography* 26:675–683, 2009.
9. Kapetanakis S, Bhan A, Murgatroyd F, et al: Real-time 3D echo in patient selection for cardiac resynchronization therapy. *JACC Cardiovasc Imag* 4:16–26, 2010.
10. Soliman O II, van Dalen BM, Nemes A, et al: Quantification of left ventricular systolic dyssynchrony by real-time three-dimensional echocardiography. *J Am Soc Echocardiogr* 22:232–239, 2009.
11. Sonne C, Sugeng L, Takeuchi M, et al: Real-time 3-dimensional echocardiographic assessment of left ventricular dyssynchrony: Pitfalls in patients with dilated cardiomyopathy. *JACC Cardiovasc Imag* 2:802–812, 2009.
12. De Castro S, Faletra F, Di Angelantonio E, et al: Tomographic left ventricular volumetric emptying analysis by real-time 3-dimensional echocardiography: Influence of left ventricular dysfunction with and without electrical dyssynchrony. *Circ Cardiovasc Imag* 1:41–49, 2008.
13. Marsan NA, Tops LF, Westenberg JJM, et al: Usefulness of multimodality imaging for detecting differences in temporal occurrence of left ventricular systolic mechanical events in healthy young adults. *Am J Cardiol* 104:440–446, 2009.
14. Conca C, Faletra FF, Miyazaki C, et al: Echocardiographic parameters of mechanical synchrony in healthy individuals. *Am J Cardiol* 103:136–142, 2009.
15. Liu W-H, Chen M-C, Chen Y-L, et al: Right ventricular apical pacing acutely impairs left ventricular function and induces mechanical dyssynchrony in patients with sick sinus syndrome: A real-time three-dimensional echocardiographic study. *J Am Soc Echocardiogr* 21:224–229, 2008.
16. Fang F, Chan JY-S, Yip GW-K, et al: Prevalence and determinants of left ventricular systolic dyssynchrony in patients with normal ejection fraction received right ventricular apical pacing: A real-time three-dimensional echocardiographic study. *Eur J Echocardiogr* 11:109–118, 2010.
17. Marsan NA, Bleeker GB, Ypenburg C, et al: Real-time three-dimensional echocardiography permits quantification of left ventricular mechanical dyssynchrony and predicts acute response to cardiac resynchronization therapy. *J Cardiovasc Electrophysiol* 19:392–399, 2008.
18. Ypenburg C, Van Bommel RJ, Marsan NA, et al: Effects of interruption of long-term cardiac resynchronization therapy on left ventricular function and dyssynchrony. *Am J Cardiol* 102:718–721, 2008.
19. Soliman O II, Geleijnse ML, Theuns DAMJ, et al: Usefulness of left ventricular systolic dyssynchrony by real-time three-dimensional echocardiography to predict long-term response to cardiac resynchronization therapy. *Am J Cardiol* 103:1586–1591, 2009.
20. van Dijk J, Knaapen P, Russel IK, et al: Mechanical dyssynchrony by 3D echo correlates with acute haemodynamic response to biventricular pacing in heart failure patients. *Europace* 10:63–68, 2008.
21. Ypenburg C, van Bommel RJ, Delgado V, et al: Optimal left ventricular lead position predicts reverse remodeling and survival after cardiac resynchronization therapy. *J Am Coll Cardiol* 52:1402–1409, 2008.
22. Johri AM, Picard MH, Newell J, et al: Can a teaching intervention reduce interobserver variability in LVEF assessment: A quality control exercise in the echocardiography lab. *J Am Coll Cardiol Cardiovasc Imag* 4:821–829, 2011.
23. Mor-Avi V, Jenkins C, Kuhl HP, et al: Real-time 3-dimensional echocardiographic quantification of left ventricular volumes: Multicenter study for validation with magnetic resonance imaging and investigation of sources of error. *J Am Coll Cardiol Cardiovasc Imag* 1:413–423, 2008.
24. Miller CA, Pearce K, Jordan P, et al: Comparison of real-time three-dimensional echocardiography with cardiovascular magnetic resonance for left ventricular volumetric assessment in unselected patients. *Eur Heart J Cardiovasc Imag* 13:187–195, 2012.
25. Kleijn SA, Aly MFA, Terwee CB, et al: Reliability of left ventricular volumes and function measurements using three-dimensional speckle tracking echocardiography. *Eur Heart J Cardiovasc Imag* 13:159–168, 2012.

Assessment of Right Ventricular Function

Florence H. Sheehan and Mary-Pierre Waiss

The right ventricle (RV) is often overlooked because most cardiologists focus their attention on the left ventricle (LV). Early work characterizing ventricular anatomy and physiology was performed on the LV and then assumed to be similar in the RV. Methods for measuring ventricular volume and function from the various imaging modalities were similarly developed for the LV and then applied to the RV. However, more recent studies have gradually revealed the differences between the two ventricles, and interest in the RV has risen because of recognition of the impact of RV dysfunction on patient prognosis, the increasing survival of patients with congenital heart disease to adulthood, and the rising incidence of pulmonary hypertension. Although the complex shape of the RV has long been recognized, it could previously only be glimpsed from two-dimensional (2D) images; the recent advent of three-dimensional (3D) surface reconstruction techniques for the RV has enabled new appreciation for the variety of phenotypes in which the RV can present in various conditions (**Figure 13-1**).

VISUALIZATION OF THE RIGHT VENTRICLE

The sector width in current ultrasound equipment is too narrow to contain both the LV and RV. Therefore, when acquiring the ultrasound study, it is necessary to ensure that the RV is completely visualized. This is easily accomplished by centering the view on the RV in both parasternal (**Figure 13-2**) and apical views (**Figure 13-3**).[1] Additional nonstandard views may be needed in patients with RV dilation. The four-chamber view can visualize the cardiac apex in normal hearts. However, centering of the RV is needed to visualize the apical bulging that may occur in hemodynamic overload states (see Figure 13-3).[2]

VOLUME MEASUREMENT
Two-Dimensional Approaches

The RV is notorious for its complex shape, which defies comparison with a geometric reference figure. In contrast, LV volume can be accurately measured from single or biplane views by comparison with an ellipsoid of revolution using the area-length method.[3] Early attempts to measure RV volume from angiograms used the formula $V = kA_1A_2/L$, where A_1 and A_2 are the areas of the RV in the two views, L is the length of the RV long axis, and k is a constant. Depending on the value of k and how L is defined, the RV was compared with a parallelepiped, ellipsoid of revolution (area-length method), triangular prism, or pyramid.[4-6] When these methods were compared with in vitro hearts or models, the disk summation method proved to be the most accurate.[7,8] The area-length method also performed well from the projection views of angiograms but proved inaccurate on 2D echocardiograms.[9]

Models that take advantage of ultrasound's tomographic, rather than projection, imaging were also developed. Levine and colleagues wrote: "A geometric structure can be constructed resembling the right ventricle with respect to its overall form and body segment, and such

Text continued on page 238

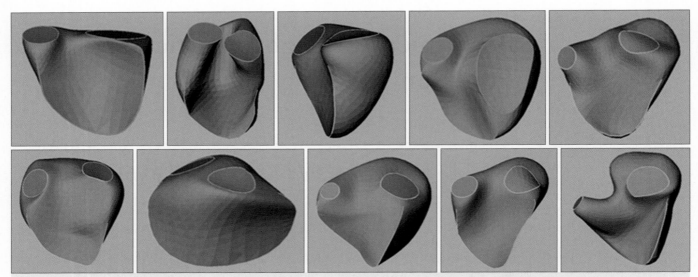

Figure 13-1   Three-dimensional reconstructions of the right ventricle showing the variety of phenotypes. *Top, right to left,* The diagnoses are normal, double-outlet right ventricle after Rastelli repair, idiopathic dilated cardiomyopathy, Ebstein's anomaly, and repaired truncus arteriosus with conduit from the right ventricle to the pulmonary artery. *Bottom, left to right,* The diagnoses are pulmonary hypertension from connective tissue disease, criss-crossed heart, repaired tetralogy of Fallot, repaired tetralogy of Fallot, and pulmonary atresia with ventricular septal defect after Rastelli repair. The view is from the septum with the pulmonary valve to the left and tricuspid valve to the right, except for an inferior view of the ventricle with the tricuspid valve in the foreground in the patient with cardiomyopathy.

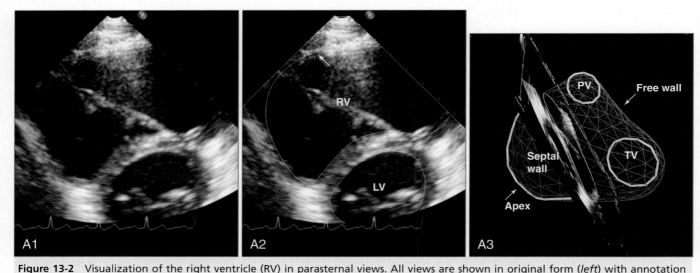

Figure 13-2   Visualization of the right ventricle (RV) in parasternal views. All views are shown in original form (*left*) with annotation (*center*), and as a three-dimensional reconstruction (*right*) of the RV illustrating the anatomic position of the view plane and the RV contour (in *yellow*). The patient has tetralogy of Fallot with wide-open pulmonary regurgitation after repair; the RV end-diastolic volume index is 132 mL/m². **A1-3,** RV-centered short-axis (SAX) view at mid-level angulated to visualize the free wall (*arrow*) within the sector.

Continued

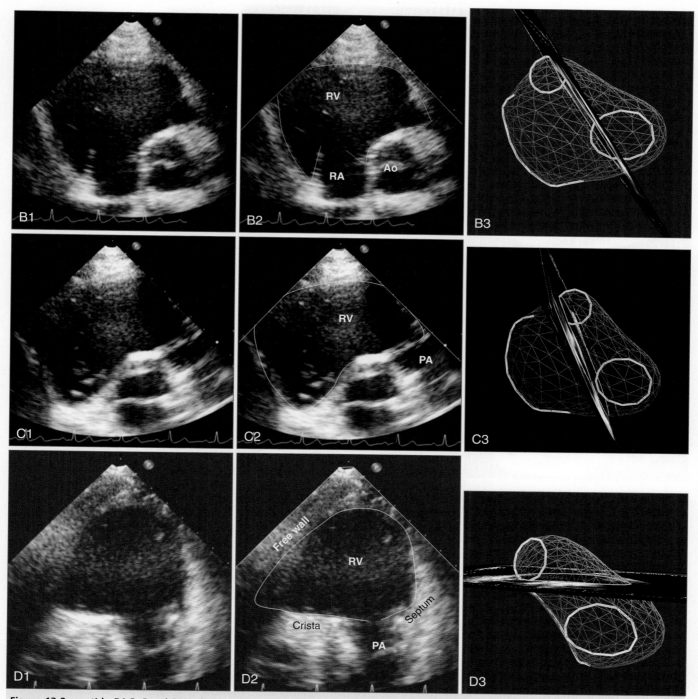

Figure 13-2, cont'd   B1-3, Basal SAX view angulated to visualize RV inflow. **C1-3,** Basal SAX view angulated to visualize RV outflow. **D1-3,** Modified SAX view to visualize RV outflow.

Continued

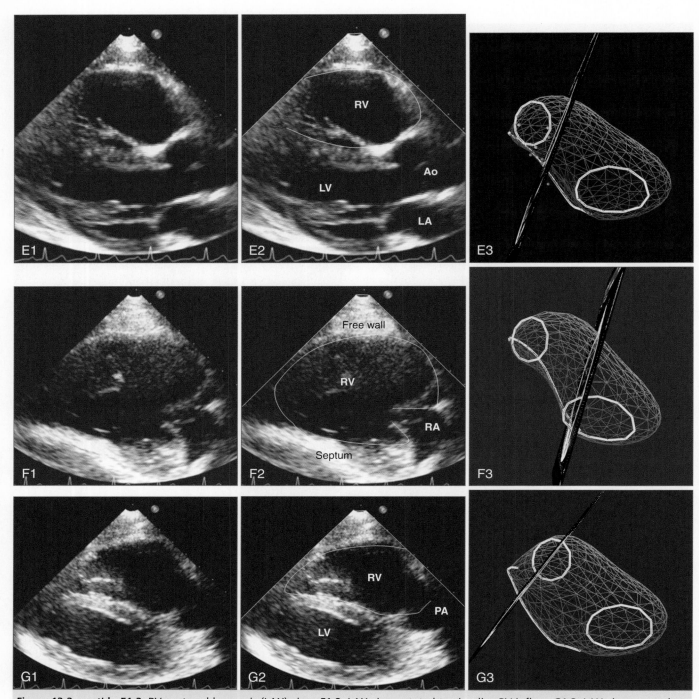

Figure 13-2, cont'd   E1-3, RV centered long-axis (LAX) view. **F1-3,** LAX view rotated to visualize RV inflow. **G1-3,** LAX view rotated to visualize RV outflow. *Ao,* aorta; *LV,* left ventricle; *PA,* pulmonary artery; *PB,* parietal band; *PV,* pulmonary valve; *TV,* tricuspid valve; *RA,* right atrium.

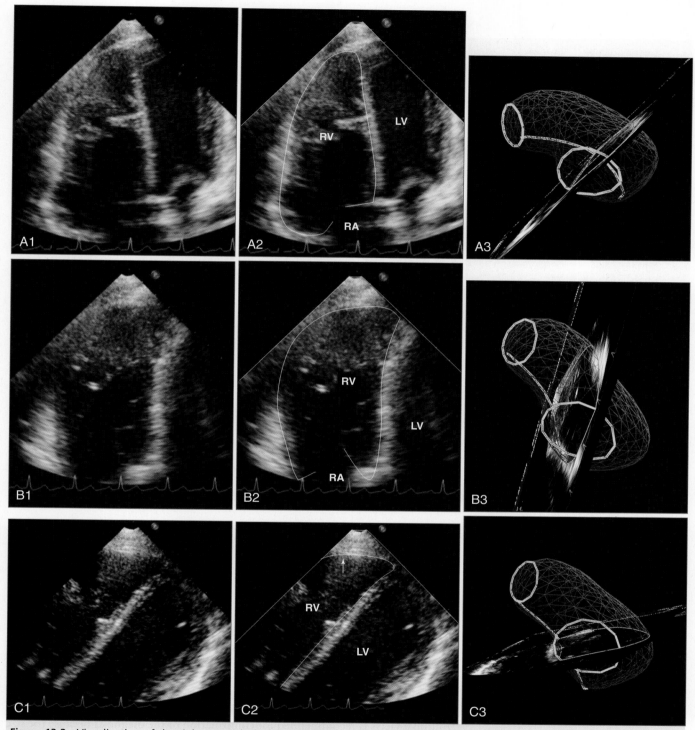

Figure 13-3 Visualization of the right ventricle (RV) in apical views shown in original form (*left*) with annotation (*center*), and as a three-dimensional reconstruction (*right*) of the RV illustrating the anatomic position of the view plane and the RV contour (in *yellow*) **A1-3,** RV-centered four-chamber (4C) view. **B1-3,** Sweeping anteriorly from the 4C view reveals the RV free wall between the valves. **C1-3,** Acquisition of the 4C view from a medial position may improve visualization of the apical free wall (*arrow*).

Continued

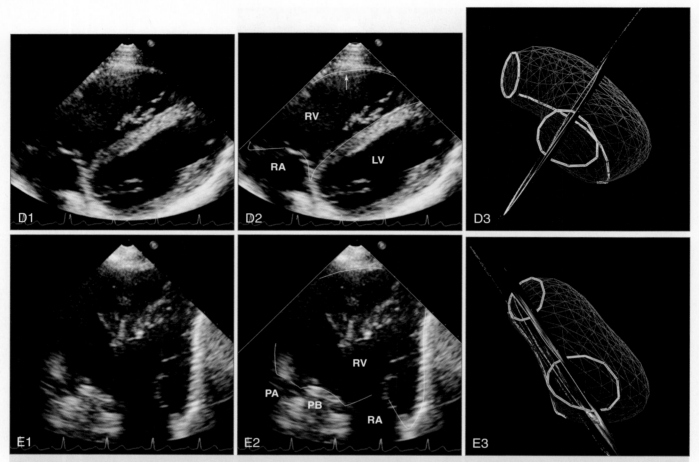

Figure 13-3, cont'd   **D1-3,** The anterior sweep from the 4C view, taken from a medial transducer position, may improve visualization of the free wall between the valves. **E1-3,** View of both inflow and outflow regions. The apex (*not seen*) is at the upper right. *LV,* left ventricle; *PA,* pulmonary artery; *PB,* parietal band; *RA,* right atrium.

a structure can have a volume equal to 2AL/3 without unreasonable restriction of its dimensions," where A is the area in one view and L spans the RV in the other, roughly orthogonal view (**Figure 13-4**).[10,11] However, these models require subcostal views that may be obtainable in only 52% of patients older than 5 years.[9]

Because of the inaccuracy in volume measurement, assessment of right ventricular ejection fraction (RVEF) based on 2D echocardiography (2DE) is not recommended.[1,9,12] Instead, visual assessment is performed to gauge RV size relative to that of the LV (**Figure 13-5; Video 13-1**).[13] Normally, the RV is only two thirds the size of the LV in the apical four-chamber view; the LV forms the apex of the heart and is round in short-axis views throughout the cardiac cycle. Deviations from this pattern may indicate RV dilation, but careful examination of multiple views is recommended for confirmation of the diagnosis because the size of the RV varies with the angle of the plane (**Figure 13-6**).[1]

Three-Dimensional Approaches

3D analysis entails delineating the RV from multiple views, a time-consuming task that is rendered more difficult by heavy trabeculations, particularly in hypertrophied RVs. For analysis of magnetic resonance imaging (MRI) scans, a recommendation has been made to trace the endocardial contour outside the trabeculations to maximize reproducibility (**Figure 13-7**).[14] Another issue is the definition of end systole. Because of the asynchronous contraction of the sinus and infundibulum, the timing of minimum chamber area will vary from region

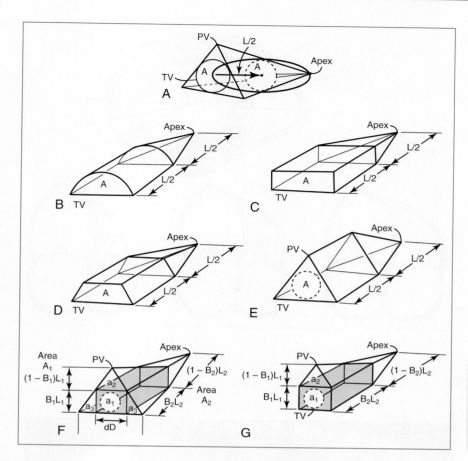

Figure 13-4   Geometric models with volume = 2AL/3. *PV,* pulmonary valve; *TV,* tricuspid valve. (From Levine RA, Gibson TC, Aretz T, et al: Echocardiographic measurement of right ventricular volume. *Circulation* 69:497–505, 1984.)

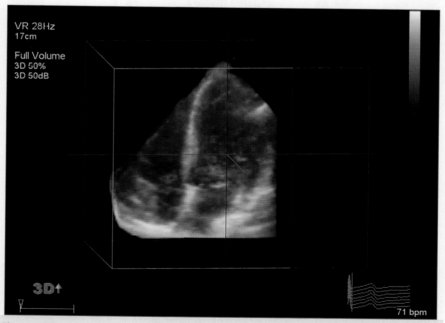

Figure 13-5   Video image of a normal echocardiogram from the apical four-chamber view. The area of the right ventricle is smaller than that of the left ventricle on visual inspection, in accordance with their end-diastolic volume indexes (86.3 mL/m^2 and 99.5 mL/m^2, respectively). The right ventricular ejection fraction is 51% (see Video 13-1).

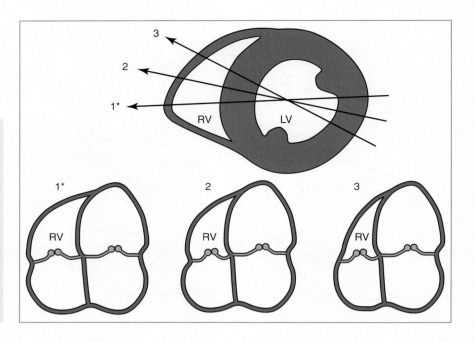

Figure 13-6 The recommended apical four-chamber (A4C) view with focus on the right ventricle (*RV, 1**) and the sensitivity of RV size with angular change (*2, 3*) despite similar size and appearance of the left ventricle (*LV*). The lines of intersection of the A4C planes (*1*, 2, 3*) with a mid–LV short axis are shown above with corresponding A4C views below. (From Rudski LG, Lai WW, Afilalo J, et al: Guidelines for the echocardiographic assessment of the right heart in adults: A report from the American Society of Echocardiography. *J Am Soc Echocardiogr* 23:685–713, 2010.)

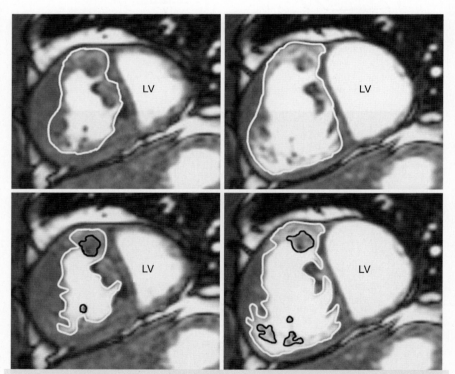

Figure 13-7 Assessment of right ventricular volume using two different protocols for analyzing the short-axis view from a multiphase steady-state free precision magnetic resonance imaging sequence in end systole (*left*) and end diastole (*right*) obtained in a patient with an atrially switched transposition of the great arteries. *Top,* Inclusion of trabeculations and papillary muscles in the ventricular cavity. *Bottom,* Exclusion of trabeculations and papillary muscles from the ventricular cavity. *LV*, left ventricle. (From Winter MM, Bernink FJP, Groenink M, et al: Evaluating the systemic right ventricle by CMR: The importance of consistent and reproducible delineation of the cavity. *J Cardiovasc Magn Res* 10:40, 2008.)

to region and from slice to slice.[15] However, frame-by-frame analysis has shown that selection of this time point from the four-chamber view and application of its systolic interval to the entire RV provide a highly accurate measurement of end-systolic volume.[16]

The disk summation method avoids assumptions concerning the shape of the RV because it does not compare the RV to a geometric figure, although it does assume that the cross-sectional contour is elliptical or hemielliptical.[17-19] Consequently, even pathologically misshapen ventricles, which are commonly found in congenital heart defects, can be accurately measured. The contours of the RV endocardium are traced from parallel views, the area of each contour is multiplied by the interplanar distance to compute the volume of each "slice," and the slice volumes are summed to compute the volume of the RV. With echocardiography, the RV is sliced into parallel short-axis views. For MRI, alternate-slice prescriptions have been advocated to more easily visualize the tricuspid annulus and define the basal limits of the RV.[20] A disadvantage of 3DE performed with a matrix array transducer is that the RV cannot be imaged in its entirety in a significant number of adult patients within the single apical scan that is most commonly used to acquire the image data. This disadvantage is particularly present when the RV is enlarged, the exact situation in which quantification of RV function is important. For both echocardiography and MRI, it is advisable to trace additional views orthogonal to the short-axis "stack" for assistance in delineating the apex, the structures in the basal slice, and the basal bulge (**Figure 13-8**).[21] Although the RV might be visualized in RV-centered images alone, this should only be done when it is certain that the LV does not need to be visualized.

An alternative to volumetric 3DE is acquisition of multiple 2D views while tracking the spatial location and orientation of the view planes for offline processing. The RV endocardial surface is reconstructed after tracing the images, and volume is computed from the 3D surface. An advantage of this approach is the use of freehand scanning so that views providing optimal image quality are acquired. As for analysis of volumetric datasets using disk summation, multiple views must be traced. Three methods have been validated for 3D reconstruction of the RV from manually traced borders. The method of Jiang and associates[22] was based on deforming a spherical template to fit traced borders (**Figure 13-9**). The method was highly accurate on in vivo testing ($r = 0.99$ for end-diastolic volume; $r = 0.98$ for end-systolic volume; $r = 0.98$ for ejection fraction (EF); and $r = 0.985$ for RV free wall mass).

Buckey and colleagues[23] swept the RV from a fixed transducer location in five-degree increments to define a series of wedges whose volumes were computed and summed to determine the RV volume. Accuracy in vitro was excellent ($r = 0.95$ and $r = 0.96$, respectively, for short-axis and apical scanning), but the entire RV had to be visualized from a single transducer position.

In the piecewise smooth subdivision surface (PSSS) method, a triangulated control mesh is designed as a model that is fit to traced borders. Parts of the control mesh can be marked as sharp around valve orifices and along the RV free wall to the septal edge (**Figure 13-10**). The PSSS method's accuracy for RV volume and mass has been validated ($r = 0.99$ and $r = 0.93$, respectively), and it is the only method shown to reproduce the 3D shape of the LV and the RV with anatomic accuracy.[24,25]

Although these three techniques are accurate for measuring RV volume, the requirement for tracing the RV border in multiple images has precluded their clinical application. One approach for reducing the human workload is to reduce the number of borders that need be traced. However, after comparing the results obtained with disk summation over 2 to 16 slices, Chen and associates[26] still found eight slices to be the "optimal choice for accurate and convenient measurement" of mass as well as volume.

Automated border detection has been stymied by the inherently noisy nature of the images, the frequent signal dropout, and the heavy trabeculation of

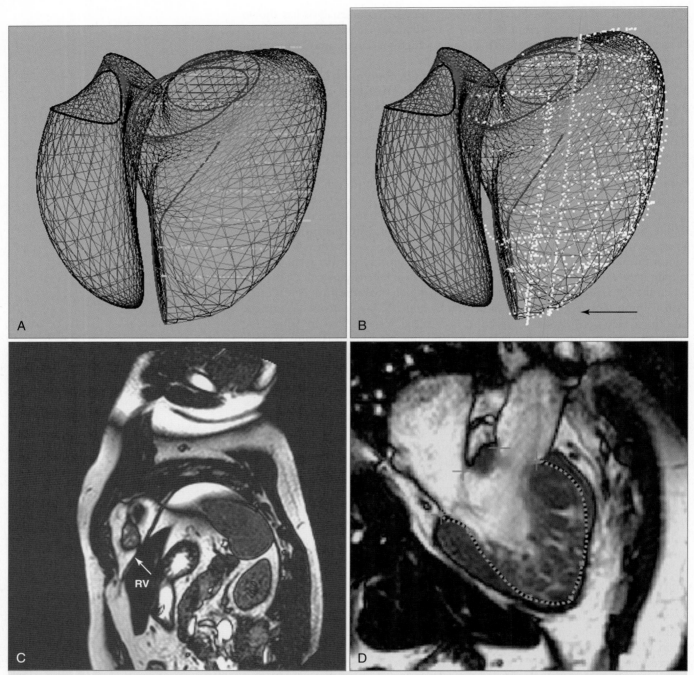

Figure 13-8   A, Reconstruction of the left ventricle (*red*) and right ventricle (*blue*) of a patient with transposition of the great arteries after atrial switch repair showing short-axis borders (*yellow*) at end diastole. **B,** Same reconstruction showing the location of the apical short-axis image (*arrow*) that was left untraced (**C**). **D,** The apical extent of the right ventricle (*RV*) is revealed by long-axis views such as this one (location in three dimensions indicated in *green*). (From Moroseos T, Mitsumori L, Kerwin WS, et al: Comparison of Simpson's method with three-dimensional reconstruction for measurement of right ventricular volume in patients with complete or corrected transposition of the great arteries. *Am J Cardiol* 105:1603–1609, 2010.)

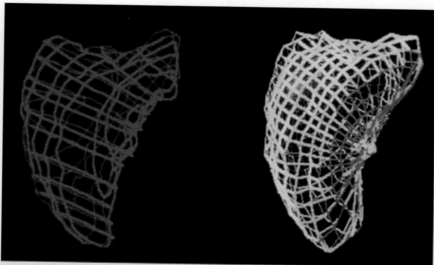

Figure 13-9   Method for three-dimensional reconstruction of the right ventricle from multiple echocardiographic views using a deformable spherical template. *Left,* Reconstructed traced borders of a right ventricular cast, with the inflow region at the upper left, apex below, and outflow at the upper right. The curved septum lies behind the anterior wall. *Right,* Corresponding surface used for volume calculation. (From Jiang L, Handschumacher MD, Hibberd MG, et al: Three-dimensional echocardiographic reconstruction of right ventricular volume: In vitro comparison with two-dimensional methods. *J Am Soc Echocardiogr* 7:150–158, 1994.)

the RV. However, TomTec Imaging Systems (Munich, Germany) markets a semi-automated method applicable to 3DE (**Figure 13-11**) that has been extensively validated.[27-29]

An alternative approach to reducing the workload of manual tracing is to use knowledge of the expected shape of the RV and the range of shapes that it can adopt in disease processes. The method marketed by VentriPoint, Inc. (Seattle, WA) is semiautomated like TomTec's, but the user traces points at anatomic landmarks (**Figure 13-12**) rather than whole borders.[30]

FUNCTION MEASUREMENT

The American Society of Echocardiography's guidelines state that "in selected patients with RV dilation or dysfunction, 3DE using the disk summation method may be used to report RVEF."[1] However, 3DE is not universally available, so surrogate parameters based on a single 2D view have been proposed for estimation of global RV function. The analysis usually is performed on the apical four-chamber view because of the predominantly longitudinal contractile pattern of the RV, which lacks the LV's middle layer of circumferential fibers.[31,32] The most commonly used parameters are fractional area change and tricuspid annular plane systolic descent (TAPSE).[33]

A major disadvantage of the single-view approach to RV function assessment is that it provides a limited perspective. The relationship between TAPSE and EF, for example, is weak if there is tricuspid regurgitation or if longitudinal shortening of the RV differs from the function of regions not visualized in the four-chamber view.[34,35] In both volume and pressure overload, analysis of short-axis contours has shown dilation and dysfunction, whereas longitudinal analysis showed poor correlation between TAPSE and EF.[36,37] Also, the function of other regions may exert a more powerful effect on patient outcome than would longitudinal contraction. For example, akinesis of the right ventricular outflow track (RVOT) is associated with a poor prognosis in repaired tetralogy of Fallot, and some advocate measuring fractional area shortening from a modified short-axis

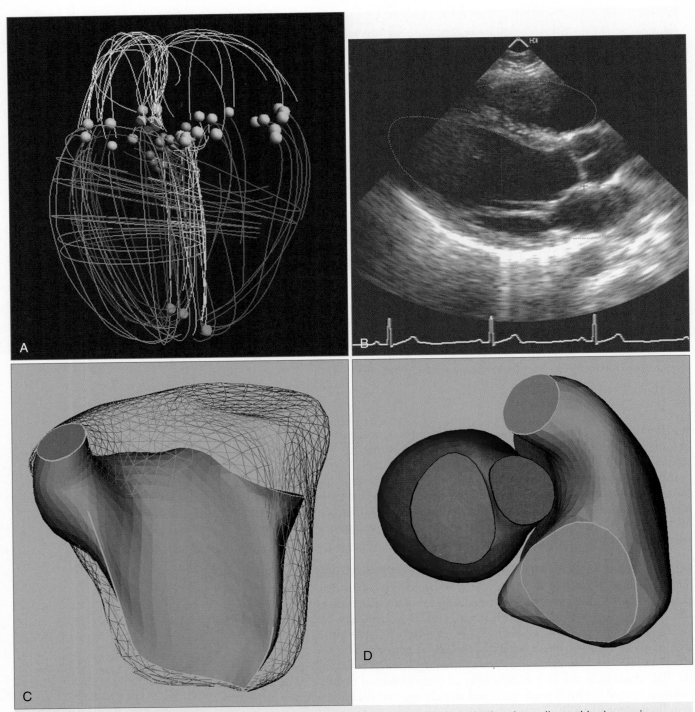

Figure 13-10   Method for three-dimensional reconstruction of the right ventricle from multiple echocardiographic views using a piecewise smooth subdivision surface. **A,** Borders of the atria and ventricles traced from multiple echocardiographic images of a normal subject. The spheres mark the valve orifices and the apex of each ventricle. **B,** Parasternal long-axis view showing traced borders. **C,** Reconstruction of the right ventricle at end diastole (*mesh*) and end systole (*surface*) displayed from the septal view. **D,** Reconstructions of the left ventricle (*red*) and right ventricle (*blue*) displayed from the atria.

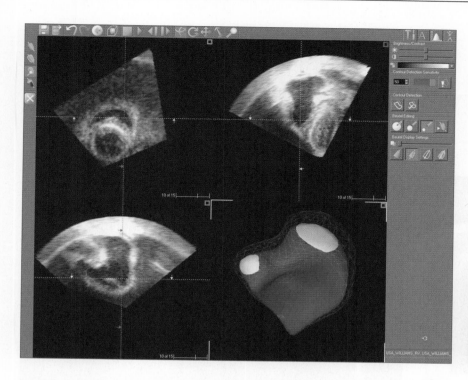

Figure 13-11 Method for three-dimensional reconstruction of the right ventricle from volumetric echocardiographic datasets using semiautomated contour detection. (Courtesy TomTec Imaging Systems, Munich, Germany.)

view that visualizes the outflow tract (**Figure 13-13**).[38,39] Another example of discordance between TAPSE and clinical outcome is a study of patients undergoing mitral valve surgery; their RVEF was unchanged after the procedure in agreement with their lack of significant complications, but TAPSE dropped significantly.[40]

Another disadvantage of the single-view approach to assessing RV function is that the reliability and reproducibility depend on the examiner's ability to acquire the specified view. One study found that 95% of apical two-chamber views were foreshortened and underestimated LV volume.[41] Another study reported that even experienced examiners achieved optimal imaging, defined as ideal plane position ±5 mm and ideal plane angle ±15 degrees, in only 32% and 48% of studies, respectively.[42] Even when care is taken to acquire a specified view correctly, such as by maximizing RV chamber area in the four-chamber view, the anatomic location of that image plane in the 3D heart cannot be verified from the 2D image. This introduces variability when assessing change in a patient's RV status between serial studies. Use of a visual guidance system to assist in locating the apical four-chamber view without foreshortening has improved accuracy in RV volume determination (**Figure 13-14**).[43]

The complex shape of the RV has made it difficult to analyze regional function. Because of the underlying assumptions concerning ventricular shape, few of the geometric models developed for 2D images of the LV can be applied to the RV. For example, radial coordinate systems do not fit short-axis views of the RV because of the sharp angles at the junction of the septal and free walls. Similarly, rectangular coordinate systems do not fit crescentic contours either. An exception is RV torsion, which can be measured using speckle tracking, as with LV torsion (**Figure 13-15**).[44] The only method that has been successfully applied for measuring regional RV function in both long-axis and short-axis views is the centerline method, which does not rely on geometric assumptions about RV shape (**Figure 13-16**); it is also applicable to multiple imaging modalities (angiograms, echo images, and MRI).[45-48]

The most accurate method for analyzing the 3D pattern of regional RV function is tagging with MRI. Studies using this modality have documented the regional heterogeneity of tagging wall motion, confirmed the greater long-axis

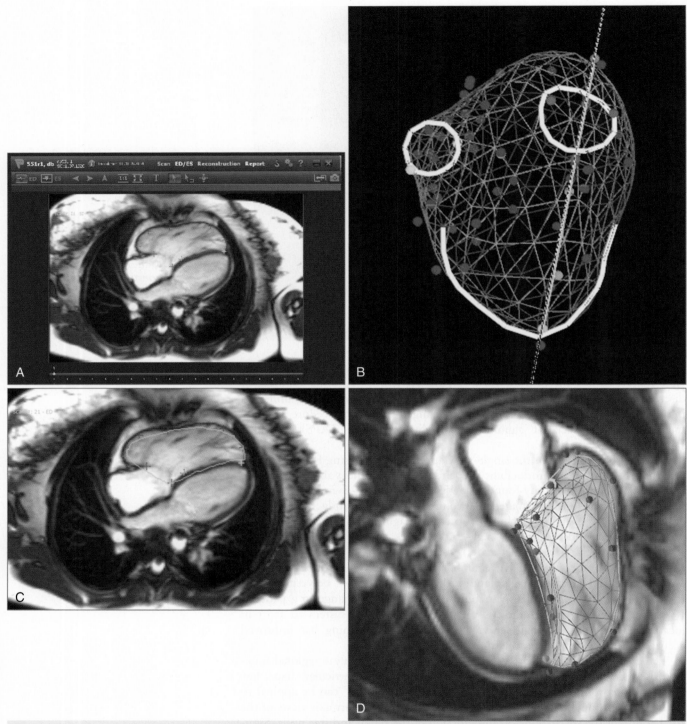

Figure 13-12 Knowledge-based method for three-dimensional (3D) reconstruction of the right ventricle from two-dimensional (2D) images. **A,** Points are entered on images instead of contours. The anatomic landmarks entered on this four-chamber view are the free wall (*red*), apex (*yellow*), septum (*blue*), tricuspid annulus (*purple*), and basal bulge (*brown*). **B,** A piecewise smooth subdivision surface is fit to a set of anatomic landmark points. The plane of the four-chamber view is indicated (*yellow line*). **C,** Intersection of the 3D surface with each 2D image produces a candidate border whose fidelity to the image can readily be evaluated. **D,** Overlay of the 3D surface on the 2D image. (Courtesy VentriPoint, Inc., Seattle, WA.)

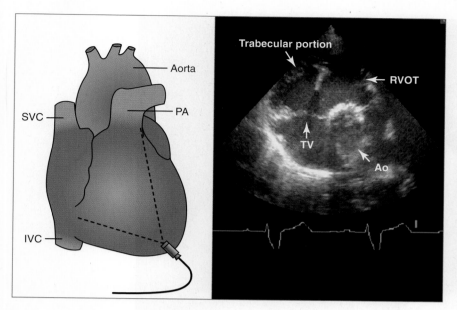

Figure 13-13 Evaluation of right ventricular systolic function using a modified short-axis view. The long axis of the aorta must be shown in the modified short-axis view. *Ao*, aorta; *IVC*, inferior vena cava; *PA*, pulmonary artery; *RA*, right atrium; *RVOT*, right ventricular outflow tract; *SVC*, superior vena cava; *TOF*, tetralogy of Fallot; *TV*, tricuspid valve. (From Hui W, El Rahman MYA, Dsebissowa F, et al: Comparison of modified short axis view and apical four chamber view in evaluating right ventricular function after repair of tetralogy of Fallot. *Int J Cardiol* 105:256–261, 2005.)

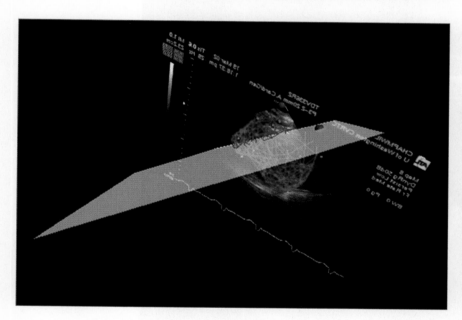

Figure 13-14 Visual guidance provides anatomic information to help users learn to scan. The display allows the location and orientation of the current image plane (*translucent area*) to be displayed and updated as the transducer is being manipulated over the patient in relation to a three-dimensional reconstruction of the right ventricle (*red mesh*) that is rapidly reconstructed from scout images. (From Dorosz J, Bolson EL, Waiss MS, Sheehan FH: Three-dimensional visual guidance improves the accuracy of calculating right ventricular volume with two-dimensional echocardiography. *J Am Soc Echocardiogr* 16:675–681, 2003.)

shortening than short-axis shortening, quantified torsion, and evaluated functional abnormality in a few disease conditions.[31,32,49-52]

For clinical imaging, investigators have developed a multiplicity of methods for assessing regional RV function from 3D image datasets. Some have applied 2D methods to multiple short-axis views.[36,48] Others have calculated regional EFs after subdividing the RV volume.[15,53] A third approach is to measure RV free wall motion from 3D surface reconstructions along vectors orthogonal to the endocardium at end diastole.[54]

The multiplicity of methods extends to segmentation. Although consensus has been reached on a segmental model corresponding to coronary artery perfusion territories, studies of regional RV function in other conditions have analyzed 2, 3, 4, 7, 9, or 12 regions.[1,15,48,50,52,53,55,56] Some studies divided the RV free wall geometrically into circumferential regions (superior, middle, inferior), vertical regions (apical, mid, basal), or both. Others used anatomic landmarks to segment the RV into inlet, trabecular, and outlet portions (**Figure 13-17**).[15,53] Thus, the study of regional RV function remains an area of active investigation.

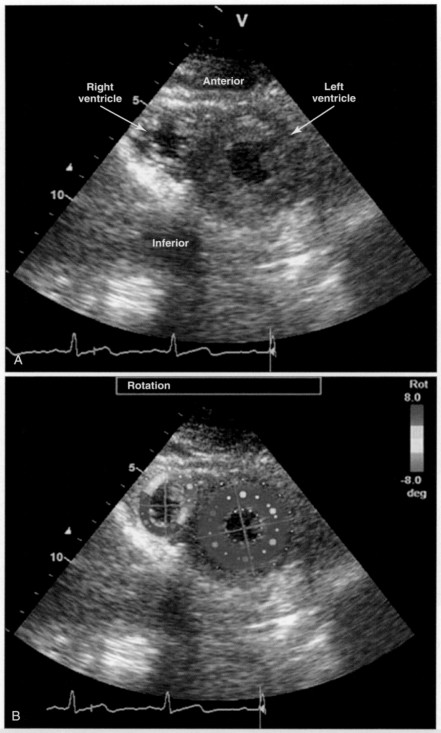

Figure 13-15   Measurement of torsion using speckle tracking. **A,** Echocardiographic image of both ventricles at the apical level. **B,** Region of interest at each ventricle. Representative image of the rotational directions in different segments of the ventricles at the time of aortic valve closure. *Blue* within the region of interest indicates counterclockwise rotation; *red* indicates clockwise rotation. (From Gustafsson U, Lindqvist P, Waldenstrom A: Apical circumferential motion of the right and left ventricles in healthy subjects described with speckle tracking. *J Am Soc Echocardiogr* 21:1326–1330, 2008.)

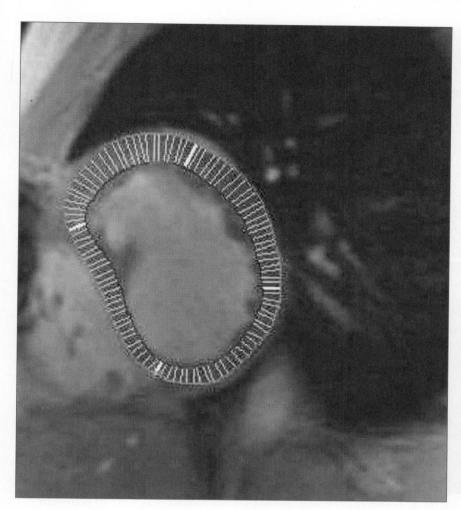

Figure 13-16 Method for measuring regional right ventricular function. Magnetic resonance imaging scan showing a slice through the middle of the morphologic right ventricle in a patient with congenitally corrected transposition. The endocardial (*red*) and epicardial (*green*) contours are shown, along with 100 centerline cords (*yellow*) of the systemic ventricle. (From Tulevski II, Zijta FM, Smeijers AS, et al: Regional and global right ventricular dysfunction in asymptomatic or minimally symptomatic patients with congenitally corrected transposition. *Cardiol Young* 14:168–174, 2004.)

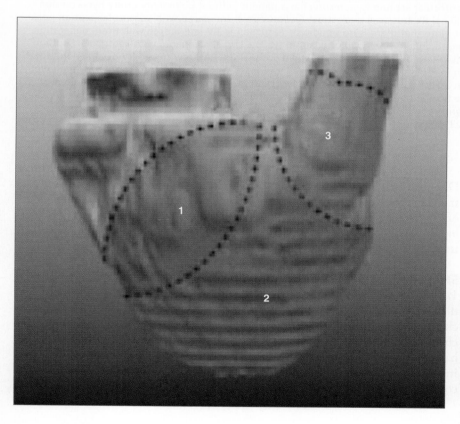

Figure 13-17 Diagram of the right ventricle illustrating its component parts. *1,* inlet; *2,* apical trabecular; *3,* outlet. (From Bodhey NK, Beerbaum P, Sarikouch S, et al: Functional analysis of the components of the right ventricle in the setting of tetralogy of Fallot. *Circ Cardiovasc Imag* 1:141–147, 2008.)

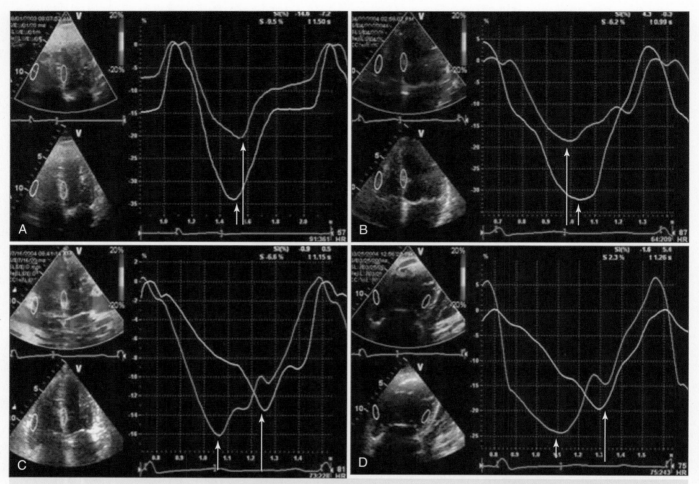

Figure 13-18   A representative tissue Doppler image. **A,** Almost synchronized time-to-peak longitudinal peak strain of both right ventricular (RV) free wall (*yellow curve*) and ventricular septum (*green curve*) in a patient without pulmonary artery hypertension (PAH). **B,** Slightly delayed time-to-peak longitudinal RV free wall peak strain (*yellow curve*) compared with ventricular septum peak strain (*green curve*) in a patient with mild PAH. Note that there is no significant reduction in RV lateral free wall strain generation. **C,** A more noticeable delayed time-to-peak longitudinal RV free wall peak strain (*yellow curve*) compared with ventricular septum peak strain (*green curve*) is evident in a patient with moderate PAH. **D,** A patient with severe PAH and severe RV dysfunction. Note that both **C** and **D** show a significant reduction in RV lateral free wall strain generation. In synchronous contraction, the *long and short arrows* are close to each other in time. In asynchronous contraction, the long and short arrows demonstrate that regions of the heart are not contracting at the same time (so the horizontal distance between them is widened). (From Lopez-Candales A, Dohi K, Rajagopalan N, et al: Right ventricular dyssynchrony in patients with pulmonary hypertension is associated with disease severity and functional class. *Cardiovasc Ultrasound* 3:23, 2005.)

An alternative to assessing endocardial excursion or wall thickening is tissue Doppler imaging for assessment of 2D strain (**Figure 13-18**). The speckle-tracking echocardiographic modality is angle independent as well as independent of interference from cardiac translation and tethering and can be applied to assess longitudinal contraction, similar to TAPSE. A promising application of speckle tracking is to assess contractile dyssynchrony (see Figure 13-18).

SHAPE MEASUREMENT

Ventricular remodeling is the term applied to the compensatory hypertrophy and dilation that maintain cardiac output in overload states. The term encompasses changes in chamber dimensions, wall thickness, and shape caused by microscopic changes in myocytes and the extracellular matrix. In the LV, the shape changes have been attributed to redistribution of stress.[57] The distribution of wall stress in the myocardium affects ventricular function, myocardial oxygen demand, coronary blood flow, vulnerability to injury, remodeling, and action potential

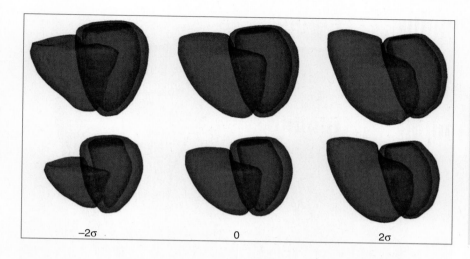

Figure 13-19 Four-dimensional shape model of the left and right ventricles. Reconstructions at phases 0 (end diastole, *top*) and 7 (rapid filling, *bottom*) produced by varying the first mode of shape variation. (From Zhang H, Thomas MT, Walker NE, et al: Four-dimensional functional analysis of left and right ventricles using MR images and active appearance models. *IEEE Trans Med Imag* 29:350–363, 2007.)

shape.[58,59] The analysis of regional ventricular stress is currently performed by using mathematical modeling of the determinants, including finite element analysis. Most of the work in this field has been performed on the more easily modeled LV, and the RV was assumed to be similar. Study of the RV has been impeded by its complex shape, which has resisted simple geometric modeling.

Most of the research on RV shape has reported on the effect of pressure overload on the curvature of the interventricular septum as viewed in 2D on a cross-sectional view, which showed that metrics of septal curvature are predictive of elevated pulmonary artery pressure.[60]

Finite element analysis techniques have been applied to characterize RV shape in 3D in the normal heart and in disease conditions.[49,61] However, these studies were performed on parallel short-axis MRI and excluded the basal portion of the RV. Principal component analysis also has been used to characterize RV shape in terms of the modes of shape variation in a population (**Figure 13-19**).[62] In addition, descriptive methods have been developed, as for 2DE, to quantify abnormalities in RV shape that are discernible from visual examination of 3D reconstructions in hemodynamic overload and intrinsic diseases (**Figure 13-20**).[2] Normal values for these and LV shape parameters have been published.[63]

CONDITIONS AFFECTING THE RIGHT VENTRICLE
Volume Overload: Tetralogy of Fallot

Tetralogy of Fallot (TOF) (**Video 13-2**) is the most common cause of cyanotic congenital heart disease. As a result of advanced surgical repair techniques, the rate of survival to adulthood now exceeds 80%. However, the procedure performed to widen the RVOT may destroy pulmonary valve competency. Over time, the volume overload from pulmonary regurgitation leads to RV dilation and dysfunction. RV volume overload has long been known to alter septal shape, as seen in the short-axis view, with changes ranging from slight flattening to curvature reversal (**Figure 13-21**, *A*).[64] In addition, the free wall bulges at the base (see Figure 13-20, *A*) and at the apex, producing an "apex-forming" RV (see Figure 13-21, *B* to *D*).[2,53] The RV cross-section is increased in area and rounded from the apex to the mid-ventricle area (**Figure 13-22**). Analysis of the RV's 3D shape reveals an additional change: tilting of the tricuspid annulus (see Figure 13-20, *B*).[2]

The changes in RV shape are accompanied by global dysfunction and altered pattern of region contraction. The EF of the outlet portion is depressed and is associated with increased risk of tachyarrhythmias.[53,54] There is hypokinesis at the mid- and apical free wall region, with relative sparing of the basal region.[36,52]

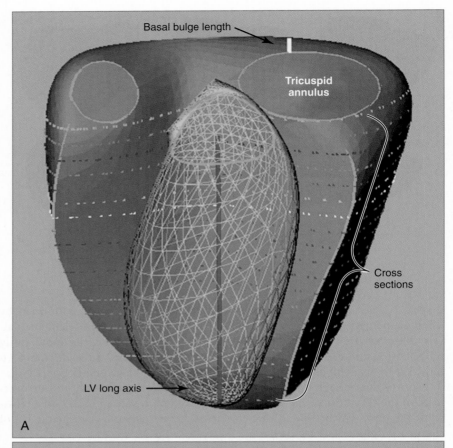

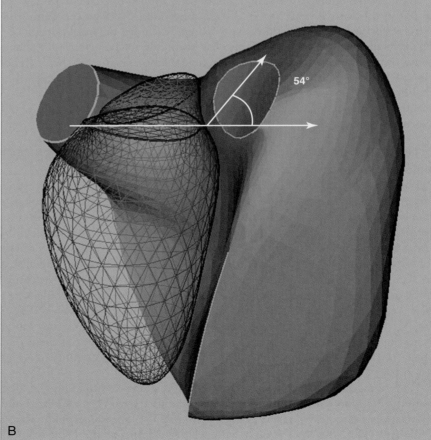

Figure 13-20 Method for quantifying right ventricular (RV) shape from three-dimensional surface reconstructions. **A,** The cross-sectional area and shape of the RV are measured in 20 parallel planes constructed orthogonal to the left ventricular (*LV*) long axis. Basal bulge length is computed parallel to the LV long axis. **B,** Tricuspid annular tilt measurement relative to the mitral annular plane. Both examples are from patients with tetralogy of Fallot and wide-open pulmonary regurgitation. (From Sheehan FH, Ge S, Vick GW, III, et al: Three-dimensional shape analysis of right ventricular remodeling in repaired tetralogy of Fallot. *Am J Cardiol* 101:107–113, 2008.)

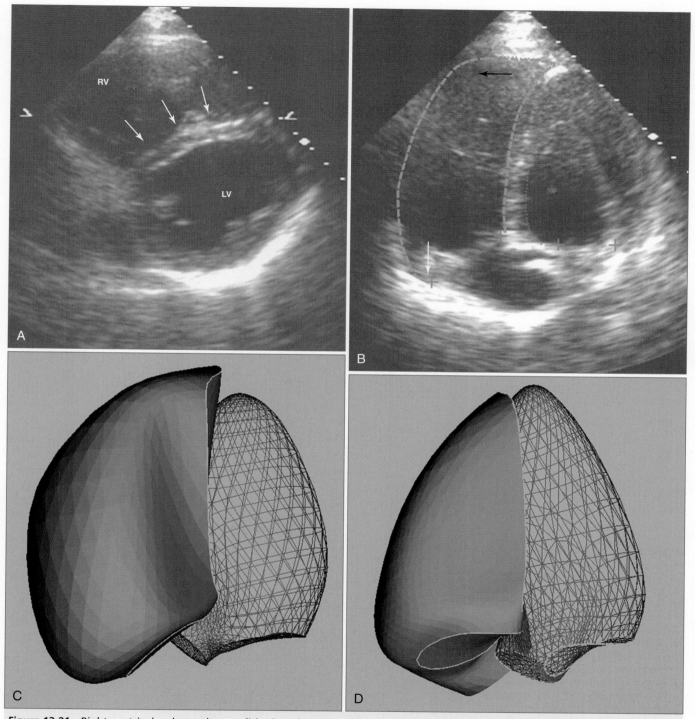

Figure 13-21   Right ventricular shape abnormalities in volume overload. **A,** Parasternal short-axis view illustrating flattening of the interventricular septum (*arrows*) in a patient with tetralogy of Fallot and wide-open pulmonary regurgitation after repair. **B,** Apical four-chamber view of the same patient illustrating apical widening (*black arrow*) and basal bulge (*white arrow*) in the right ventricle. **C,** Reconstructions of the right (*blue surface*) and left (*red mesh*) ventricles in the same orientation as in **B** showing the apical widening and basal bulge in three dimensions. **D,** Reconstructions of the left and right ventricles of a normal subject for comparison. LV, left ventricle; RV, right ventricle.

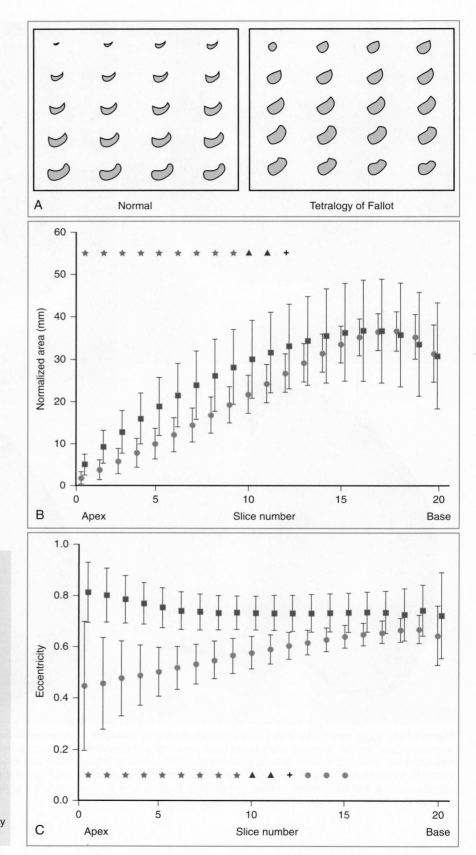

Figure 13-22 Quantitative three-dimensional analysis of right ventricular (RV) shape in tetralogy of Fallot (TOF). **A,** RV shape at 20 cross-sections created by the method shown in Figure 13-20 in a normal subject and in a patient with TOF. RV dilation and apical rounding in TOF are illustrated. The septal surface is above, the free wall below, the tricuspid valve to the left, and the pulmonary valve to the right. **B,** Normalized end-diastolic cross-sectional area is significantly (*$P < .01$) greater in patients with TOF (*squares*) than normal (*circles*) in the apical half of the RV. **C,** Eccentricity of the end-diastolic cross-section. The RV cross-section was more circular in patients with TOF (*squares*) (*$P < .05$) than in normal subjects (*circles*). (From Sheehan FH, Ge S, Vick GW, III, et al: Three-dimensional shape analysis of right ventricular remodeling in repaired tetralogy of Fallot. *Am J Cardiol* 101:107–113, 2008.)

Both the severity of regional dysfunction and the area of dysfunction contribute to depressing the global EF.[54] The alteration in regional contraction pattern may explain the weak correlation of TAPSE with RVEF.[36]

Pressure Overload: Pulmonary Hypertension

The response of the RV to chronic pressure overload is initial compensatory hypertrophy with preserved function, but continued pressure overload leads to RV and right atrial dilation, tricuspid regurgitation, and failure. Findings seen on 2DE are septal flattening or curvature reversal (**Figures 13-23 to 13-25; Videos 13-3 and 13-4**), diminished longitudinal contraction (**Figure 13-26**), and increased dependence of the global EF on transverse contraction.[37,60] In the apical four-chamber view, broadening of the apical angle correlates with RV dysfunction measured in terms of fractional area change in the same view (**Figure 13-27**).[65] The observations on RV shape and function from 2DE have been confirmed by 3D analyses showing reduced global RVEF and rounding of the RV in cross-section (**Figure 13-28**).[66]

More recent studies have sought to assess the prognostic power of parameters of shape, function, or both. In a serial study following diagnosis, it was found that patients who died within 4 years had RV dilation and decreased EF; however, the drop in function was caused by diminution of transverse contraction—not of TAPSE—from progressive septal bowing.[67] Thus, analysis of RV shape helps elucidate the mechanism of the RV response.

ISCHEMIC HEART DISEASE AND HEART FAILURE

Attention usually is focused solely on the LV in ischemic heart disease and heart failure. RV dysfunction in ischemic heart disease usually is secondary to elevated filling pressure, but the RV may develop regional hypokinesis from coronary occlusion. Experimental studies have shown that a more proximal occlusion of the right coronary artery produces a larger wall motion defect, but the size of the defect in RV ischemia is excessive for the size of the infarction.[68] Despite severe free wall dysfunction, global RV function recovers early after occlusion because of stiffening of the free wall. Clinically, most patients recover, whether or not the right coronary artery is reperfused.[69]

A segmentation plan has recently been developed on the basis of ischemic dysfunction patterns for the RV (**Figure 13-29**).[1] This plan differs completely from segmentation based on muscle anatomy (see Figure 13-17). RV remodeling appears to follow the former; pulmonary hypertension secondary to LV dysfunction is associated with RV dilation in the basal region, with relative apical sparing (**Figure 13-30**).[70]

In heart failure, the RV may be involved either directly or secondarily. In a study of patients with acute class III or IV LV failure, 42% had RV failure and were more likely to have right atrial enlargement, elevated pulmonary artery systolic pressure, and tricuspid regurgitation.[71] RVEF is lower in nonischemic cardiomyopathy, presumably because both ventricles are involved in the primary condition.[72]

Many studies have shown that involvement of the RV in ischemic heart disease, heart failure, and other conditions denotes a poorer prognosis.[73] The use of imaging to help with identification of those at risk of developing RV failure may be useful in their management. For example, the development of RV failure in patients receiving an LV assist device is a major contributor of morbidity and mortality.[74] Also, preoperative assessment of RV function may help predict which patients are likely to require additional resources after bypass surgery.[75]

As methods for quantitative analysis of the RV from 3DE datasets become more accurate and clinically feasible, it will be easier to apply measurements of global and regional RV function and shape to understand and manage patients with conditions affecting the right heart.

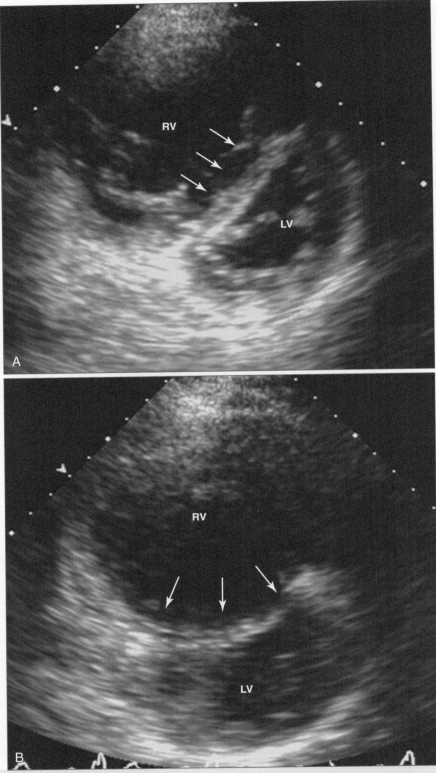

Figure 13-23   The right ventricle under pressure overload. **A,** Septal flattening (*arrows*) in a patient with pulmonary hypertension. **B,** Reverse septal curvature (*arrows*) in pulmonary hypertension. *LV*, left ventricle; *RV*, right ventricle.

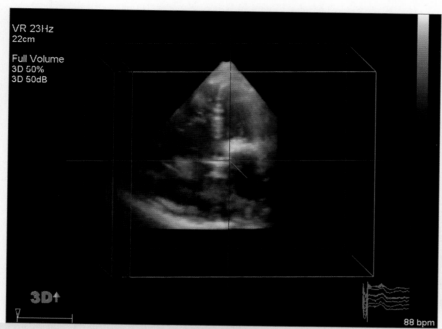

Figure 13-24 Video image in the apical four-chamber view of a patient with rheumatic mitral stenosis evidenced by calcification of the mitral leaflets and chordal thickening. The left atrium is severely enlarged. Left ventricular size (volume index = 68.4 mL/m^2) and function are normal. There is severe right ventricular enlargement (volume index = 128.1 mL/m^2), severely reduced systolic function, and septal flattening consistent with right ventricular pressure overload (see Video 13-2).

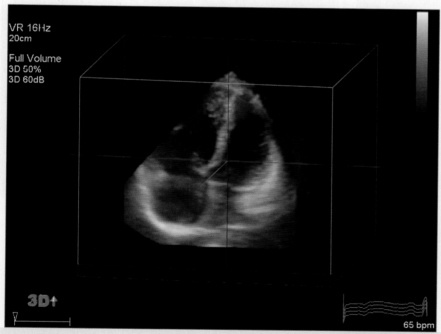

Figure 13-25 Video image in the apical four-chamber view of a patient with idiopathic pulmonary artery hypertension evidenced by the septal bowing to the left. The right ventricle is severely enlarged (volume index = 142.4 mL/m^2), with severely decreased systolic function (ejection fraction = 18%). Left ventricular size is normal (volume index = 93.4 mL/m^2) and function is normal. Biatrial size is severely increased (see Video 13-3).

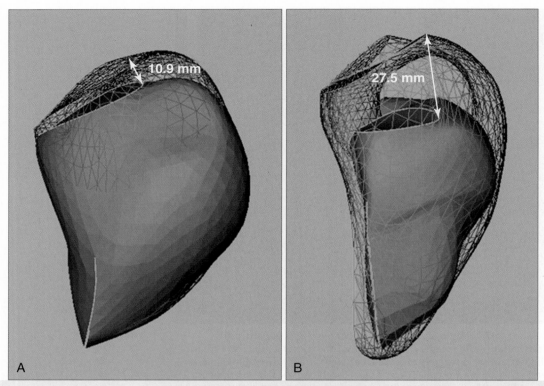

Figure 13-26 Reduced longitudinal contraction in a patient with pulmonary hypertension (**A**) compared with normal (**B**).

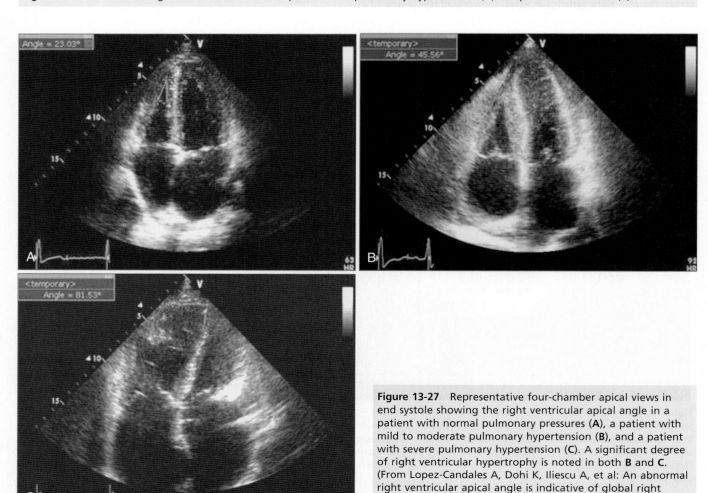

Figure 13-27 Representative four-chamber apical views in end systole showing the right ventricular apical angle in a patient with normal pulmonary pressures (**A**), a patient with mild to moderate pulmonary hypertension (**B**), and a patient with severe pulmonary hypertension (**C**). A significant degree of right ventricular hypertrophy is noted in both **B** and **C**. (From Lopez-Candales A, Dohi K, Iliescu A, et al: An abnormal right ventricular apical angle is indicative of global right ventricular impairment. *Echocardiography* 23:361–368, 2006.)

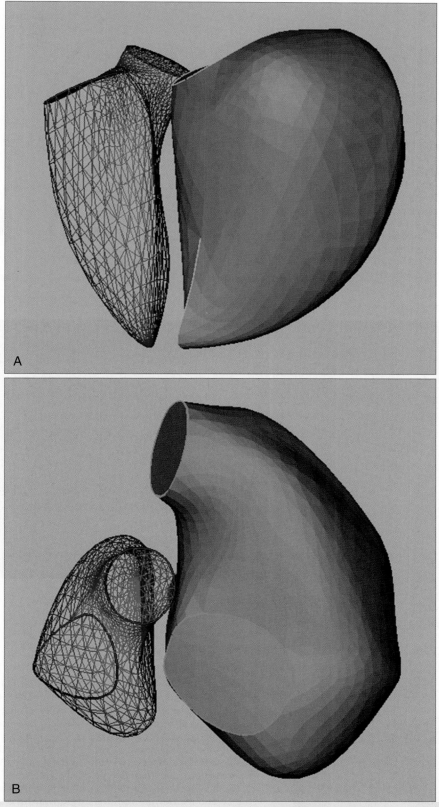

Figure 13-28   The right ventricle (RV) in pulmonary hypertension. **A,** Rounding of the RV as seen from reconstructions of the left ventricle (LV, *red mesh*) and RV (*blue surface*) in the same patient as in Figure 13-3 and in the same orientation. The RV end-diastolic volume index is 134 mL/m², and the ejection fraction is 10%. **B,** Reconstructions of the same patient as seen from the atria looking toward the apex. Septal flattening is clear from the shape of the LV.

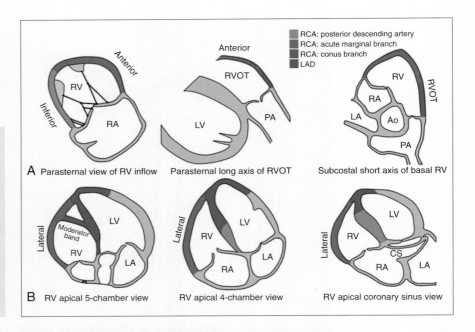

Figure 13-29 Segmental nomenclature of the right ventricular walls, along with their coronary supply. *Ao,* Aorta; *CS,* coronary sinus; *LA,* left atrium; *LAD,* left anterior descending artery; *LV,* left ventricle; *PA,* pulmonary artery; *RA,* right atrium; *RCA,* right coronary artery; *RV,* right ventricle; *RVOT,* right ventricular outflow tract. (From Rudski LG, Lai WW, Afilalo J, et al: Guidelines for the echocardiographic assessment of the right heart in adults: A report from the American Society of Echocardiography. *J Am Soc Echocardiogr* 23:685–713, 2010.)

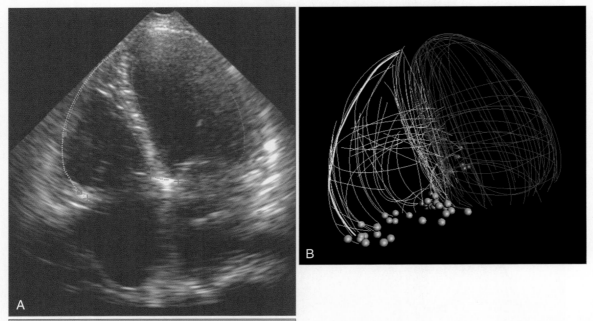

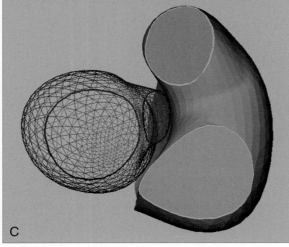

Figure 13-30 The right ventricle (*RV*) in heart failure. **A,** Four-chamber view of a patient with ischemic cardiomyopathy. RV dilation (end-diastolic volume index [*EDVI*] of 122 mL/m² vs. 93 ± 20 mL/m² in normal subjects[63]) is difficult to appreciate visually because the left ventricle (*LV*) is also dilated (EDVI of 89 mL/m² vs. 77 ± 17 mL/m² in normal subjects). **B,** Wire mesh display of the borders of the RV and LV traced from multiple echocardiographic views in the same patient showing that the four-chamber view (*highlighted*) is representative of LV and RV areas. **C,** RV dilation is more evident in three-dimensional reconstructions of the LV and RV viewed from the atria toward the apex. The patient's RV ejection fraction was 35% (normal, 47% ± 8%); LV ejection fraction was 33% (normal, 56% ± 10%). *Ao,* aorta; *CS,* coronary sinus; *LA,* left atrium; *LAD,* left anterior descending artery; *LV,* left ventricle; *PA,* pulmonary artery; *RA,* right atrium; *RCA,* right coronary artery; *RVOT,* right ventricular outflow tract.

References

1. Rudski LG, Lai WW, Afilalo J, et al: Guidelines for the echocardiographic assessment of the right heart in adults: A report from the American Society of Echocardiography. *J Am Soc Echocardiogr* 23:685–713, 2010.

2. Sheehan FH, Ge S, Vick GW, III, et al: Three-dimensional shape analysis of right ventricular remodeling in repaired tetralogy of Fallot. *Am J Cardiol* 101:107–113, 2008.

3. Dodge HT, Sandler H, Ballew DW, Lord JD, Jr: The use of biplane angiocardiography for the measurement of left ventricular volume in man. *Am Heart J* 60:762–776, 1960.

4. Arcilla RA, Tsai P, Thilenius O, Ranniger K: Angiographic method for volume estimation of right and left ventricles. *Chest* 60:446–454, 1971.

5. Fisher EA, DuBrow IW, Hastreiter AR: Right ventricular volume in congenital heart disease. *Am J Cardiol* 36:67–75, 1975.

6. Ferlinz J, Gorlin R, Cohn PF, Herman MW: Right ventricular performance in patients with coronary artery disease. *Circulation* 52:608–615, 1975.

7. Wellnhofer E, Ewart P, Hug J, et al: Evaluation of new software for angiographic determination of right ventricular volumes. *Int J Cardiovasc Imag* 21:575–585, 2005.

8. Sheehan FH, Bolson EL: Measurement of right ventricular volume from contrast ventriculograms: In vitro validation by cast and 3 dimensional echo. *Cathet Cardiovasc Interven* 62:46–51, 2004.

9. Helbing WA, Bosch HG, Maliepaard C, et al: Comparison of echocardiographic methods with magnetic resonance imaging for assessment of right ventricular function in children. *Am J Cardiol* 76:589–594, 1995.

10. Levine RA, Gibson TC, Aretz T, et al: Echocardiographic measurement of right ventricular volume. *Circulation* 69:497–505, 1984.

11. Denslow S: An ellipsoidal shell model for volume estimation of the right ventricle from magnetic resonance images. *Acad Radiol* 1:345–351, 1994.

12. Aebischer N, Meuli R, Jeanrenaud X, et al: An echocardiographic and magnetic resonance imaging comparative study of right ventricular volume determination. *Int J Card Imag* 14:271–278, 1998.

13. Lang RM, Bierig M, Devereux RB, et al: Recommendations for chamber quantification: A report from the American Society of Echocardiography's guidelines and standards committee and the chamber quantification writing group, developed in conjunction with the European Association of Echocardiography, a branch of the European Society of Echocardiography. *J Am Soc Echocardiogr* 18:1440–1463, 2005.

14. Winter MM, Bernink FJP, Groenink M, et al: Evaluating the systemic right ventricle by CMR: the importance of consistent and reproducible delineation of the cavity. *J Cardiovasc Magn Res* 10:40, 2008.

15. Geva T, Powell AJ, Crawford EC, et al: Evaluation of regional differences in right ventricular systolic function by acoustic quantification echocardiography and cine magnetic resonance imaging. *Circulation* 98:339–345, 1998.

16. Edwards R, Shurman AJ, Sahn DJ, et al: Determination of right ventricular end systole by cardiovascular magnetic resonance imaging: A standard method of selection. *Int J Cardiovasc Imag* 25:791–796, 2009.

17. Graham TP, Jarmakani JM, Atwood GF, Canent RV: Right ventricular volume determinations in children: Normal values and observations with volume or pressure overload. *Circulation* 47:144–153, 1973.

18. Gentzler RD, Briselli MF, Gault JH: Angiographic estimation of right ventricular volume in man. *Circulation* 50:324–330, 1974.

19. Boak JG, Bove AA, Kreulen T, Spann JF: A geometric basis for calculation of right ventricular volume in man. *Cathet Cardiovas Diagn* 3:217–230, 1977.

20. Strugnell WE, Slaughter RE, Riley RA, et al: Modified RV short axis series—a new method for cardiac MRI measurement of right ventricular volumes. *J Cardiovasc Magn Res* 7:769–774, 2005.

21. Moroseos T, Mitsumori L, Kerwin WS, et al: Comparison of Simpson's method with three-dimensional reconstruction for measurement of right ventricular volume in patients with complete or corrected transposition of the great arteries. *Am J Cardiol* 105:1603–1609, 2010.

22. Jiang L, de Prada JAV, Handschumacher MD, et al: Three-dimensional echocardiography: In vivo validation for right ventricular free wall mass as an index of hypertrophy. *J Am Coll Cardiol* 23:1715–1722, 1994.

23. Buckey JC, Beattie JM, Nixon JV, et al: Right and left ventricular volumes in vitro by a new nongeometric method. *Am J Cardiac Imag* 1:227–233, 1987.

24. Legget ME, Leotta DF, Bolson EL, et al: System for quantitative three dimensional echocardiography of the left ventricle based on a magnetic field position and orientation sensing system. *IEEE Trans Biomed Eng* 45:494–504, 1998.

25. Hubka M, Bolson EL, McDonald JA, et al: Three-dimensional echocardiographic measurement of left and right ventricular mass and volume: In vitro validation. *Int J Cardiovasc Imag* 18:111–118, 2002.

26. Chen G, Sun K, Huang G: In vitro validation of right ventricular volume and mass measurement by real-time three-dimensional echocardiography. *Echocardiography* 23:395–399, 2006.

27. Lu X, Nadvoretskiy V, Bu L, et al: Accuracy and reproducibility of real-time three dimensional echocardiography for assessment of right ventricular volumes and ejection fraction in children. *J Am Soc Echocardiogr* 21:84–89, 2008.

28. Niemann PS, Pinho L, Balbach T, et al: Anatomically oriented right ventricular volume measurements with dynamic three-dimensional echocardiography validated by 3-tesla magnetic resonance imaging. *J Am Coll Cardiol* 50:1668–1676, 2007.

29. Johnson TR, Hoch M, Huber A, et al: Quantification of right ventricular function in congenital heart disease: Correlation of 3D echocardiography and MRI as complementary methods. *Fortschr Roentgenstr* 178:1014–1021, 2006.

30. Sheehan FH, Kilner P, Sahn D, et al: *Accuracy of right ventricular volume and function analysis in tetralogy of Fallot using Knowledge Based Reconstruction [abstract]*. Presented at the American Heart Association annual meeting, New Orleans, LA, 2008.

31. Fayad ZA, Ferrari VA, Kraitchman DL, et al: Right ventricular regional function using MR tagging: Normals versus chronic pulmonary hypertension. *Magn Reson Med* 39:116–123, 1998.

32. Naito H, Arisawa J, Harada K, et al: Assessment of right ventricular regional contraction and comparison with the left ventricle in normal humans: A cine magnetic resonance study with presaturation myocardial tagging. *Br Heart J* 74:186–191, 1995.

33. Kaul S, Tei C, Hopkins J, Shah P: Assessment of right ventricular function using two-dimensional echocardiography. *Am Heart J* 107:526–531, 1984.

34. Hsiao S-H, Lin S-K, Wang W-C, et al: Severe tricuspid regurgitation shows significant impact in the relationship among peak systolic tricuspid annular velocity, tricuspid annular plane systolic excursion, and right ventricular ejection fraction. *J Am Soc Echocardiogr* 19:902–919, 2006.

35. Smith JL, Bolson EL, Wong SP, et al: Three-dimensional assessment of two-dimensional technique for evaluation of right ventricular function by tricuspid annulus motion. *Int J Card Imag* 19:189–197, 2003.

36. Morcos P, Vick GW, Sahn D, et al: Correlation of right ventricular ejection fraction and tricuspid annular plane systolic excursion in tetralogy of Fallot by magnetic resonance imaging. *Int J Cardiovasc Imaging* 25:263–270, 2008.

37. Kind T, Mauritz G-J, Marcus T, et al: Right ventricular ejection fraction is better reflected by transverse rather than longitudinal wall motion in pulmonary hypertension. *J Cardiovasc Magn Res* 12:35, 2010.

38. Davlouros PA, Kilner PJ, Hornung TS, et al: Right ventricular function in adults with repaired tetralogy of Fallot assessed with cardiovascular magnetic resonance imaging: Detrimental role of right ventricular outflow aneurysms or akinesia and adverse right-to-left ventricular interaction. *J Am Coll Cardiol* 40:2044–2052, 2002.

39. Hui W, El Rahman MYA, Dsebissowa F, et al: Comparison of modified short axis view and apical four chamber view in evaluating right ventricular function after repair of tetralogy of Fallot. *Int J Cardiol* 105:256–261, 2005.

40. Tamborini G, Muratori M, Brusoni D, et al: Is right ventricular systolic function reduced after cardiac surgery? A two- and three-dimensional echocardiographic study. *Eur J Echocardiogr* 10:630–634, 2009.

41. Erbel R, Schweizer P, Lambertz H, et al: Echoventriculography—a simultaneous analysis of two-dimensional echocardiography and cineventriculography. *Circulation* 67:205–215, 1983.

42. King DL, Harrison MR, King DL, Jr, et al: Ultrasound beam orientation during standard two-dimensional imaging: Assessment by three-dimensional echocardiography. *J Am Soc Echocardiogr* 5:569–576, 1992.

43. Dorosz J, Bolson EL, Waiss MS, Sheehan FH: Three-dimensional visual guidance improves the accuracy of calculating right ventricular volume with two-dimensional echocardiography. *J Am Soc Echocardiogr* 16:675–681, 2003.

44. Gustafsson U, Lindqvist P, Waldenstrom A: Apical circumferential motion of the right and left ventricles in healthy subjects described with speckle tracking. *J Am Soc Echocardiogr* 21:1326–1330, 2009.

45. Sheehan FH, Mathey DG, Wygant J, et al: Measurement of regional right ventricular wall motion from biplane contrast angiograms using the centerline method. In *Computers in cardiology*, Long Beach, CA, 1985, IEEE Computer Society, pp 149–152.

46. Nakasato M, Akiba T, Sato S, et al: Right and left ventricular function assessed by regional wall motion analysis in patients with tetralogy of Fallot. *Int J Cardiol* 58:127–134, 1997.

47. Yang P, Otto C, Sheehan F: The effect of normalization in reducing variability in regional wall thickening. *J Am Soc Echocardiogr* 10:197–204, 1997.

48. Tulevski, II, Zijta FM, Smeijers AS, et al: Regional and global right ventricular dysfunction in asymptomatic or minimally symptomatic patients with congenitally corrected transposition. *Cardiol Young* 14:168–174, 2004.

49. Haber I, Metaxas DN, Geva T, Axel L: Three-dimensional systolic kinematics of the right ventricle. *Am J Physiol* 289:H1826–H1833, 2005.

50. Klein SS, Graham TPJ, Lorenz CH: Noninvasive delineation of normal right ventricular contractile motion with magnetic resonance imaging myocardial tagging. *Ann Biomed Eng* 26:756–763, 1998.

51. Young AA, Fayad ZA, Axel L: Right ventricular midwall surface motion and deformation using magnetic resonance tagging. *Am J Physiol* 271:H2677–H2688, 1996.

52. Menteer J, Weinberg PM, Fogel MA: Quantifying regional right ventricular function in tetralogy of Fallot. *J Cardiovasc Magn Res* 7:753–761, 2005.

53. Bodhey NK, Beerbaum P, Sarikouch S, et al: Functional analysis of the components of the right ventricle in the setting of Tetralogy *of Fallot. Circ Cardiovasc Imag* 1:141–147, 2008.

54. Wald RM, Haber I, Wald R, et al: Effects of regional dysfunction and late gadolinium enhancement on global right ventricular function and exercise capacity in patients with repaired tetralogy of Fallot. *Circulation* 119:1370–1377, 2009.

55. Yoerger DM, Marcus F, Sherrill D, et al: Echocardiographic findings in patients meeting Task Force criteria for arrhythmogenic right ventricular dysplasia. *J Am Coll Cardiol* 45:860–865, 2005.

56. Bomma C, Dal D, Tandri H, et al: Regional differences in systolic and diastolic function in arrhythmogenic right ventricular dysplasia/cardiomyopathy using magnetic resonance imaging. *Am J Cardiol* 95:1507–1511, 2005.

57. Dodge HT, Frimer M, Stewart DK: Functional evaluation of the hypertrophied heart in man. *Circ Res* 34-35(Suppl II):II-122–II-127, 1974.

58. McCulloch AD: Cardiac biomechanics. In Bronzino JD, editor: *Biomedical engineering handbook*, Boca Raton, FL, 1995, CRC Press, pp 149–152.

59. McCulloch AD, Omens JH: Factors affecting the regional mechanics of the diastolic heart. In Glass L, Hunter R, Mcculloch AD, editors: *Theory of heart: Biomechanics, biophysics, and nonlinear dynamics of cardiac function*, New York, 1991, Springer-Verlag, pp 87–119.

60. King ME, Braun H, Goldblatt A, et al: Interventricular septal configuration as a predictor of right ventricular systolic hypertension in children: A cross-sectional echocardiographic study. *Circulation* 68:68–75, 1983.

61. Young AA, Orr R, Smaill BH, Dell'Italia LJ: Three-dimensional changes in left and right ventricular geometry in chronic mitral regurgitation. *Am J Physiol* 271:H2689–H2700, 1996.

62. Zhang H, Thomas MT, Walker NE, et al: Four-dimensional functional analysis of left and right ventricles using MR images and active appearance models. *IEEE Trans Med Imag* 29:350–363, 2007.

63. Clark TJ, Sheehan FH, Bolson EL: Characterizing the normal heart using quantitative three-dimensional echocardiography. *Physiol Meas* 27:467–508, 2006.

64. Weyman AE, Wann S, Feigenbaum H, Dillon JC: Mechanism of abnormal septal motion in patients with right ventricular overload: a cross-sectional echocardiographic study. *Circulation* 54:179–186, 1976.

65. Lopez-Candales A, Dohi K, Iliescu A, et al: An abnormal right ventricular apical angle is indicative of global right ventricular impairment. *Echocardiography* 23:361–368, 2006.

66. Kurtz CE, Sheehan FH: Characterization of right ventricular shape and function in pulmonary hypertension with 3D-echocardiography [abstract]. *J Am Soc Echocardiogr* 23:B-68, 2010.

67. Mauritz G-J, Kind T, Marcus JT, et al: Progressive changes in right ventricular geometric shortening and long-term survival in pulmonary arterial hypertension. *Chest* 141(4):935–943, 2011.

68. Laster SB, Shelton TJ, Barzilai B, Goldstein JA: Determinants of the recovery of right ventricular performance following experimental chronic right coronary artery occlusion. *Circulation* 88:696–708, 1993.

69. Goldstein JA: Right heart ischemia: Pathophysiology, natural history, and clinical management. *Prog Cardiovasc Dis* 40:325–341, 1998.

70. Sukmawan R, Akasaka T, Watanabe N, et al: Quantitative assessment of right ventricular geometric remodeling in pulmonary hypertension secondary to left-sided heart disease using real-time three-dimensional echocardiography. *Am J Cardiol* 94:1096–1099, 2004.

71. Berkowitz R, Alhaj E, Manchikalapudi RB, et al: Determinants of right ventricular failure in patients admitted with acute left heart failure. *Congest Heart Fail* 16:243–248, 2010.

72. Guglin M, Verma S: Right side of heart failure. *Heart Fail Rev* 17(3):511–527, 2012.

73. Hesse B, Asher CR: Time to move to the right: The study of right ventricular performance: Too long neglected. *Clin Cardiol* 28:8–12, 2005.

74. John R, Lee S, Eckman P, Liao K: Right ventricular failure—a continuing problem in patients with left ventricular assist device support. *J Cardiovasc Transl Res* 3:604–611, 2010.

75. Maslow AD, Regan MM, Panzica P, et al: Precardiopulmonary bypass right ventricular function is associated with poor outcome after coronary artery bypass grafting in patients with severe left ventricular systolic dysfunction. *Anesth Analg* 95:1507–1518, 2002.

Guidance of Catheter-Based Cardiac Interventions

Nicole M. Bhave and Roberto M. Lang

Over the past 2 decades, percutaneous interventions for structural heart disease have become increasingly common. Interventional cardiologists are now treating a variety of lesions that previously required surgery, and these interventions have become more technically complex over time. Although fluoroscopy, two-dimensional transesophageal echocardiography (2DTEE), and intracardiac echocardiography (ICE) are most typically used for procedural guidance, real-time three-dimensional TEE (RT3DTEE) offers several important advantages over these modalities (**Figure 14-1**).[1]

First and foremost, RT3DTEE represents the anatomy and pathology of interest in an intuitive manner. Although the echocardiographer's expertise is required for image acquisition, those with relatively little training in cardiac imaging can understand 3DTEE images with little difficulty. For example, simultaneous visualization of all six mitral valve scallops is possible in one view in the vast majority of patients, making RT3DTEE ideal for transcutaneous mitral valve repair using the Mitra Clip device (Abbott Vascular, Abbott Park, IL).[2-4] In this procedure, the "clip" is delivered to the left atrium via transseptal puncture. RT3DTEE can facilitate this portion of the procedure by demonstrating tenting of the interatrial septum, allowing optimal positioning of the Brockenbrough needle for the septal puncture. For this particular procedure, it is optimal to be slightly superior and posterior to the center of the fossa ovalis. Once the mitral valve clip has been passed into the left atrium, it must then be positioned perpendicular to the line of leaflet coaptation, in the center of the valvular orifice. The clip is deployed to grasp the A2 and P2 scallops. Because spatial relationships on RT3DTEE closely mirror the actual anatomy, an interventionalist can use RT3DTEE to guide catheter movements, verify device placement, and confirm that the mitral valve orifice has been appropriately cleaved in two (**Figures 14-2 to 14-8; Videos 14-1 and 14-2**).

RT3DTEE is invaluable in preprocedural planning, particularly when device sizing is a concern. For instance, when a device must be selected for atrial septal defect (ASD), ventricular septal defect (VSD), or patent foramen ovale closure, 3DTEE can provide a true en face view of the defect so that its dimensions can be accurately measured. Such a defect often is elliptical or fenestrated such that 2D imaging cannot fully capture its complex shape.[5] Furthermore, the relationship of a defect to vital structures such as the aortic root (in ASD closure) or mitral valve (in VSD closure) is easier to appreciate on RT3DTEE. This may help the interventionalist avoid complications during device deployment (**Figure 14-9**).

Because RT3DTEE can accurately characterize orifice areas and shapes, it also is well suited for catheter-based left atrial appendage (LAA) closure. RT3DTEE allows optimal visualization of the LAA in the vast majority of patients. 2DTEE tends to underestimate orifice area values, but RT3DTEE findings were shown to correlate well with computed tomography in one small study.[6] Accurate device sizing and positioning are critical

Text continued on page 269

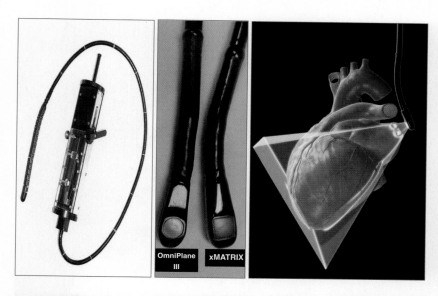

Figure 14-1   The first three-dimensional transesophageal echocardiography (3DTEE) probe, termed the "lobster" (*left*), had multiple piezoelectric crystals distributed along its length that obtained images as the probe was withdrawn from the esophagus. The subsequent OmniPlane III probe (Philips Healthcare, Andover, MA) (*middle, left*) required a rotational technique for sequential data acquisition, followed by offline processing. The xMATRIX TEE (*MTEE*) probe (Philips Healthcare) (*middle, right*) allows rapid, automated acquisition and display of 3D images in real time. In full-volume mode, the matrix TEE probe can be used to visualize the left ventricle, as shown (*right*). The zoom mode allows more detailed imaging of structures such as valves and the left atrial appendage.

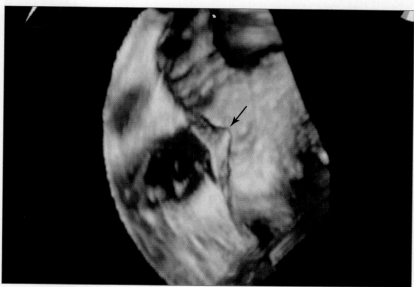

Figure 14-2   Real-time three-dimensional transesophageal echocardiography can be used to guide interatrial septal puncture, a technique commonly required for percutaneous electrophysiologic and valvular procedures. Tenting of the interatrial septum by the needle (*arrow*) confirms that the needle is passing appropriately from the right atrium to the left atrium (see Video 14-1).

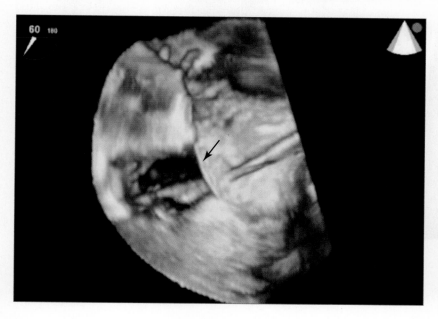

Figure 14-3   Shown is a continuation of the procedure in Figure 14-2. The catheter can then safely traverse the interatrial septum (*arrow*) to gain access to the left atrium, the mitral valve, or both. In Video 14-2, it is clear that two catheters are present.

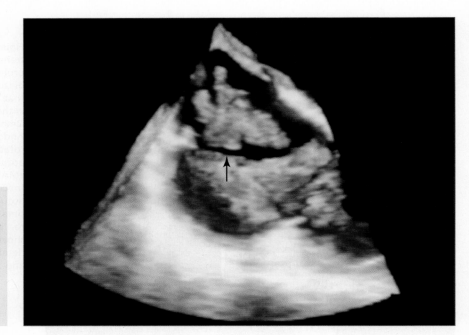

Figure 14-4 In lengthy catheter-based procedures, thrombus formation on the tip of the catheter can have significant adverse consequences, such as myocardial infarction and stroke. Thrombi attached to catheters, such as the one seen here (*arrow*), often are easier to appreciate with three-dimensional transesophageal echocardiography compared with two-dimensional echocardiography.

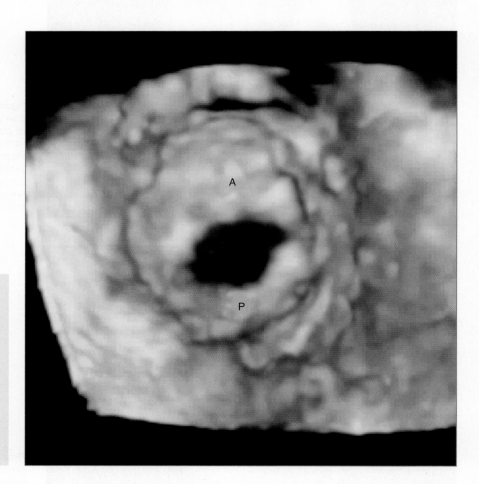

Figure 14-5 Visualization of the mitral valve leaflets is more intuitive with three-dimensional echocardiography than with two-dimensional echocardiography. In the left atrial, or "surgeon's" view, the anterior leaflet (*A*) and posterior leaflet (*P*) are clearly seen as distinct structures. In this example of rheumatic mitral stenosis, commissural fusion and reduced leaflet excursion can be appreciated. For accurate quantitation of the mitral orifice area, real-time three-dimensional transesophageal echocardiography is the method of choice.

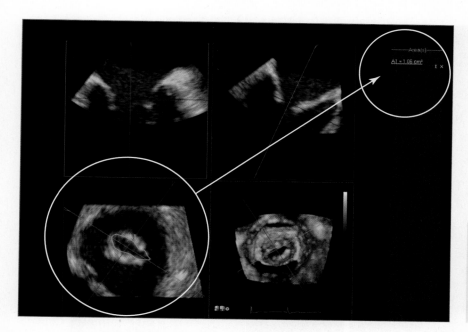

Figure 14-6 The use of multiplanar reconstruction allows accurate measurement of the mitral orifice area. With real-time three-dimensional echocardiography, it is possible to perform planimetry truly at the tips of the mitral valve leaflets in the zoom mode, en face view (*bottom right*).

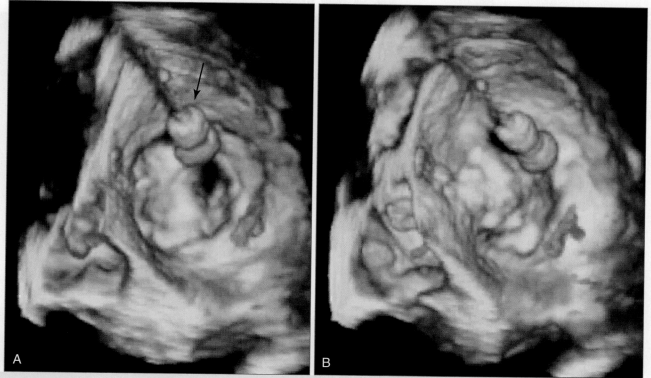

Figure 14-7 A, In percutaneous balloon mitral valvuloplasty, an hourglass-shaped Inoue balloon (*arrow*) is used. This series of images from the left atrial view shows the balloon before it crosses the valve (**A** and **B**), as it crosses the valve from left atrium to right ventricle (**C** and **D**), during inflation (**E**), and immediately following inflation (**F**). (Courtesy Dr. Vahanian and Dr. Brochet, Bichat Hospital, Paris.)

Continued

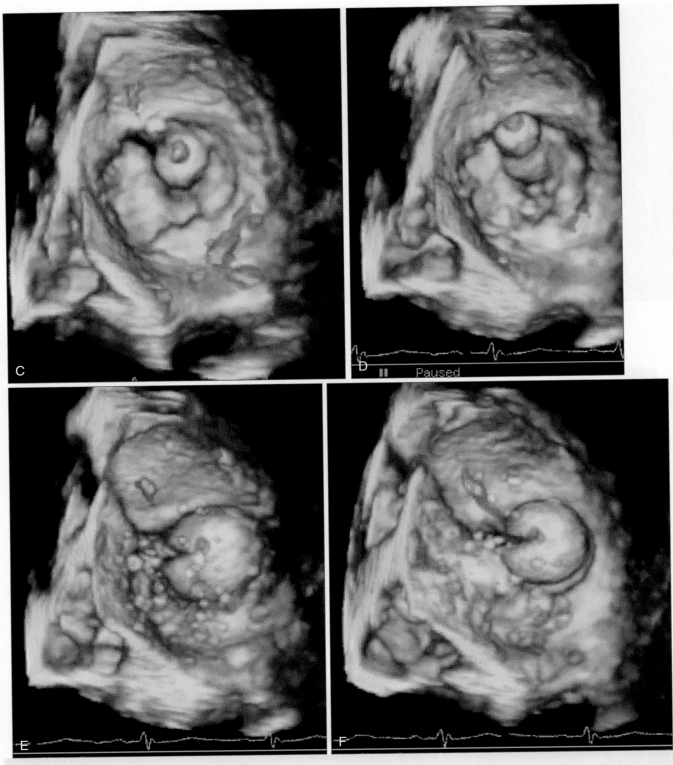

Figure 14-7, cont'd

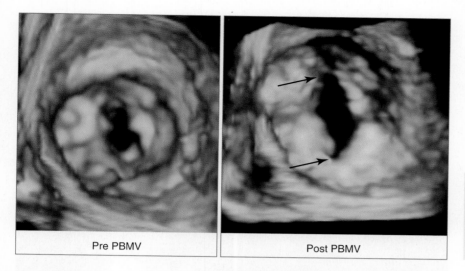

Pre PBMV

Post PBMV

Figure 14-8 After percutaneous balloon mitral valvuloplasty (*PBMV*), the mitral valve orifice is clearly larger. The *arrows* indicate the splitting of the commissures. (Courtesy Dr. Vahanian and Dr. Brochet, Bichat Hospital, Paris.)

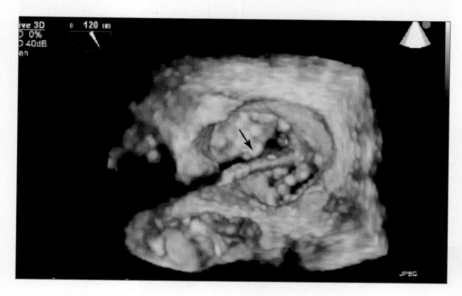

Figure 14-9 Percutaneous mitral valve repair, performed for severe mitral regurgitation, requires catheter-based delivery of a clip that grasps both valve leaflets. In this left atrial view, the clip delivery catheter (*arrow*) passes through the mitral valve orifice. Performance of this percutaneous procedure has been greatly facilitated by the use of real-time three-dimensional transesophageal echocardiography. (Courtesy Dr. Kronzon, Lennox Hill Hospital, New York.)

in this procedure to avoid complications such as device embolization, stroke, and hemopericardium from appendage laceration. RT3DTEE is used to guide transseptal puncture, catheter manipulation in the left atrium, and device deployment. Prior to the conclusion of the procedure, RT3DTEE confirms stability of the device.

Perhaps the most spatially complex lesions addressed in the catheterization laboratory are periprosthetic valvular leaks. Dehiscence of a mitral valve annuloplasty ring or prosthesis, for instance, often results in a single elliptical defect, but multiple defects also may be present. Before starting such an intervention, a thorough evaluation of the relationship between the mitral annulus and the implant is essential to identify the site of the largest defect and the most significant periprosthetic regurgitation. In this setting, RT3DTEE provides significant additional detail that 2DTEE cannot.[7,8] During the intervention, RT3DTEE facilitates positioning of wires, catheters, and the closure device. In a patient with a mechanical valve, this modality can help ensure that device deployment does not restrict prosthetic disk motion. Finally, RT3DTEE can be used to reevaluate mitral regurgitation at the conclusion of the intervention. In summary, transcatheter repair of periprosthetic regurgitation is very difficult, if not impossible, to perform effectively without the use of RT3DTEE guidance (**Figures 14-10** to **14-16; Video 14-3**).

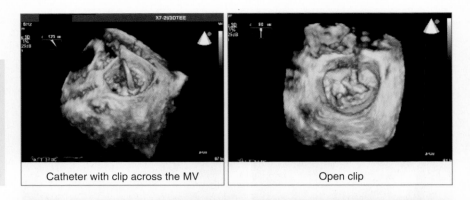

Catheter with clip across the MV | Open clip

Figure 14-10 Before clip deployment, three-dimensional transesophageal echocardiography facilitates clip positioning perpendicular to the line of leaflet coaptation (*right*). This ensures that the clip can simultaneously grasp the anterior and posterior leaflets. *MV,* mitral valve. (Courtesy Dr. Kronzon, Lennox Hill Hospital, New York.)

Figure 14-11 On two-dimensional transesophageal echocardiography with color Doppler in the apical long-axis view, dehiscence of a mechanical mitral valve prosthesis is suggested by the echo-free space between the valve leaflets and the native annulus (**A,** *arrow*) as well as an eccentric mitral regurgitation jet external to the ring (**B**). With two-dimensional echocardiography, it is difficult to define the true location and extent of the prosthetic dehiscence.

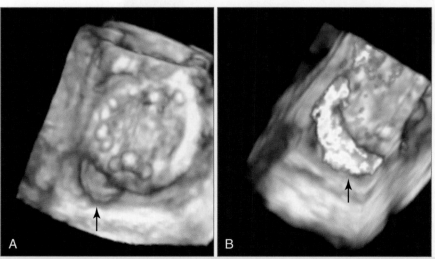

Figure 14-12 In this zoom mode, three-dimensional transesophageal echocardiography image from the left atrial view, the precise location of a mechanical mitral valve dehiscence—in this case, at the posterolateral aspect of the annulus—can be appreciated (**A,** *arrow*). Color Doppler confirms the presence of mitral regurgitation at this site (**B,** *arrow*). Interestingly, most mitral valve dehiscences occur along the posterior aspect of the annulus. There are two potential explanations for this phenomenon. First, the anteriorly located aortic-mitral curtain, a fibrous structure providing continuity between the anterior mitral valve leaflet and the aortic valve in the roof of the left ventricle, serves as a secure anchor for the anterior aspect of the valve. The posterior aspect of the annulus, in contrast, contains more adipose tissue. Second, because the left circumflex coronary artery is close to the posterior aspect of the annulus, it is technically difficult to suture the corresponding portion of the valve securely without damaging the artery (see Video 14-3).

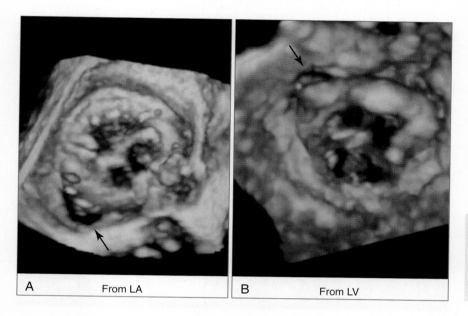

A From LA	**B** From LV

Figure 14-13 This mitral valve annuloplasty ring, seen on three-dimensional transesophageal echocardiography from the left atrial (*LA*) (**A**) and left ventricular (*LV*) (**B**) views, is dehisced along its posterolateral aspect (*arrows*).

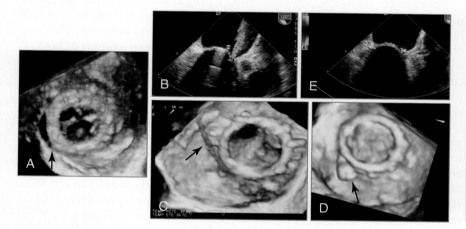

Figure 14-14 Percutaneous repair of this bioprosthetic mitral valve dehiscence is guided by three-dimensional transesophageal echocardiography (3DTEE). The site of dehiscence is along the posterior aspect (**A**). Whereas conventional two-dimensional (2D) TEE with color Doppler demonstrates periprosthetic mitral regurgitation (**B**), the precise location and extent of the dehiscence is best appreciated with 3DTEE, which can guide placement of an interventional catheter within the area of dehiscence (**C**, *arrow*). After placement of an Amplatzer (St. Jude Medical, St. Paul, MN) occluder device (**D**, *arrow*), the mitral regurgitation is considerably lessened (**E**). (Courtesy Dr. Garcia Fernandez.)

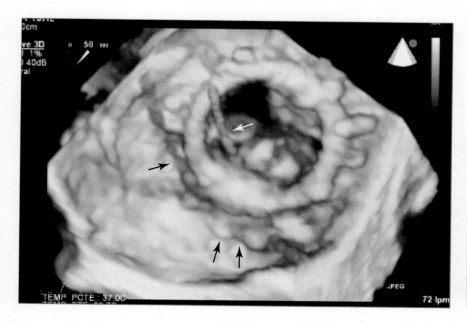

Figure 14-15 This bioprosthetic mitral valve, visualized from the left atrium on zoom mode three-dimensional (3D) transesophageal echocardiography (TEE), is dehisced posteriorly (*double arrow*). With live 3D imaging guidance, interventional catheters have been placed within the valve orifice (*white arrow*) and through the site of dehiscence (*single black arrow*). With two-dimensional TEE or fluoroscopy, this would be an extremely difficult task, even if biplane imaging were used. (Courtesy Dr. Garcia Fernandez.)

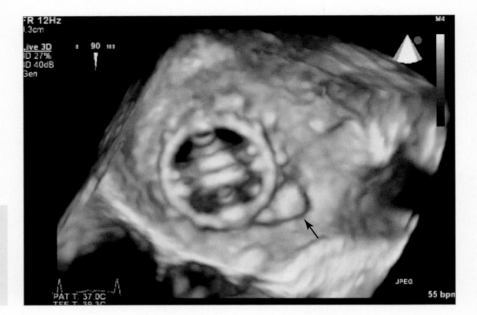

Figure 14-16 This mechanical bileaflet valve, visualized from the left atrium at mid-diastole, was dehisced along its posterior aspect and has been repaired by percutaneous placement of an Amplatzer device (St. Jude Medical, St. Paul, MN) (*arrow*). (Courtesy Dr. Garcia Fernandez.)

Immediately following any catheter-based intervention, RT3DTEE can be used to confirm procedural success. After a device is deployed, it can be examined in multiple views while the patient is still in the interventional suite. This may obviate the need for follow-up imaging studies, repeat intervention, or both. If subsequent imaging is indicated on the basis of changes in clinical status or concerns regarding device stability, subsequent 3D transthoracic echocardiography (3DTTE) may be performed, and the images may be compared with those obtained during the procedure.

In addition to interventions for structural heart disease, RT3DTEE also shows promise for guidance of catheter-based arrhythmia ablation. In pulmonary vein isolation for atrial fibrillation, RT3DTEE can identify the orifices of the veins and confirm appropriate catheter tip placement. Unlike 2DTEE or ICE, it clearly demonstrates the relationship of the catheters to the endocardial surface. With RT3DTEE, it often is possible to see the entire length of a catheter within a region of interest, facilitating precise catheter manipulation (**Figures 14-17 to 14-32**).[9] The utility of RT3DTEE in electrophysiologic procedures is an area that deserves further study.

Because image acquisition is relatively rapid with current technology, RT3DTEE does not appear to lengthen procedure times. One small, retrospective study of interatrial communication closures found that RT3DTEE, when added to 2DTEE, was associated with a reduction in fluoroscopy times.[10] In a catheterization laboratory where many complex interventions are performed, such a finding could translate into a meaningful reduction in radiation exposure for staff and patients.

RT3DTEE imaging requires a multiplane TEE probe, which also is capable of 2D imaging, so no probe exchange is required during a procedure. Typically, the echocardiographer uses 2D imaging to find the appropriate window, then switches to 3D full-volume mode for initial 3D imaging. Cardiac structures of interest can then be selectively examined with zoom mode imaging. Compared with ICE, TEE requires additional sedation for patient comfort and closer airway monitoring, but it does not require placement of a large-bore intravenous catheter, potentially reducing the risk of bleeding complications. Furthermore, the TEE probe is reusable, whereas an ICE catheter is single use and quite costly.

Current limitations of RT3DTEE include motion artifacts, which are worsened by respiratory motion; tissue dropout, which can result in blurred images;

Text continued on page 279

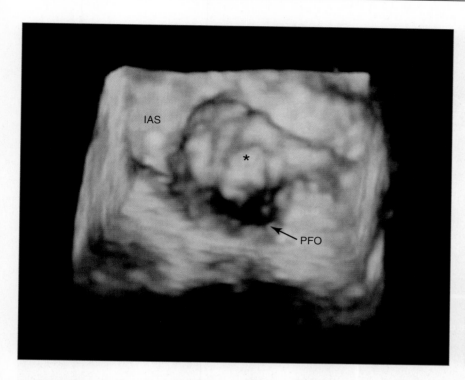

Figure 14-17 Real-time three-dimensional, zoom mode transesophageal echocardiography provides an en face view of this patent foramen ovale (*PFO, arrow*) from the left atrium. The flap of the septum secundum (*asterisk*) is partially in contact with the septum primum, but a defect remains. *IAS*, interatrial septum.

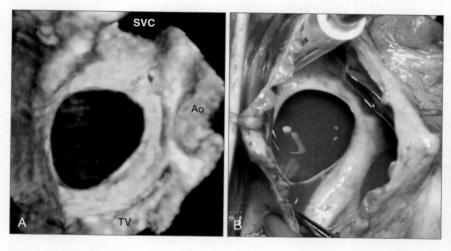

Figure 14-18 In the assessment of this large ostium secundum atrial septal defect, three-dimensional transesophageal echocardiography (**A**) closely replicates the surgeon's view from the right atrium (**B**). *Ao*, aorta; *SVC*, superior vena cava; *TV*, tricuspid valve.

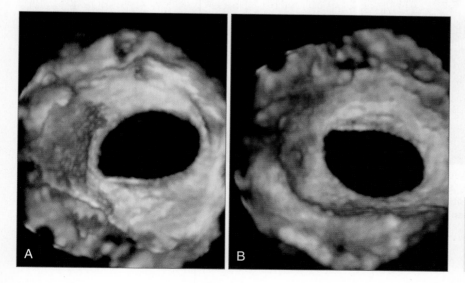

Figure 14-19 This ostium secundum atrial septal defect can be viewed from either the right (**A**) or left atrial (**B**) view with three-dimensional transesophageal echocardiography in zoom mode.

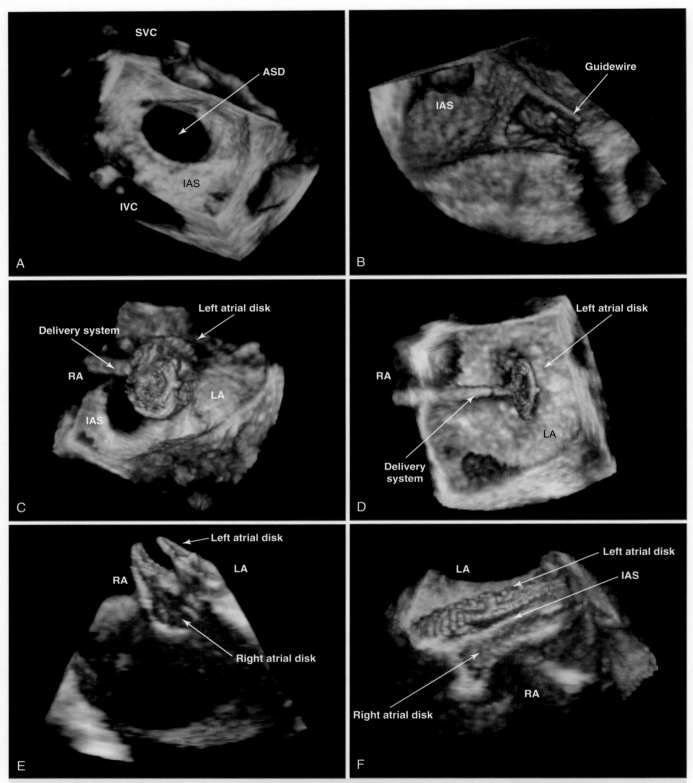

Figure 14-20 Real-time three-dimensional transesophageal echocardiography guidance assists in initial visualization of the atrial septal defect (*ASD*) from the right atrium (*RA*, **A**), passage of a guidewire (**B**) and occluder delivery catheter (**C**) through the defect, deployment of the left atrial disk (**D**), and positioning (**E**) and deployment (**F**) of the right atrial disk. With this method, good apposition of both disks with the interatrial septum (*IAS*) can be confirmed before the end of the procedure. *IVC*, inferior vena cava; *LA*, left atrium; *SVC*, superior vena cava.

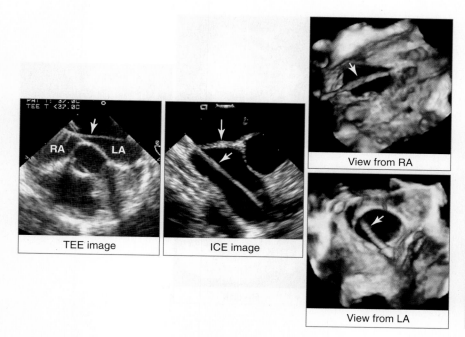

View from RA

View from LA

TEE image

ICE image

Figure 14-21 In this modified four-chamber two-dimensional transesophageal echocardiography (TEE) image (*left*), the guide catheter (*arrow*) crosses the interatrial septum from the right atrium (*RA*) to the left atrium (*LA*). Intracardiac echocardiography (*ICE, middle*) also demonstrates this (*upper arrow*, interatrial septum; *lower arrow*, guide catheter). However, only real-time three-dimensional TEE (*right, top* and *bottom*) clearly demonstrates that the guide catheter (*arrows*) is truly crossing through the atrial septal defect.

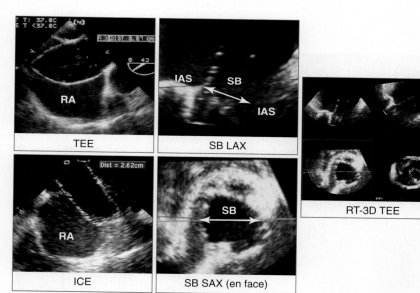

TEE

SB LAX

ICE

SB SAX (en face)

RT-3D TEE

Figure 14-22 Sizing balloons (*SB*) typically are used to evaluate atrial septal defect dimensions before selection of an appropriately sized Amplatzer occluder device (St. Jude Medical, St. Paul, MN). With two-dimensional transesophageal echocardiography (TEE) (modified bicaval view, *top left*) and intracardiac echocardiography (*ICE, lower left*), the sizing balloon is viewed obliquely, as in the real-time three-dimensional (3D) TEE long-axis (*LAX*) view (*middle, top*). Only the 3DTEE short-axis (*SAX*) view from the right atrium (*middle, bottom*) clearly depicts the true diameter of the balloon, allowing for more accurate Amplatzer sizing. It is also possible to calculate the volume of an atrial septal defect using full-volume acquisition with offline processing and specialized quantitative software (*right*). *IAS*, interatrial septum; *RA*, right atrium.

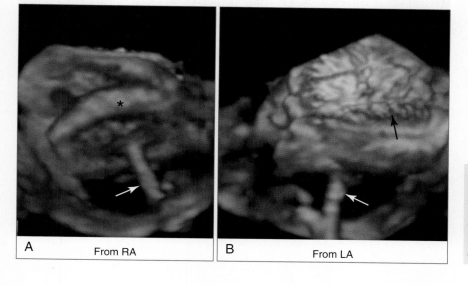

A   From RA

B   From LA

Figure 14-23 Appropriate positioning of the right atrial (*RA*) disk (**A,** *asterisk*) and left atrial (*LA*) disk (**B,** *black arrow*) can be confirmed by real-time three-dimensional transesophageal echocardiography prior to removal of the delivery catheter (*white arrows*).

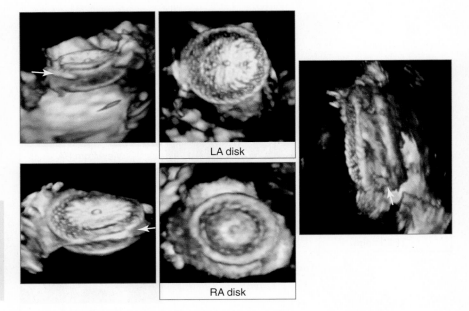

LA disk

RA disk

Figure 14-24 Real-time three-dimensional transesophageal echocardiography in multiple views demonstrating good apposition of both disks of the Amplatzer device (St. Jude Medical, St. Paul, MN) with the interatrial septum (*arrows*). *LA,* left atrial; *RA,* right atrial.

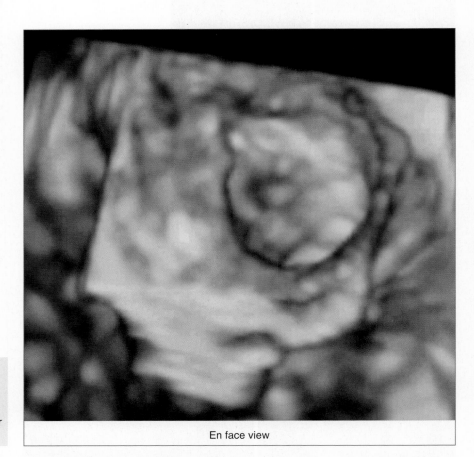

En face view

Figure 14-25 Before percutaneous closure of the left atrial appendage (LAA), this zoom mode real-time three-dimensional transesophageal echocardiography image allows quantification of LAA dimensions for proper device sizing.

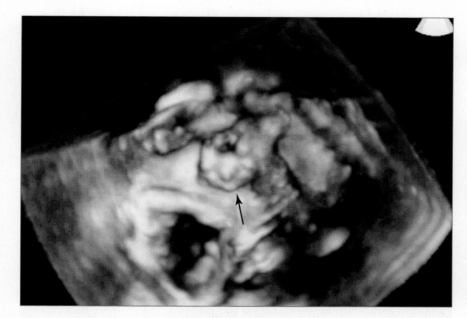

Figure 14-26 As in percutaneous mitral valve repair, real-time three-dimensional transesophageal echocardiography is an excellent means of guiding transseptal puncture and visualizing catheter placement for a percutaneous left atrial appendage (LAA) occlusion procedure. After deployment of an LAA occluder device (*arrow*), this view from the left atrium demonstrates appropriate device position. Superimposed color Doppler also may be used to confirm the absence of communication between the LAA and the left atrium.

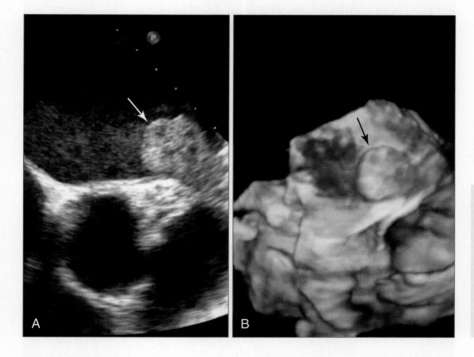

Figure 14-27 A large left atrial appendage (LAA) thrombus is seen on this two-dimensional transesophageal echocardiography (TEE) image (**A**, *arrow*), along with spontaneous echocardiographic contrast in the left atrium suggesting stasis. With real-time three-dimensional TEE (**B**, *arrow*), it is easier to appreciate the volume of the thrombus. This is an example of a complication of percutaneous closure of the LAA.

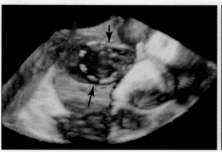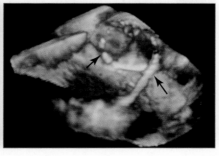

Figure 14-28 Real-time three-dimensional transesophageal echocardiography can be used to guide the positioning of a lasso catheter (*arrows*) at the site of the right upper pulmonic vein prior to an atrial fibrillation ablation procedure.

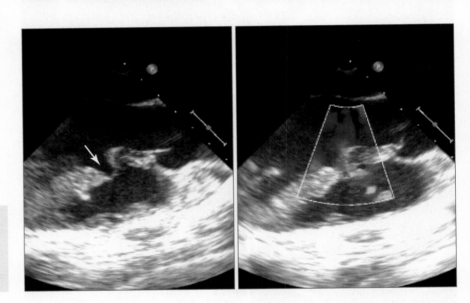

Figure 14-29 A large thrombus is noted in a dilated pulmonic vein by two-dimensional (**A**) and three-dimensional (**B**) echocardiography. Note the ridge separating the pulmonic vein from the left atrial appendage (*arrows*).

Figure 14-30 These two-dimensional transesophageal echocardiography images show thinning of the interventricular septum (*arrow*) and color flow across the septum consistent with a muscular ventricular septal defect.

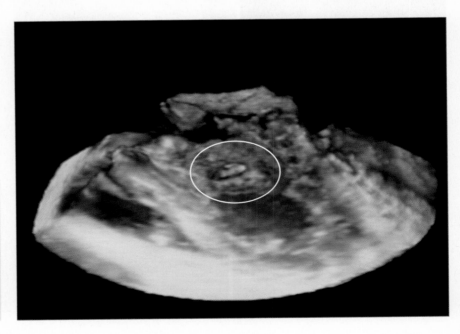

Figure 14-31 This real-time three-dimensional transesophageal echocardiography zoom mode image, obtained from the mid-esophageal window, shows the ventricular septal defect (VSD) in Figure 14-30 en face (*oval*) from the left ventricle. It is possible to measure the VSD's dimensions precisely to facilitate selection of a repair device. Color Doppler could be used to illustrate flow across the defect.

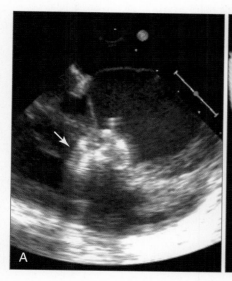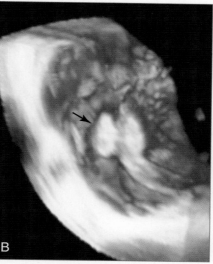

Figure 14-32 Deployment of a ventricular septal defect closure device can be guided by real-time three-dimensional (3D) transesophageal echocardiography (TEE). A two-dimensional TEE four-chamber image (**A**) shows the closure device, but the right ventricular half of the device (*arrow*) appears somewhat hazy, making it difficult to determine whether it is appropriately deployed. With 3DTEE, the edge of the device is clearly delineated (**B**, *arrow*).

and visual delay with moving structures. Anterior cardiac structures, such as the tricuspid and aortic valves, may be less well visualized than more posterior structures, such as the mitral valve and left atrial appendage.[4] Larger, controlled trials are needed to determine definitively whether RT3DTEE can improve procedural outcomes.

References

1. Perk G, Lang RM, Garcia-Fernandez MA, et al: Use of real-time three-dimensional transesophageal echocardiography in intracardiac catheter based interventions. *J Am Soc Echocardiogr* 22:865–882, 2009.
2. Sugeng L, Shernan SK, Salgo IS, et al: Live 3-dimensional transesophageal echocardiography initial experience using the fully-sampled matrix array probe. *J Am Coll Cardiol* 52:446–449, 2008.
3. Lee PW, Lam YY, Yip GWK, et al: Role of real-time three-dimensional transesophageal echocardiography in guidance of interventional procedures in cardiology. *Heart* 96(18):1485–1493, 2010.
4. Altiok E, Becker M, Hamada S, et al: Optimized guidance of percutaneous edge-to-edge repair of the mitral valve using real-time 3-D transesophageal echocardiography. *Clin Res Cardiol* 100(8):675–681, 2011.
5. Lodato JA, Cao QL, Weinert L, et al: Feasibility of real-time three-dimensional transoesophageal echocardiography for guidance of percutaneous atrial septal defect closure. *Eur J Echocardiogr* 10:543–548, 2009.
6. Shah SJ, Bardo DM, Sugeng L, et al: Real time three-dimensional transesophageal echocardiography of the left atrial appendage: Initial experience in the clinical setting. *J Am Soc Echocardiogr* 21:1362–1368, 2008.
7. Kronzon K, Sugeng L, Perk G, et al: Real-time 3-dimensional transesophageal echocardiography in the evaluation of postoperative mitral annuloplasty ring and prosthetic valve dehiscence. *J Am Coll Cardiol* 53:1543–1547, 2009.
8. Kim MS, Casserly IP, Garcia JA, et al: Percutaneous transcatheter closure of prosthetic mitral paravalvular leaks: Are we there yet? *J Am Coll Cardiol Interven* 2:81–90, 2009.
9. Yang HS, Srivathsan K, Wissner E, Chandrasekaran K: Images in cardiovascular medicine: Real-time 3-dimensional transesophageal echocardiography: Novel utility in atrial fibrillation ablation with a prosthetic mitral valve. *Circulation* 117:e304–e305, 2008.
10. Balzer J, van Hall S, Rassaf T, et al: Feasibility, safety, and efficacy of real-time three-dimensional echocardiography for guiding device closure of interatrial communications: Initial clinical experience and impact on radiation exposure. *Eur J Echocardiogr* 11:1–8, 2010.

Congenital Heart Disease

Tara Bharucha and Luc Mertens

In patients with congenital heart disease, a complete and accurate description of the morphologic abnormalities is crucial for determining appropriate management strategies. Currently, two-dimensional echocardiography (2DE) allows a complete description of the intracardiac anatomy of different congenital lesions. Because of its high spatial and temporal resolution, 2DE is still the mainstay technique for the diagnosis and follow-up of patients with congenital defects. However, the representation of a three-dimensional (3D) structure by a 2D technique has intrinsic limitations, which explains why 3DE, particularly real-time (RT) 3DE, has potential applications in congenital heart disease. The development of RT3DE with matrix transducers and a high-frequency pediatric matrix 3D transducer has especially sparked growth and interest in the congenital field. RT3DE has emerged as a valuable additional tool because it provides a direct representation of morphology and volumetric calculations. The real additional diagnostic value still remains to be proven, but recently published data suggest potential use in the following three areas[1]:

1. Improved visualization and understanding of the 3D nature of congenital heart defects
2. Measurement of cardiac mass and volumes
3. Aid in planning and guiding therapeutic interventions

In each of these three areas, RT3DE provides possibly useful additional information that is more difficult to appreciate by 2D imaging alone and can be helpful in clinical management.

THREE-DIMENSIONAL VISUALIZATION OF ANATOMY

Instead of 2D tomographic images, current 3D techniques allow real-time representation of intracardiac structures, which aids in the understanding of cardiac morphology even in simple heart defects. By combining cropping and the multiplanar review modes, the operator can "slice" the heart in an anatomically appropriate plane to view the structures of interest in an appropriate orientation. Views that help in surgical understanding and planning can be created.

Atrial and Ventricular Septa

Atrial and ventricular septal defects typically are not circular "holes," but instead are complex structures, often irregularly shaped or fenestrated, that are difficult to visualize in two dimensions. RT3DE enables improved visualization of septal defects using unique en face representations of the interatrial and interventricular septa. The interatrial septum can be represented as viewed from the left or right atrium and the interventricular septum as viewed from the left or right ventricular side. This allows the creation of surgical views of the defects as well as improved understanding of their shape and relationships to surrounding intracardiac structures. These views also allow a more accurate measurement of defect size, including their dynamic shape change during the cardiac cycle.[2-4] The importance of viewing the

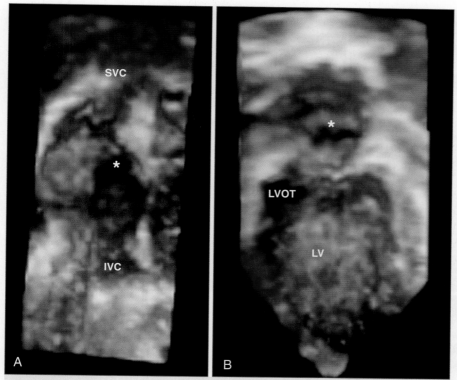

Figure 15-1 **A,** Atrial septal defect viewed from the right atrium. Three-dimensional echocardiography more clearly demonstrates the defect's margins and shape. The *asterisk* notes the septal defect. **B,** Atrial septal defect in a 4-year-old girl. The defect is viewed en face from the left atrial side, demonstrating its irregular margins. Both patients presented with incidental findings of murmurs and were asymptomatic but had significant right ventricular dilation. Both proceeded to elective closure of the defect via cardiac catheterization (see Video 15-1). *IVC,* inferior vena cava; *LV:* left ventricle; *LVOT:* left ventricular outflow tract; *SVC,* superior vena cava.

defects from both sides of the septum cannot be overemphasized; this aids in understanding their anatomy and particularly facilitates the determination of both the right and left border edges and shapes.[5] These measurements are useful for surgical or interventional planning in the catheterization laboratory (**Figures 15-1** and **15-2**; **Videos 15-1** to **15-3**).

Atrioventricular Valves

Transthoracic RT3DE is complementary to 2D transesophageal echocardiography (2DTEE) and 2D transthoracic echocardiography (2DTTE) in detecting anatomic and functional abnormalities of atrioventricular (AV) valves in patients with congenital heart disease.[6-8] This is mainly due to the unique 3D visualization and representation of the AV valves. RT3DE facilitates viewing of the mitral valve with its complex annular shape and interactions with the left ventricular shape and function and the subchordal apparatus.[7,9] RT3DE also facilitates increased understanding of the maturation of the dynamic function of the mitral valve. The mitral valve is saddle shaped, and its motion and dynamic function during the cardiac cycle are complex. In adults, the mitral valve annulus has its largest dimension at end systole and is smallest at end diastole.[10,11] However, RT3DE has demonstrated that in children, the mitral annular motion is somewhat different and that it has its largest area in systole and decreases in diastole.[12,13] The main advantage of 3DE is that the individual scallops of the mitral valve can be imaged in the same view, which helps define the surgical anatomy and enhances communication between the echocardiographer and the surgeon.

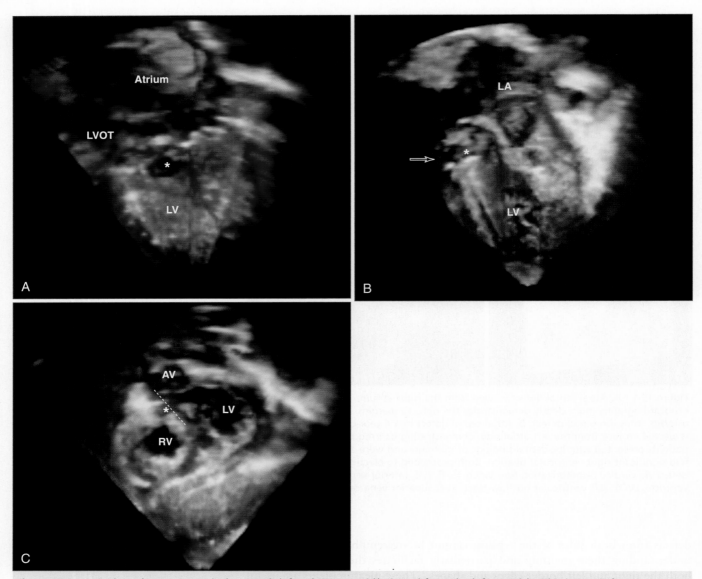

Figure 15-2 **A,** Perimembranous ventricular septal defect (VSD; *asterisk*) viewed from the left ventricle. This image is from a 6-month-old infant who had a routine echocardiogram performed as part of an investigation for dysmorphism with a possible genetic cause. This defect is small and does not cause symptoms or heart failure; a conservative management approach was therefore taken (see Video 15-2). **B,** Perimembranous VSD (*asterisk*) from a 2-year-old boy born prematurely at 34 weeks' gestation who had a murmur detected while in the neonatal unit. This image demonstrates the relationship of the VSD to the tricuspid valve, by which it is partially shrouded (*arrow,* tricuspid valve tissue). The patient was asymptomatic and the VSD restrictive. Surgery is currently not planned (see Video 15-3). **C,** Subcostal view of a VSD (*asterisk*) with partial override of the aortic valve (*AV*) in a 4-month-old infant with tetralogy of Fallot diagnosed after birth. The *dotted line* marks the plane of the ventricular septum. This patient had elective surgical repair at the age of 5 months without complications (see Video 15-4). *LA,* left atrium; *LV,* left ventricle; *LVOT,* left ventricular outflow tract; *RV,* right ventricle.

RT3DE has a clear advantage for imaging the tricuspid valve because the three leaflets are very difficult to view together by cross-sectional imaging. For congenital abnormalities of the tricuspid valve, RT3DE can be useful for a better representation of the valvar anatomy. A typical example is imaging of the tricuspid valve in Ebstein's anomaly. In this lesion, RT3DE can provide better visualization of the morphology of the tricuspid valve leaflets, their attachments, their degree of coaptation, and the mechanism of regurgitation.[14] The multiplanar review mode also facilitates appreciation of the degree of displacement and rotation of the tricuspid valve annulus, which is the key feature of this anomaly.[7] Potentially, RT3DE could also help determine the right ventricular stroke volume,

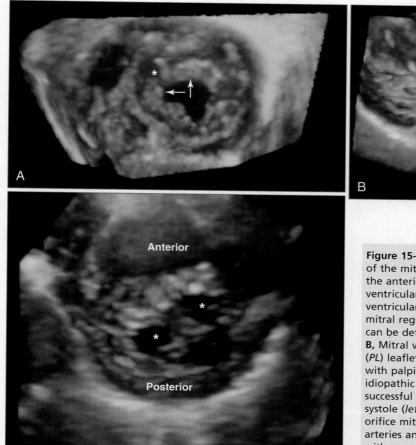

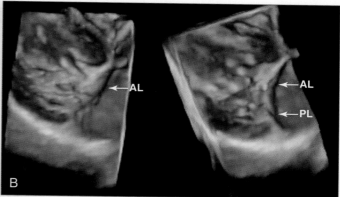

Figure 15-3   A, Isolated cleft (*asterisk*) in the anterior leaflet of the mitral valve. The *arrows* demonstrate the free edges of the anterior leaflet. This patient also had large complex apical ventricular septal defects that were detected antenatally. The ventricular septal defects rapidly became restrictive and the mitral regurgitation was mild and well tolerated, so surgery can be deferred until the child is older (see Video 15-5). **B,** Mitral valve with prolapsing anterior (*AL*) and posterior (*PL*) leaflets from a 12-year-old boy. This patient presented with palpitations of unknown cause. He was found to have idiopathic dysplasia of the mitral valve and underwent successful mitral valve repair. The mitral valve is viewed in systole (*left*) and diastole (*right*) (see Video 15-6). **C,** Double-orifice mitral valve in a patient with transposition of the great arteries and a ventricular septal defect. This patient presented with cyanosis and tachypnea at 1 week of age. The *asterisks* mark the two orifices (see Video 15-7).

although no validation data on right ventricular volumes have been published yet in this disease (**Figures** 15-2 to **15-5; Videos** 15-2 to **15-9**).

Atrioventricular Septal Defects

Patients with AV septal defects have a common AV junction with a single AV valve at the entrance of both ventricles. RT3DE can provide clear visualization of the anatomic variability, which is crucial in the preoperative planning. Studies have demonstrated that RT3DE can provide additional anatomic information to cross-sectional imaging in patients before and after surgical repair.[15-17] In preoperative assessment, the anatomy of the superior and inferior bridging leaflets, as well as that of the left-sided mural leaflet, provides useful clinical information. In postoperative patients with residual AV valve regurgitation, the mechanisms contributing to the regurgitation can be complex, and RT3DE can be useful in clarifying the origin of the regurgitant jets and in guiding surgical decision making by demonstrating defects such as residual cleft, central regurgitation, leaflet prolapse, dysplasia, annular dilation, and so on (**Figures** 15-6 and **15-7; Videos 15-10** to **15-12**).

Outflow Tracts

RT3DE allows accurate anatomic visualization of both left and right outflow tracts and is helpful in defining the mechanisms contributing to complex outflow tract obstruction.[18] In both outflow tracts, the obstruction can be present at different levels (subvalvar, valvar, and supravalvar). In the left ventricular outflow tract, a subvalvar obstruction can be caused by a subvalvar membrane, abnormal

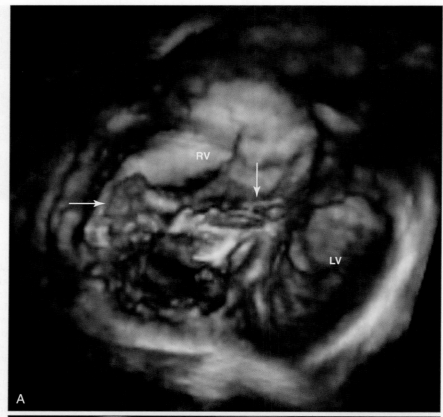

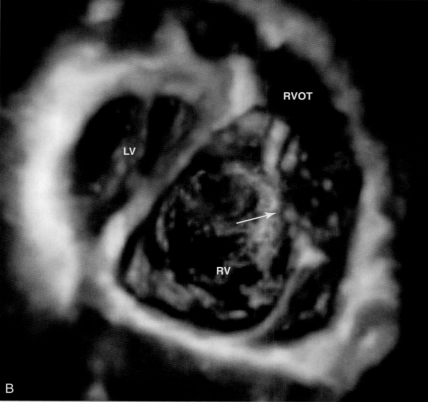

Figure 15-4 Ebstein's anomaly of the tricuspid valve in a 13-year-old boy who presented with supraventricular tachycardia. Regurgitation was mild and the patient tolerated it well. **A,** A short-axis cut from the ventricular apex. The *vertical arrow* points to the septal leaflet, which has multiple abnormal attachments to the septum. The *horizontal arrow* points the anterosuperior leaflet, which has additional redundant tissue. The left ventricle (*LV*) is small (see Video 15-8). **B,** Displacement and rotation of the tricuspid valve toward the right ventricular outflow tract (*RVOT*); the *arrow* indicates the plane of opening of the valve (see Video 15-9). *RV,* right ventricle.

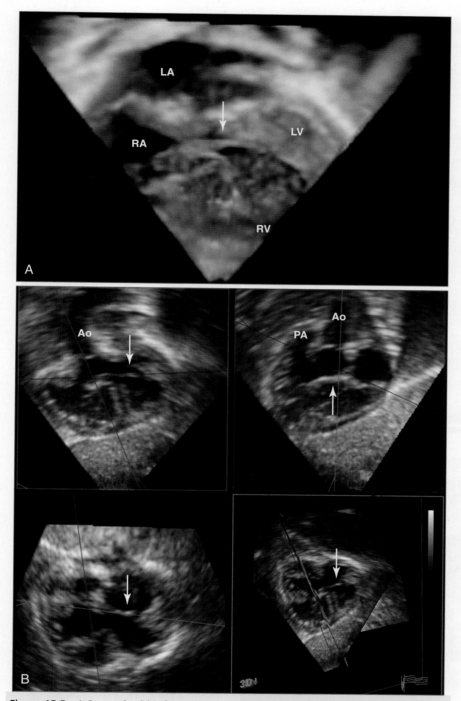

Figure 15-5 A 3-month-old infant presented with a double-outlet right ventricle and a large perimembranous ventricular septal defect (VSD) extending to the inlet septum and a straddling tricuspid valve. The great arteries are normally related. Because of the significant attachments of the tricuspid valve through the VSD into the left ventricle (*LV, arrow*), this patient was unable to have a two-ventricle repair and instead underwent successful single-ventricle palliation. In **A,** the three-dimensional dataset has been cropped to show the straddling valve. In **B,** the dataset has been cropped with the multiplanar review mode. *Ao,* aorta; *LA,* left atrium; *PA,* pulmonary artery; *RA,* right atrium; *RV,* right ventricle.

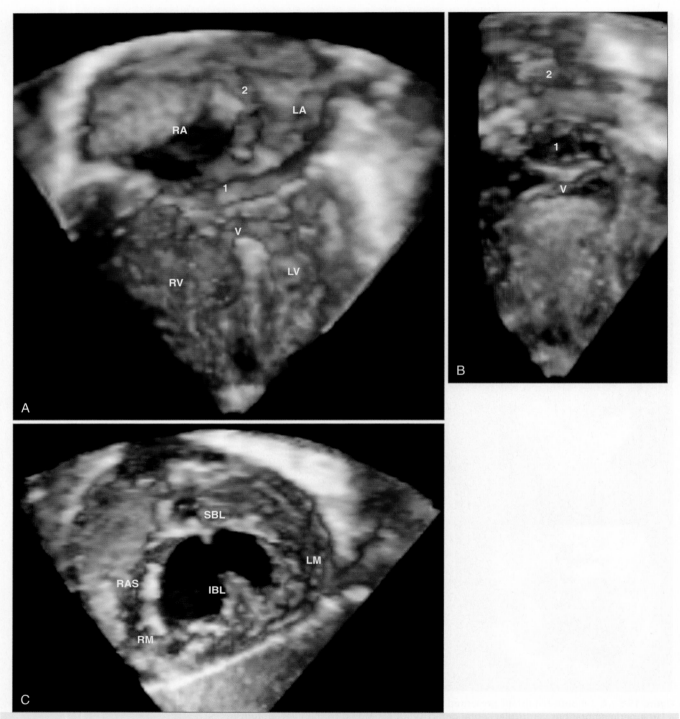

Figure 15-6 This patient had a balanced atrioventricular septal defect and trisomy 21 (Down syndrome). **A,** Four cardiac chambers with a deficient atrioventricular septum causing the ventricular septal defect (*V*) and primum atrial septal defect (*1*). There is an additional secundum atrial septal defect (*2*) (see Video 15-10). **B,** A view of the atrial and ventricular septa from the left ventricle. **C,** Subcostal view of the common atrioventricular valve. The common valve is composed of five leaflets, the superior and inferior bridging (*SBL* and *IBL*), left mural (*LM*), right mural (*RM*), and right anterior superior (*RAS*). This patient underwent echocardiography as screening for congenital heart disease when a postnatal diagnosis of trisomy 21 was made (see Video 15-11). *LA,* left atrium; *LV,* left ventricle; *RA,* right atrium; *RV,* right ventricle.

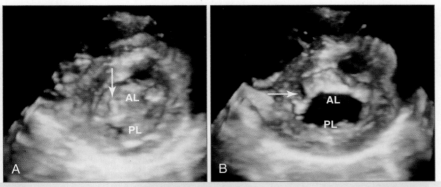

Figure 15-7   This 12-year-old patient had left atrioventricular valve regurgitation following atrioventricular septal defect repair. **A,** The valve is closed. Note the thickening and rolling of both anterior (*AL*) and posterior (*PL*) leaflets. The *arrow* indicates the stitch line where the surgeon closed the zone of apposition between the superior and inferior bridging leaflets to create a bifoliate left atrioventricular valve. **B,** With the valve open, there is a tear in the leaflet (*arrow*) adjacent to the stitch line, which was an unusual source of valvar regurgitation in this patient. This echocardiographic study contributed to preoperative planning, and the patient was able to undergo successful repeat repair of the left atrioventricular valve (see Video 15-12).

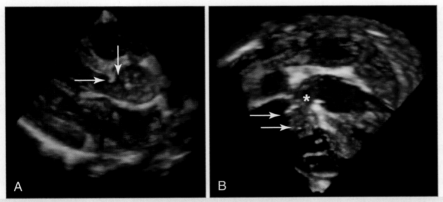

Figure 15-8   A 2-year-old child with subaortic stenosis and ventricular septal defect. There is a discrete subaortic ridge (**A,** *horizontal arrow*). In addition, there is a perimembranous ventricular septal defect (*asterisk*) partially occluded by tricuspid valve tissue (**B,** *arrows*) and minor prolapse of the right coronary cusp of the aortic valve (**A,** *vertical arrow*). This patient presented after premature birth with a murmur. Although he has remained asymptomatic, he requires careful echocardiographic follow-up to monitor for any progression of either the subaortic ridge or the aortic cusp prolapse (see Videos 15-13 and 15-14).

AV valve tissue with septal attachments, or a tunnel-like obstruction. Here, RT3DE with multiplanar reconstructions can be helpful in defining the exact anatomic mechanisms. Semilunar valve abnormalities may, however, be well delineated by RT3DE, which has been demonstrated to correlate well with surgical findings.[19]

Subaortic obstructions usually are incompletely visualized by the surgeon, who approaches the lesion through the aortic valve. Therefore, accurate preoperative imaging is beneficial for surgical planning and may demonstrate additional lesions, such as abnormal mitral chordal attachments in subaortic stenosis.[20]

The right ventricular outflow tract can be more difficult to visualize with RT3DE because of its anterior position. Right ventricular outflow tract obstruction also can be complex with subvalvar, valvar, and supravalvar components. The additional value of RT3DE still remains to be proven for this indication (**Figures 15-8** to **15-11**; **Videos 15-13** to **15-18**).

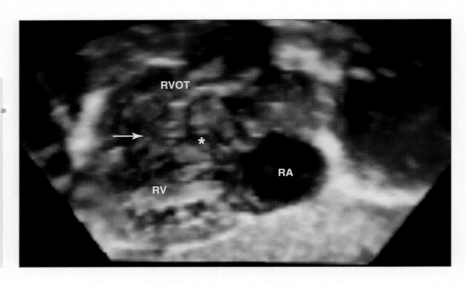

Figure 15-9 Tetralogy of Fallot in an unoperated 2-month-old patient, viewed from the subcostal position. There is anterior deviation of the outlet septum (*arrow*) causing a perimembranous ventricular septal defect (*asterisk*) and narrowing of the right ventricular outflow tract (*RVOT*). This patient presented at birth with dysmorphic features suggestive of 22q11 deletion, commonly associated with conotruncal cardiac defects, and underwent elective repair of the tetralogy of Fallot (see Video 15-15). *RA*, right atrium; *RV*, right ventricle.

MEASUREMENT OF SIZE AND FUNCTION

RT3DE can provide useful functional information on valvar and ventricular size and function in patients with congenital heart defects.

Valve Orifice

In certain congenital heart diseases, accurate assessment of valve size may be important in determining surgical management. RT3DE enables the operator to view the true plane of the valve orifice more accurately. For stenotic lesions, this allows direct measurement of the effective orifice using planimetry on 3D images.[21] RT3DE for area calculation has been shown to be more reliable, with a lower interobserver variability, compared with cross-sectional imaging (**Figure 15-12**).[22]

Regurgitant Jets

Valvar regurgitation in patients with congenital heart disease may have complex mechanisms that are difficult to evaluate fully by 2DE; RT3DE helps elucidate these details. The regurgitant jet may have an irregular shape, which makes it more readily appreciated in 3D than in 2D (**Figures 15-13** and **15-14**; **Video 15-19**).

Ventricular Volume and Mass Quantification

There are many congenital lesions in which quantification of left ventricular volume or mass is important. RT3DE demonstrates excellent intraobserver and interobserver reproducibility in left ventricular quantification.[23,24] This can be a useful adjunctive investigation in patients in whom determination of left ventricular adequacy is important for clinical decision making, such as in those with borderline left ventricles when the choice is either two-ventricle repair or single-ventricle palliation. In patients with a functional single ventricle, RT3DE measurements of mass and volume correlate well with cardiac magnetic resonance imaging (MRI) measurement and allow monitoring of ventricular size and function over time.[25]

Evaluation of right ventricular function is extremely important in congenital heart disease, particularly in patients with right-sided lesions, such as tetralogy of Fallot, or in patients in whom the right ventricle is the systemic ventricle, such as in congenitally corrected transposition of the great arteries, or after an atrial switch procedure. 3DE has been demonstrated to be a sensitive tool to identify right ventricular dysfunction and also may be useful to assess which patients would benefit from quantitative analysis, for which cardiac MRI remains the gold standard.[26-28]

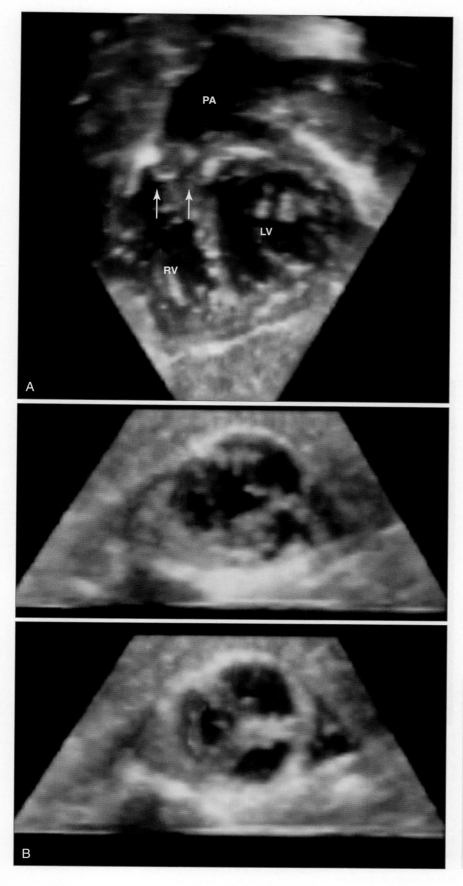

Figure 15-10 Pulmonary valvar stenosis with thickening of the valve leaflets (*arrows*). **A,** Right ventricular (*RV*) outflow tract cropped from a three-dimensional dataset acquired from the subcostal position (see Video 15-16). *LV,* left ventricle; *PA,* pulmonary artery. **B,** A dataset acquired from the parasternal position showing an en face view of the valve with the leaflets open (*top*) and closed (*bottom*). This 6-month-old patient presented with a cardiac murmur and was found to have moderate pulmonary stenosis (see Video 15-17).

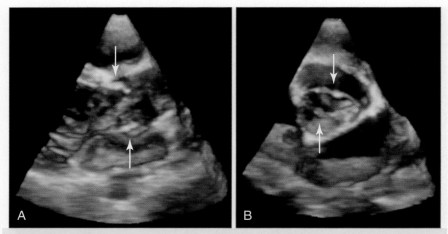

Figure 15-11 This 8-year-old boy has a bicuspid aortic valve. The *arrows* indicate the valve leaflets, shown in long-axis (**A**) and short-axis (**B**) views. He was referred in early childhood for screening because of a family history positive for significant cardiac abnormalities; his father had marfanoid aortic root dilation, and his sister had mitral valve prolapse. Genetic testing in the family was negative (see Video 15-18).

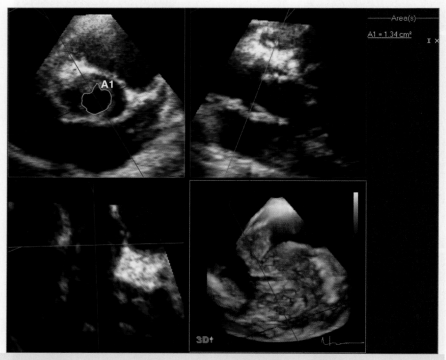

Figure 15-12 A patient with aortic stenosis. In the multiplanar review mode, the aortic valvar annulus has been transected in three planes, positioned such that two planes were in the valve's long axis and perpendicular to each other and the third plane was in the true short axis of the valve. These three planes were used to define the hinge points of the valve; the short-axis plane was then slid to the leaflet tips to determine the valve's effective orifice area, maintaining reference to the other two planes and tilting the plane, if necessary, to account for eccentric valve opening. The perimeter of the orifice was then planimetered to determine the area. This patient had two previous balloon aortic valvoplasties, the first at age 6 months and the second at age 13 years. This echocardiogram was performed just prior to his third valvoplasty at age 15 years, which yielded an excellent result, with significant relief of the transvalvar gradient.

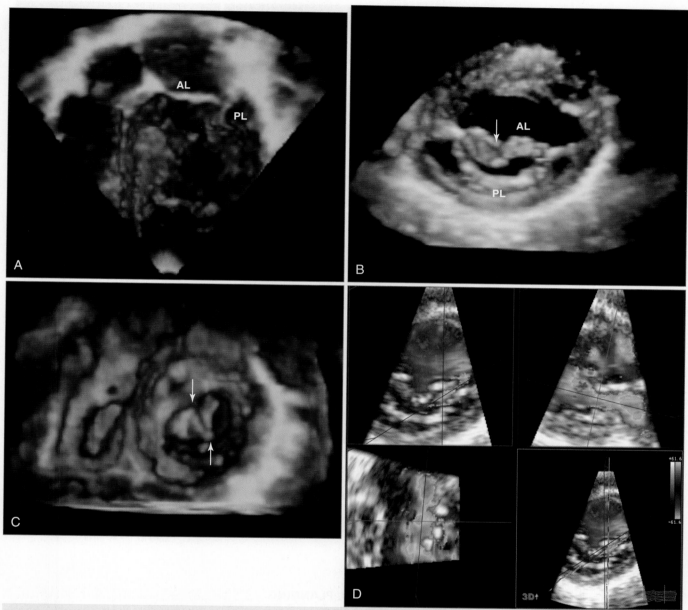

Figure 15-13 This patient has ulcerative colitis and presented at the age of 8 years with infective endocarditis affecting his mitral valve. After full resolution of the endocarditis, he had significant mitral regurgitation requiring surgical repair. **A,** Prolapse of the anterior leaflet (*AL*) of the mitral valve and restriction of movement of the posterior leaflet (*PL*) caused failure of coaptation. There is "folding" of the anterior leaflet (*arrow*) seen from the atrial aspect in **B** and the ventricular aspect in **C. D,** The multiplanar review allows more complete visualization of the complex shape of the regurgitant jet.

RT3DE also allows excellent visualization of intracardiac masses, which may be monitored by RT3DE assessment of the volume of the mass (**Figures 15-15 to 15-17; Videos 15-20 and 15-21**).

Dyssynchrony Assessment: Regional Left Ventricular Volumes

As in adults, RT3DE has been used to demonstrate left ventricular dyssynchrony in children with left ventricular dysfunction.[29] In congenital heart disease, dyssynchrony is an important mechanism that can contribute to ventricular dysfunction. Data on the potential use of timing of the regional volume changes for the diagnosis of dyssynchrony in patients with congenital heart disease are still limited.

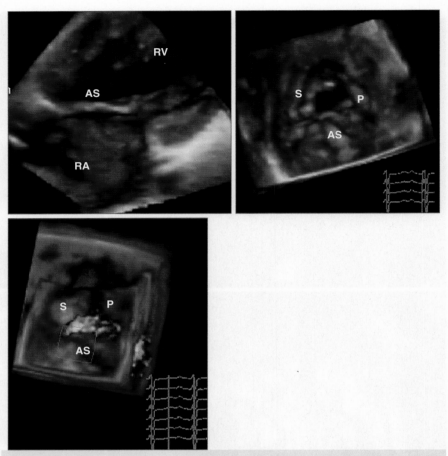

Figure 15-14 This 6-month-old patient with hypoplastic left heart syndrome, which was antenatally diagnosed, has had palliation in the form of a Norwood procedure, with the right ventricle (*RV*) acting as the systemic ventricle. There is significant tricuspid regurgitation. Note the thickening of the anterosuperior leaflet and the failure of coaptation of all three leaflets, with the regurgitant jet arising along all three commissures (see Video 15-19). *AS*, anterosuperior leaflet; *P*, posterior leaflet; *RA*, right atrium; *S*, septal leaflet.

INTERVENTIONAL PLANNING
Presurgical Imaging

RT3DE can be used to enhance preoperative planning of procedures by enhancing understanding of intracardiac anatomy. RT3DE reduces operation time by giving improved anatomic detail before surgery in some patients, such as those with complex outflow tract obstruction.[18] Findings on RT3DE correlate well with anatomic and surgical findings in congenital heart disease in both simple and complex defects.[18,20,30] New, clinically important information that substantially alters the course of management may be discovered with RT3DE analysis in a small subset of patients.[20]

Intraprocedural Imaging

Both intraoperative epicardial RT3DE and intraoperative RT3DTEE have been demonstrated to be useful in the immediate postbypass evaluation of surgical repair of congenital heart defects.[31] Both techniques may provide particular additive value in the intraoperative imaging of AV valves.[32] Transcatheter closure of atrial septal defects has traditionally been guided by 2DTEE or intracardiac echocardiography, but RT3DE is increasingly being used either alone or as an adjunct to 2DE. RT3DE may minimize the use of fluoroscopy in some

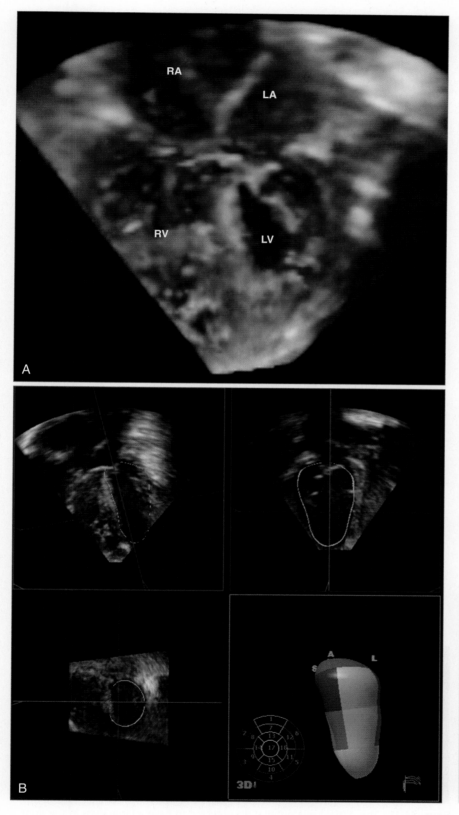

Figure 15-15 A, This 18-month-old patient has a complete atrioventricular septal defect that is slightly unbalanced, with the left heart structures being smaller than those of the right heart. **B,** Left ventricular volume analysis, which can be helpful in borderline cases such as this, can be used to determine suitability for biventricular repair versus single-ventricle palliation. This patient underwent biventricular repair, which resulted in some left atrioventricular valve stenosis in the postoperative period; it resolved over time with somatic growth (see Video 15-20). *LA,* left atrium; *LV,* left ventricle; *RA,* right atrium; *RV,* right ventricle.

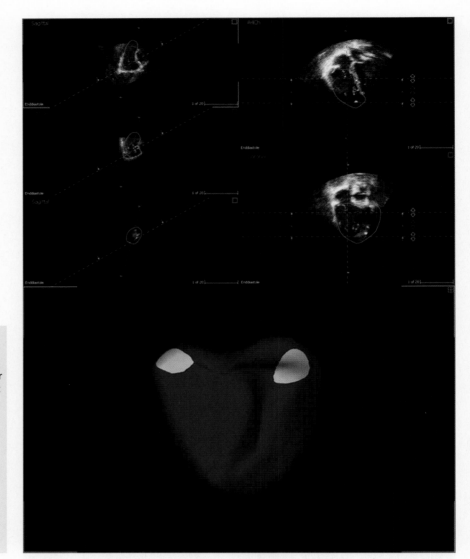

Figure 15-16 This 16-year-old patient had surgical repair of tetralogy of Fallot in infancy, with a patch across the hypoplastic pulmonary valve annulus, which has left her with free pulmonary insufficiency. The right ventricle is progressively becoming dilated and is being carefully monitored by echocardiography and cardiac magnetic resonance imaging to determine the optimal time for pulmonary valve replacement. Commercially available software allows the operator to trace the right ventricular endocardial border in several planes (*top panels*) and then generates a three-dimensional model (*bottom*) and calculations of right ventricular volume and function.

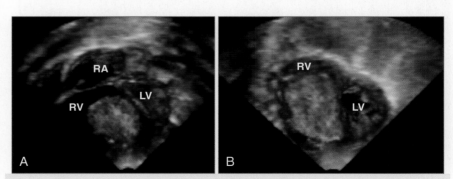

Figure 15-17 This patient was antenatally detected to have a large mass in the right ventricle but was asymptomatic at birth. There is a large mass in the right ventricle (*RV*) that is not obstructing the tricuspid valve. This is a rhabdomyoma, which has a benign course. Because there is no obstruction to inflow or outflow, conservative management was chosen. **A,** A three-dimensional dataset acquired from the apex (see Video 15-21). **B,** Image acquired subcostally. *RV*, right ventricle; *LV*, left ventricle.

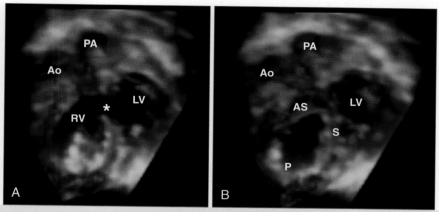

Figure 15-18 This 2-year-old patient has double-outlet right ventricle, with the aorta (*Ao*) rightwards of the pulmonary artery (*PA*). **A,** A subcostal image with the tricuspid valve closed. The *asterisk* marks the ventricular septal defect. **B,** The tricuspid valve opening toward the outflow tract, an important view for planning surgical repair. The patient initially had been directed toward single-ventricle palliation but after this assessment had a successful biventricular repair (see Video 15-22). *AS,* Anterosuperior leaflet; *LV,* left ventricle; *P,* posterior leaflet; *RV,* right ventricle; *S,* superior leaflet.

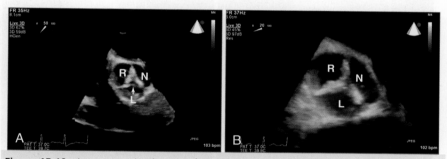

Figure 15-19 Intraoperative live three-dimensional transoesophageal echocardiography from a 13-year-old patient with aortic regurgitation undergoing surgical repair. **A,** After the first bypass run and attempted repair, there was still a significant residual coaptation defect (*arrow*) causing significant aortic insufficiency. **B,** After the second bypass run, guided by this image, excellent coaptation of all three leaflets was seen, and there was no significant regurgitation. The patient made an excellent recovery from surgery and is now asymptomatic. *L,* Left coronary cusp; *N,* noncoronary cusp; *R,* right coronary cusp.

procedures; for example, it has been successfully used in guiding endomyocardial biopsy of the right ventricle in children (**Figures 15-18 to 15-20; Videos 15-22 to 15-24**).[33]

FETAL ECHOCARDIOGRAPHY

Although 2DE remains the primary imaging modality for antenatal diagnosis of congenital heart disease, 3DE may provide additional information in a small subgroup of patients (**Figure 15-21**).[34-36]

SUMMARY

3DE is feasible in congenital heart disease, even in small patients, and aids in the diagnosis of complex anatomy. It provides additional information to 2DE, which significantly assists management planning both before and during procedures.

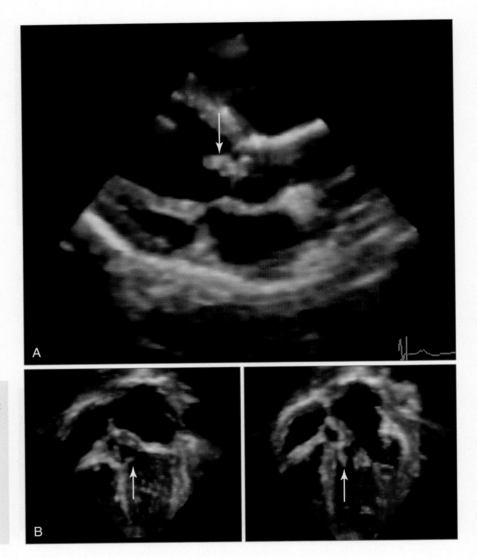

Figure 15-20 While undergoing balloon dilation of the aortic valve for severe aortic stenosis, this 5-year-old patient developed severe aortic insufficiency after the second inflation of the balloon. **A,** A dataset acquired from the parasternal position shows the right coronary cusp (*arrow*) to be flailing (see Video 15-23). **B,** View from the apical position in systole (*left*) and diastole (*right*). The patient proceeded to a successful Ross procedure a few weeks later (see Video 15-24).

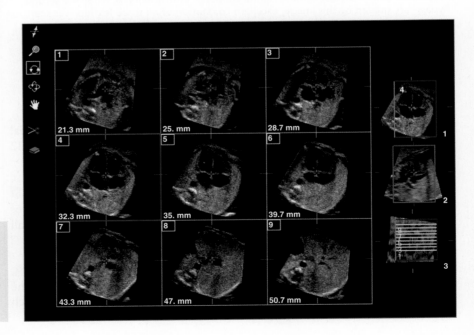

Figure 15-21 Three-dimensional echocardiography allows rapid acquisition of a full volume of a fetal heart, which can be analyzed offline. Demonstrated here is a series of axial slices allowing analysis of the intracardiac anatomy and great vessels, in this case of a normal fetal heart.

References

1. Shirali GS: Three dimensional echocardiography in congenital heart defects. *Ann Pediatr Cardiol* 1(1):8–17, 2008.

2. Cheng TO, Xie MX, Wang XF, et al: Real-time 3-dimensional echocardiography in assessing atrial and ventricular septal defects: an echocardiographic-surgical correlative study. *Am Heart J* 148(6):1091–1095, 2004.

3. Maeno YV, Benson LN, McLaughlin PR, Boutin C: Dynamic morphology of the secundum atrial septal defect evaluated by three dimensional transoesophageal echocardiography. *Heart* 83(6):673–677, 2000.

4. Handke M, Schafer DM, Muller G, et al: Dynamic changes of atrial septal defect area: New insights by three-dimensional volume-rendered echocardiography with high temporal resolution. *Eur J Echocardiogr* 2(1):46–51, 2001.

5. Saric M, Perk G, Purgess JR, Kronzon I: Imaging atrial septal defects by real-time three-dimensional transesophageal echocardiography: Step-by-step approach. *J Am Soc Echocardiogr* 23(11):1128–1135, 2010.

6. Takahashi K, Mackie AS, Rebeyka IM, et al: Two-dimensional versus transthoracic real-time three-dimensional echocardiography in the evaluation of the mechanisms and sites of atrioventricular valve regurgitation in a congenital heart disease population. *J Am Soc Echocardiogr* 23(7):726–734, 2010.

7. Bharucha T, Anderson RH, Lim ZS, Vettukattil JJ: Multiplanar review of three-dimensional echocardiography gives new insights into the morphology of Ebstein's malformation. *Cardiol Young* 20(1):49–53, 2010.

8. van den Bosch AE, van Dijk VF, McGhie JS, et al: Real-time transthoracic three-dimensional echocardiography provides additional information of left-sided AV valve morphology after AVSD repair. *Int J Cardiol* 106(3):360–364, 2006.

9. Barrea C, Levasseur S, Roman K, et al: Three-dimensional echocardiography improves the understanding of left atrioventricular valve morphology and function in atrioventricular septal defects undergoing patch augmentation. *J Thorac Cardiovasc Surg* 129(4):746–753, 2005.

10. Pai RG, Jintapakorn W, Tanimoto M, Shah PM: Role of papillary muscle position and mitral valve structure in systolic anterior motion of the mitral leaflets in hyperdynamic left ventricular function. *Am J Cardiol* 76(8):623–628, 1995.

11. Salgo IS, Gorman JH, 3rd, Gorman RC, et al: Effect of annular shape on leaflet curvature in reducing mitral leaflet stress. *Circulation* 106(6):711–717, 2002.

12. Bharucha T, Sivaprakasam MC, Roman KS, Vettukattil JJ: A multiplanar three dimensional echocardiographic study of mitral valvar annular function in children with normal and regurgitant valves. *Cardiol Young* 18(4):379–385, 2008.

13. Nii M, Roman KS, Macgowan CK, Smallhorn JF: Insight into normal mitral and tricuspid annular dynamics in pediatrics: A real-time three-dimensional echocardiographic study. *J Am Soc Echocardiogr* 18(8):805–814, 2005.

14. Vettukattil JJ, Bharucha T, Anderson RH: Defining Ebstein's malformation using three-dimensional echocardiography. *Interact Cardiovasc Thorac Surg* 6(6):685–690, 2007.

15. Singh A, Romp RL, Nanda NC, et al: Usefulness of live/real time three-dimensional transthoracic echocardiography in the assessment of atrioventricular septal defects. *Echocardiography* 23(7):598–608, 2006.

16. Hlavacek AM, Crawford FA, Jr, Chessa KS, Shirali GS: Real-time three-dimensional echocardiography is useful in the evaluation of patients with atrioventricular septal defects. *Echocardiography* 23(3):225–231, 2006.

17. Miller AP, Nanda NC, Aaluri S, et al: Three-dimensional transesophageal echocardiographic demonstration of anatomical defects in AV septal defect patients presenting for reoperation. *Echocardiography* 20(1):105–109, 2003.

18. Dall'Agata A, Cromme-Dijkhuis AH, Meijboom FJ, et al: Use of three-dimensional echocardiography for analysis of outflow obstruction in congenital heart disease. *Am J Cardiol* 83(6):921–925, 1999.

19. Sadagopan SN, Veldtman GR, Sivaprakasam MC, et al: Correlations with operative anatomy of real time three-dimensional echocardiographic imaging of congenital aortic valvar stenosis. *Cardiol Young* 16(5):490–494, 2006.

20. Bharucha T, Ho SY, Vettukattil JJ: Multiplanar review analysis of three-dimensional echocardiographic datasets gives new insights into the morphology of subaortic stenosis. *Eur J Echocardiogr* 9(5):614–620, 2008.

21. Poh KK, Levine RA, Solis J, et al: Assessing aortic valve area in aortic stenosis by continuity equation: A novel approach using real-time three-dimensional echocardiography. *Eur Heart J* 29(20):2526–2535, 2008.

22. Binder TM, Rosenhek R, Porenta G, et al: Improved assessment of mitral valve stenosis by volumetric real-time three-dimensional echocardiography. *J Am Coll Cardiol* 36(4):1355–1361, 2000.

23. Baker G, Flack E, Hlavacek A, et al: Variability and resource utilization of bedside three-dimensional echocardiographic quantitative measurements of left ventricular volume in congenital heart disease. *Congenit Heart Dis* 1(6):309–314, 2006.

24. Hascoet S, Brierre G, Caudron G, et al: Assessment of left ventricular volumes and function by real time three-dimensional echocardiography in a pediatric population: A TomTec versus QLAB comparison. *Echocardiography* 27(10):1263–1273, 2010.

25. Soriano BD, Hoch M, Ithuralde A, et al: Matrix-array 3-dimensional echocardiographic assessment of volumes, mass, and ejection fraction in young pediatric patients with a functional single ventricle: A comparison study with cardiac magnetic resonance. *Circulation* 117(14):1842–1848, 2008.

26. van der Zwaan HB, Helbing WA, Boersma E, et al: Usefulness of real-time three-dimensional echocardiography to identify right ventricular dysfunction in patients with congenital heart disease. *Am J Cardiol* 106(6):843–850, 2010.

27. van der Zwaan HB, Helbing WA, McGhie JS, et al: Clinical value of real-time three-dimensional echocardiography for right ventricular quantification in congenital heart disease: Validation with cardiac magnetic resonance imaging. *J Am Soc Echocardiogr* 23(2):134–140, 2010.

28. Mertens LL, Friedberg MK: Imaging the right ventricle-current state of the art. *Nat Rev Cardiol* 7(10):551–563, 2010.

29. Baker GH, Hlavacek AM, Chessa KS, et al: Left ventricular dysfunction is associated with intraventricular dyssynchrony by 3-dimensional echocardiography in children. *J Am Soc Echocardiogr* 21(3):230–233, 2008.

30. van den Bosch AE, Ten Harkel DJ, McGhie JS, et al: Surgical validation of real-time transthoracic 3D echocardiographic assessment of atrioventricular septal defects. *Int J Cardiol* 112(2):213–218, 2006.

31. Suradi H, Byers S, Green-Hess D, et al: Feasibility of using real time "live 3D" echocardiography to visualize the stenotic aortic valve. *Echocardiography* 27(8):1011–1020, 2010.

32. Rawlins DB, Austin C, Simpson JM: Live three-dimensional paediatric intraoperative epicardial echocardiography as a guide to surgical repair of atrioventricular valves. *Cardiol Young* 16(1):34–39, 2006.

33. Scheurer M, Bandisode V, Ruff P, et al: Early experience with real-time three-dimensional echocardiographic guidance of right ventricular biopsy in children. *Echocardiography* 23(1):45–49, 2006.

34. Meyer-Wittkopf M, Cooper S, Vaughan J, Sholler G: Three-dimensional (3D) echocardiographic analysis of congenital heart disease in the fetus: Comparison with cross-sectional (2D) fetal echocardiography. *Ultrasound Obstet Gynecol* 17(6):485–492, 2001.

35. Cohen L, Mangers K, Grobman WA, et al: Three-dimensional fast acquisition with sonographically based volume computer-aided analysis for imaging of the fetal heart at 18 to 22 weeks' gestation. *J Ultrasound Med* 29(5):751–757, 2010.

36. Nelson TR, Pretorius DH, Sklansky M, Hagen-Ansert S: Three-dimensional echocardiographic evaluation of fetal heart anatomy and function: Acquisition, analysis, and display. *J Ultrasound Med* 15(1):1–9, 1996.

CHAPTER 16

Evaluation of Intracardiac Masses

Elisa Zaragosa-Macias and Edward A. Gill

INTRODUCTION

Perhaps no finding on echocardiography creates a bigger diagnostic challenge than the presence of an intracardiac mass. This is because tissue characterization by any imaging modality is limited. The advent of tomographic imaging in general, including computed tomography (CT), magnetic resonance imaging, and echocardiography, has dramatically improved the detection of intracardiac masses, but mass characterization remains challenging. The diagnosis of some masses, particularly thrombi, can be reasonably certain on the basis of the company that they keep, such as the association of thrombi and regional wall motion abnormalities. Likewise, papillary fibroelastomas are classically seen on the ventricular side of the semilunar valves, and atrial myxomas frequently attach to the interatrial septum. Angiosarcomas typically originate from a vascular structure, particularly the inferior or superior vena cava.

Beyond these generalities, additional deductive reasoning is limited when it comes to the diagnosis of an intracardiac mass. Although real-time three-dimensional echocardiography (RT3DE) can add some information about the tissue characterization of cardiac masses, its true strengths are accurate assessment of size and volume of the mass as well as the relationship of the mass to adjacent cardiac structures. Both RT3D transthoracic echocardiography (TTE) and more recently RT3D transesophageal echocardiography (TEE) have been extensively used, even within the brief time of their existence, for imaging cardiac masses.

TYPES OF REAL-TIME THREE-DIMENSIONAL ECHOCARDIOGRAPHY IMAGING

3DE imaging took a major step in 2002, when previous gated methods of 3DE acquisition were replaced with RT3DTTE. In 2007, RT3DTEE imaging became available, revolutionizing the evaluation of intracardiac masses.

GENERAL BENEFITS OF THREE-DIMENSIONAL ECHOCARDIOGRAPHY OVER TWO-DIMENSIONAL ECHOCARDIOGRAPHY

The potential and realized benefits of 3DE for mass evaluation include (1) improved spatial relationships to adjacent anatomic structures; (2) improved accuracy of size and volume of the masses; (3) improved detail of the homogeneity (or lack thereof) of the mass using the cropping function of 3D software; (4) involvement or noninvolvement of adjacent structures, such as interatrial or interventricular septum, valves, or myocardium; and (5) mobility in 3D space and, as a correlate, identification of the stalk of the mass, if present.

Intracardiac Masses: Generalities

The differential diagnosis of an intracardiac mass includes thrombus, vegetation, tumor, iatrogenic material, extracardiac tissue, and normal variant. Narrowing the diagnosis down by 2DE and then 3DE should be and is the goal of imaging. As mentioned, tissue characterization remains the holy grail of imaging and, as such, remains challenging. However, characteristics such as inhomogeneity suggest tumor, whereas a highly homogeneous sessile mass is more characteristic of a thrombus. However, clot lysis does exist, presenting a highly inhomogeneous look, and thrombi can be quite mobile. A clear stalk has been believed to suggest tumor, but thrombi occasionally are attached to clear stalks as well. Further details are provided with each individual discussion of masses that follows.

Tumors: Generalities

Primary tumors of the heart are extremely rare, with a reported prevalence of 0.001% to 0.03% by autopsy series.[1] The most common primary cardiac tumor is the myxoma, even though myxoma is relatively uncommon. Myxomas are most common in the atria, particularly the left atrium. They often have a clear stalk attached to the interatrial septum and clearly visualized with 3DE. Myxomas typically are benign, but the most common primary malignant tumors are sarcomas, which are highly invasive and uniformly fatal tumors. Angiosarcoma is the most common of this group. Metastatic tumors to the heart are much more common than are primary tumors, with the most common being breast and lung tumors; the usual cardiac site of metastasis is the pericardium. In fact, secondary involvement of the heart by extracardiac tumors is 20 to 40 times more common compared with primary cardiac tumors.[1-3] Melanoma is a tumor that has particular propensity to metastasize to the heart.[4]

Individual Tumors: Myxomas

As mentioned, myxomas are the most common primary cardiac tumors (**Figures 16-1 to 16-3; Videos 16-1 to 16-6**). 3D imaging of atrial myxomas has been reported by transthoracic and transesophageal methods. The main benefits of 3DE over 2DE for myxomas are (1) identification of the stalk of the tumor and (2) evaluation of the heterogeneity of the mass. In fact, both characteristics often are seen with 2DE. The first case of imaging a right atrial myxoma by RT3DTEE was reported by Scohy et al (**Figure 16-4**).[5] At the time of surgical excision, it was noted that the size of the mass correlated extremely well with the estimate by RT3DTEE. In fact, the volume of 6.4 mL was the same as shown by 3DTEE and by ex vivo measurement. Butz et al[6] also measured a left atrial myxoma preoperatively by using 3DTEE and determined excellent correlation with the excised mass at the time of surgery. In another case study, a right ventricular and tricuspid valve myxoma was identified by 2DTTE; it measured 5.5 × 3.8 cm but was remarkably larger as shown by 3DTTE (12 × 6 cm). 3DTTE improved the visualization of the special relationship with surrounding structures and identified the involvement of the tricuspid valve, which was not appreciated by 2DTTE (**Figure 16-5**).[7] Two cases of giant myxoma resulting in significant mitral valve obstruction were described by Culp et al.[8] RT3DTEE volume measurement coordinated well with the ex vivo measurement. 2DTEE underestimated the volume (**Figure 16-6**).

Prior to these publications, incremental value for the characterization of internal composition of masses and volume calculation had been appreciated with RT3DTTE imaging for myxomas and a hemangioma. In this small series, four left atrial tumors, including three myxomas and one hemangioma, were imaged by RT3D and correlated with histopathology specimens. Echolucencies suggestive of intramass hemorrhage were more frequently seen with 3D imaging compared with 2DE. In addition, 3DTTE detected more extensive and closely packed echolucencies involving the whole extent of the tumor in the hemangioma compared with more scattered echolucencies in myxomas (**Figure 16-7**).[9]

Text continued on page 305

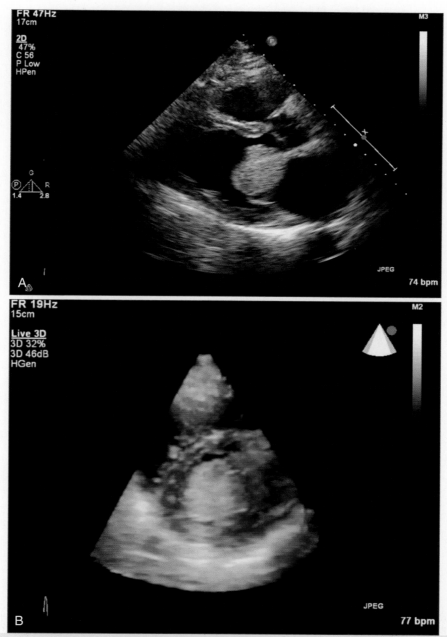

Figure 16-1   Left atrial myxoma imaging with two-dimensional echocardiography (**A**) and three-dimensional echocardiography (**B**) in the short-axis view (see Videos 16-1 and 16-2).

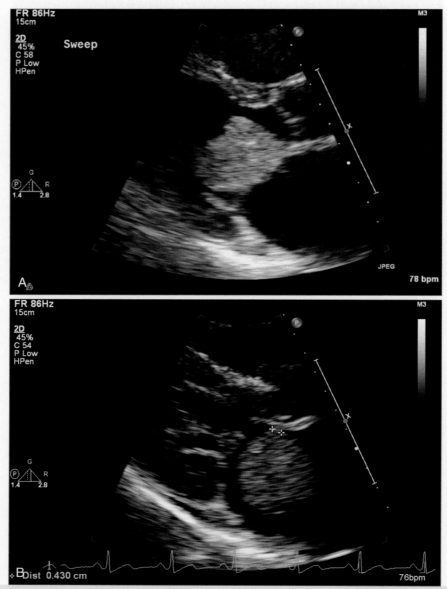

Figure 16-2   A, Zoom of two-dimensional echocardiography view of left atrial myxoma showing the attachment point of the mass to the left atrial wall **(B).** Note the attachment point to the left atrial wall has a close relationship to the anterior leaflet of the mitral valve and the posterior portion of the aortic annulus (see Video 16-3).

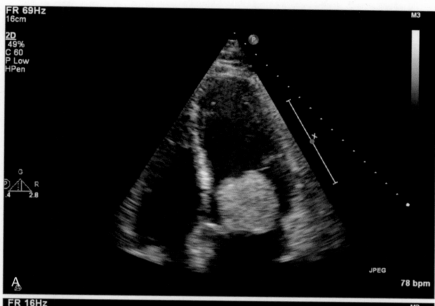

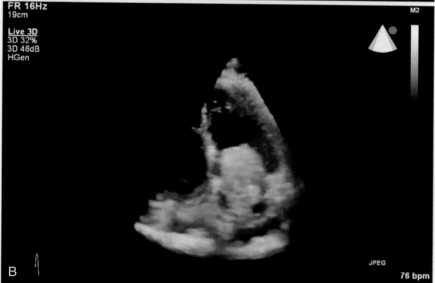

Figure 16-3   Two-dimensional (2D) (**A**) and three-dimensional (3D) echocardiography (**B**) of the apical four-chamber view of left atrial myxoma. The volume perspective and size are appreciated in the 3D view. Note that in these particular views, the stalk of the mass, attached to the interatrial septum, is more easily visualized in the 2D image, although cropping of the 3D image was possible and identified the stalk (see Videos 16-4 to 16-6).

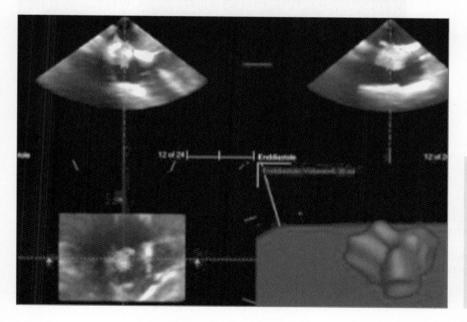

Figure 16-4   Volume rendering of the right atrial mass offline by TomTec (Munich, Germany) four-dimensional imaging showing that volume measurement can be performed. The result was 6.36 mL, comparable with the in vitro measurement of 6.4 mL. (From Scohy TV, Lecomte PV, McGhie J, et al: Intraoperative real time three-dimensional transesophageal echocardiographic evaluation of right atrial tumor. *Echocardiography* 25:646–649, 2008.)

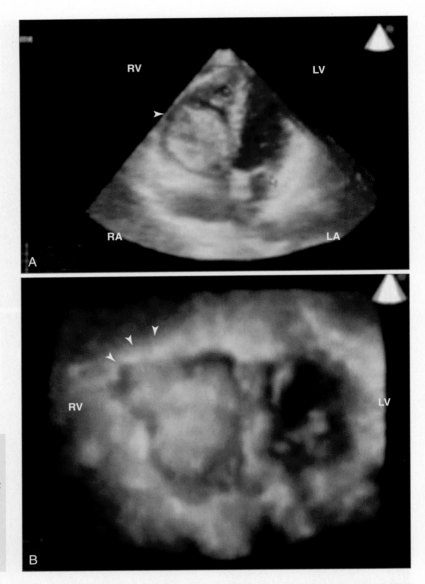

Figure 16-5 **A** and **B,** A right ventricular myxoma with involvement of the tricuspid valve. The tricuspid valve involvement was not appreciated by two-dimensional echocardiography. *LV,* left ventricle; *RA,* right atrium; *RV,* right ventricle. (From Reddy VK, Faulkner M, Bandarupalli N, et al: Incremental value of live/real time three-dimensional transthoracic echocardiography in the assessment of right ventricular masses. *Echocardiography* 26:598–609, 2009.)

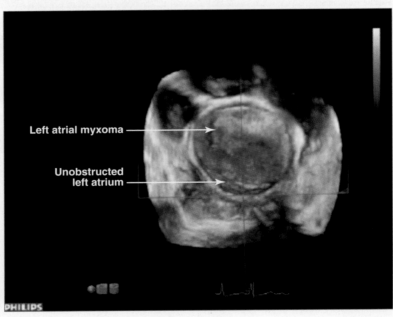

Figure 16-6 A giant myxoma of the left atrium causing obstruction of the mitral orifice. (From Culp WC Jr, Ball TR, Armstrong CS, et al: Three-dimensional transesophageal echocardiographic imaging and volumetry of giant left atrial myxomas. *J Cardiothorac Vasc Anesth* 23:66–68, 2009.)

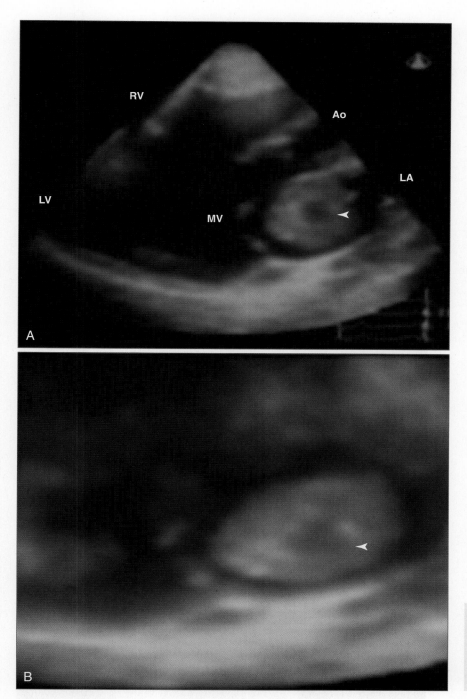

Figure 16-7 **A** and **B**, Example of echolucencies seen with cardiac masses suggesting intramass hemorrhage or necrosis of the tumor (*arrowhead*). *Ao,* aorta; *LA,* left atrium; *LV,* left ventricle; *MV,* mitral valve; *RV,* right ventricle.

Fibroma

Fibroma is a congenital neoplasm that usually affects children. A right ventricular fibroma was diagnosed by 2DTTE in a patient with previous incomplete resection of the same. The fibroma (**Figure 16-8**) was dramatically larger (9.0 × 2.8 cm) by RT3DTTE compared with 2DE (2.6 × 2.7 cm).[7] A left atrial fibroma (**Figure 16-9**) was associated with Gardner syndrome.[10]

Papillary Fibroelastoma

Papillary fibroelastoma is the third most common tumor of the heart, with an incidence of 0.33% among autopsy series.[11] It is the most common tumor of the heart valves and is most frequently identified on the aortic valve (**Figure 16-10**),

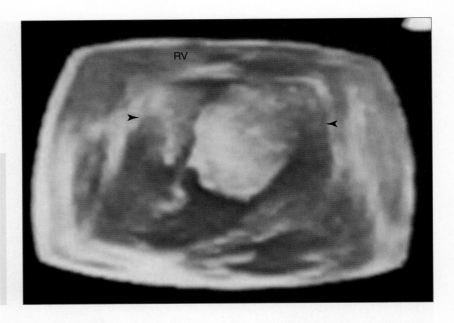

Figure 16-8 A right ventricular fibroma in a patient with history of previous incomplete resection of the same. The fibroma was much larger by three-dimensional compared with two-dimensional transthoracic echocardiography. *RV,* right ventricle. (From Reddy VK, Faulkner M, Bandarupalli N, et al: Incremental value of live/real time three-dimensional transthoracic echocardiography in the assessment of right ventricular masses. *Echocardiography* 26:598–609, 2009.)

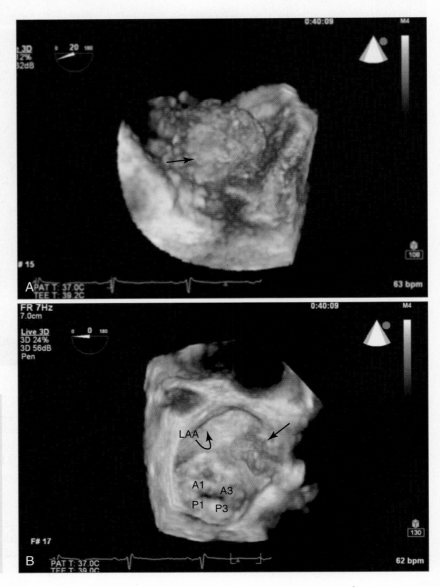

Figure 16-9 **A,** A left atrial fibroma (*arrow*) is shown by three-dimensional transesophageal echocardiography. This mass was associated with Gardner syndrome with familial adenomatous polyposis and associated extracolonic growths, including fibromas. **B,** Left atrial fibroma. *LAA,* left atrial appendage; *A1, A3,* anterior scallops 1 and 3; *P1, P3,* posterior scallops 1 and 3. (From Yang HS, Arabia FA, Chaliki HP, et al: Images in cardiovascular medicine. Left atrial fibroma in Gardner syndrome: Real-time 3-dimensional transesophageal echo imaging. *Circulation* 118:e692–e696, 2008.)

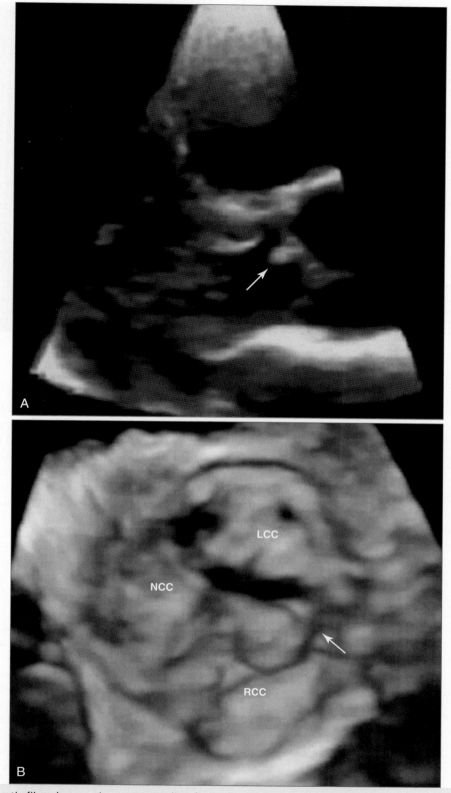

Figure 16-10   **A,** An aortic fibroelastoma is seen protruding from the ventricular side of the aortic valve (*arrow*). **B,** Aortic fibroelastoma. *LCC,* left coronary cusp; *NCC,* noncoronary cusp; *RCC,* right coronary cusp. (From Le Tourneau T, Polge AS, Gautier C, Deklunder G: Three-dimensional echography: cardiovascular applications. *J Radiol* 87:1993–2004, 2006.)

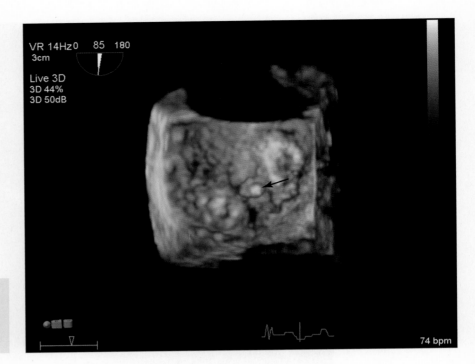

Figure 16-11 Papillary fibroelastoma (*arrow*) is shown on the tip of the anterior leaflet of the mitral valve. This patient had been asymptomatic; this was an incidental finding (see Video 16-7).

although all valves have been described (**Figure 16-11; Video 16-7**). The value of RT3DTTE was illustrated in a case presented by Singh and colleagues[12] with a papillary fibroelastoma of the pulmonary valve. RT3DTTE pinpointed the attachment point, which was helpful in planning valve-sparing surgery. Also, 3D cropping through multiple orthogonal planes revealed frondlike projections and no echolucencies, which helped differentiate the mass from a myxoma or thrombus (**Figure 16-12**). Le Tourneau and associates[13] studied seven consecutive patients with this lesion who had surgical resection of the lesion and found feasibility of imaging the mass to be 100%. Correlation of the 3D volume size with the actual resected tumor was very good. They believed RT3DTTE helped with surgical planning in three of the seven patients; surgical planning is key when valve-sparing surgery is planned. Most of the lesions (five of seven) were on the aortic valve.[13]

Sarcomas

Sarcomas are quite rare primary tumors of the heart but are, in fact, the most common type of primary malignant cardiac tumor, at least in the adult population. Angiosarcoma is the most common among cardiac sarcomas and typically arises in the right atrium, often adjacent to the inferior or superior vena cava. These tumors often are large and aggressive, sometimes occupying much of the right atrium (**Figures 16-13 to 16-16; Videos 16-8 to 16-10**). Suwanjutah et al[14] described a case of leiomyosarcoma imaged by RT3DTTE (**Figure 16-17**). The notable incremental value of RT3DTTE was the composition of the mass. RT3DTTE, again, thanks to its cropping capability, allowed imaging of an area of echolucency, suggesting necrosis or hemorrhage surrounded by bandlike structures consistent with collagen. This image created a "donut" appearance. Excision and evaluation of the resultant histopathology revealed the same pattern of necrosis and vascular channels within the fibrotic tumor. The morphology seen in this case of the tumor by RT3DTTE was suggestive of tumor as opposed to a thrombus. Just as important, the size of the mass by RT3DTTE was significantly larger than when measured by 2DTTE.

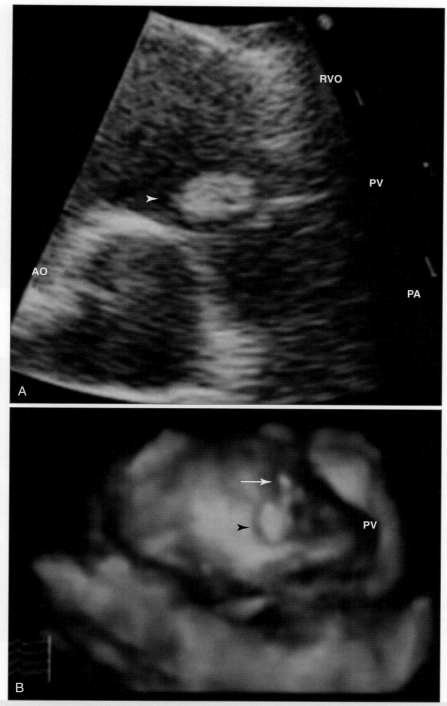

Figure 16-12 Papillary fibroelastoma of the pulmonary valve. **A,** The mass (*arrowhead*), imaged by two-dimensional echocardiography, is attached to the pulmonary valve. **B,** The same mass imaged by three-dimensional echocardiography (*arrowhead*). The *arrow* shows frondlike attachment to the valve. AO, aorta; PA, pulmonary artery; PV, pulmonary valve; RVO, right ventricular outflow tract. (From Singh A, Miller AP, Nanda NC, et al: Papillary fibroelastoma of the pulmonary valve: Assessment by live/real time three-dimensional transthoracic echocardiography. *Echocardiography* 23:880–883, 2006.)

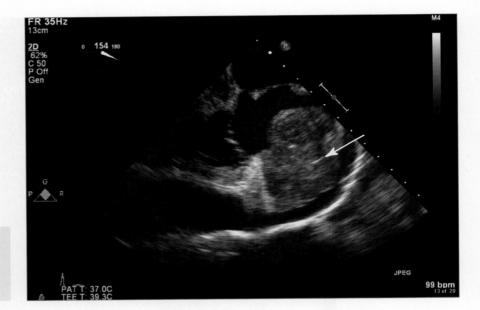

Figure 16-13 Two-dimensional transesophageal echocardiography of a right atrial mass (*arrow*) found by biopsy to be angiosarcoma. Note the pericardial effusion.

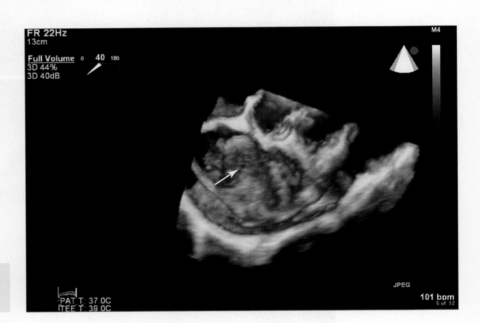

Figure 16-14 Three-dimensional transesophageal echocardiography of a right atrial angiosarcoma (*arrow*).

Lymphomas

Lymphomas represent 5% of primary cardiac malignancies, although diagnosis is not commonly made during life due to nonspecific presenting symptoms. A case of non-Hodgkin lymphoma in the right atrium that presented as atrial fibrillation was described and imaged by RT3DTTE. Follow-up imaging was useful for chemotherapy cleanup and showed marked shrinkage of the mass.[15]

Carcinoid Syndrome

Cardiac involvement occurs in more than 50% of patients with carcinoid syndrome. The right-sided heart valves are characteristically involved, with the tricuspid valve particularly affected. As previously mentioned, the pulmonary valve

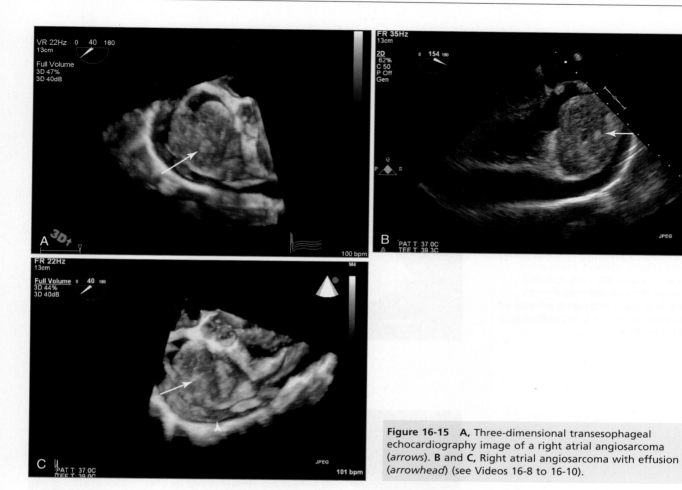

Figure 16-15 **A,** Three-dimensional transesophageal echocardiography image of a right atrial angiosarcoma (*arrows*). **B** and **C,** Right atrial angiosarcoma with effusion (*arrowhead*) (see Videos 16-8 to 16-10).

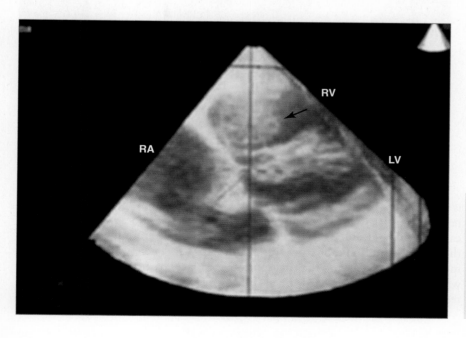

Figure 16-16 Right ventricular sarcoma (*arrow*). *LV,* left ventricle; *RA,* right atrium; *RV,* right ventricle. (From Reddy VK, Faulkner M, Bandarupalli N, et al: Incremental value of live/real time three-dimensional transthoracic echocardiography in the assessment of right ventricular masses. *Echocardiography* 26:598–609, 2009.)

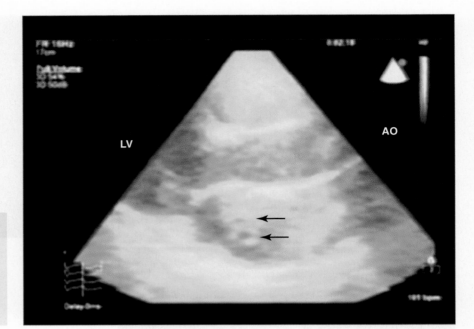

Figure 16-17   Leiomyosarcoma. *Arrows* depict area of tumor necrosis. AO, aorta; LV, left ventricle. (From Suwanjutah T, Singh H, Plaisance BR, et al: Live/real time three-dimensional transthoracic echocardiographic findings in primary left atrial leiomyosarcoma. *Echocardiography* 25:337–339, 2008.)

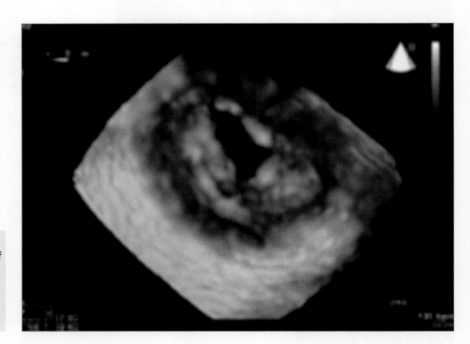

Figure 16-18   Three-dimensional transesophageal echocardiography image of the tricuspid valve showing carcinoid involvement of the valve with thickening of all three leaflets. The valve leaflets stayed in the open position, even during systole, resulting in severe tricuspid regurgitation.

is particularly challenging to image by echocardiography. In a series of cases reported by Nalawadi and colleagues[16] in three patients who were diagnosed with cardiac carcinoid, RT3DTEE performed well when determining involvement of the tricuspid and pulmonary valves (**Figure 16-18**). There was particular incremental value for viewing the tricuspid valve en face, particularly by RT3DTTE, which demonstrated a fixed, open-orifice tricuspid valve with severe tricuspid regurgitation. The pulmonary valve was seen well in only one of the four cases, and notable RT3DTEE findings were not visible in the images provided. However, the authors state that "RT3D was particularly helpful in showing carcinoid involvement of the pulmonic valve with thickening, retraction, and distortion, as well as, if present, identifying a mass on the valve." Our own experience with RT3DTEE in carcinoid syndrome has been limited, but it is clear that the aortic arch view of the pulmonary valve would be useful in this setting (see Chapter 10).

Rarer Metastatic Tumors

A case of renal cell carcinoma metastatic to the inferior vena cava was imaged by the RT3DTEE probe. The significant incremental value over 2D image was in the en face view, which showed the tumor adherent to the os of the inferior vena cava–right atrial junction. RT3DTEE provided an en face view of the tumor that was causing intermittent obstruction of the inferior vena cava.[17]

Chordomas and melanomas are relatively rare tumors, but melanoma has a known unique propensity to localize to the heart.[1] Conversely, chordoma rarely metastasizes to the heart. Despite these paradoxic facts, both melanoma and chordoma metastatic to the right atrium and right ventricle, respectively, have been identified and imaged by RT3DTEE (**Figure 16-19**).[18,19] In one report, the chordoma volume by 3DE (45 mL) correlated well with the excised volume of 40 mL. Echodense areas by 3DE correlated with fibrotic areas of the tumor and echolucencies likewise correlated with areas of necrosis.[19]

Cardiomyopathy or Noncompaction

In a series by Reddy and associates,[7] three cases of right ventricular noncompaction were identified. RT3DTTE was believed to have incremental value in that the certainty of noncompaction was increased by identifying the lack of expansion of the muscle at the right ventricular apex. In another case described by Nemes et al,[20] 2DTTE diagnosed left ventricular noncompaction with a reduced ejection fraction of 38%, but only the addition of RT3DTTE yielded the

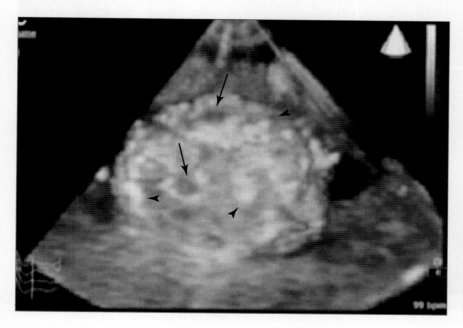

Figure 16-19 Chordoma. *Arrows* represent hemorrhage and/or cystic areas. *Arrowheads* represent fibrous bands. (From Pothineni KR, Nanda NC, Burri MV, et al: Live/real time three-dimensional transthoracic echocardiographic description of chordoma metastatic to the heart. *Echocardiography* 25:440–442, 2008.)

diagnosis of right ventricular noncompaction. The additional benefits derived from using 3DE in addition to 2D imaging to assess for noncompaction syndrome also were described by Rajdev and associates.[21] In their substantial review of 21 patients with left ventricular noncompaction syndrome, 2DTTE underestimated left ventricular trabecular mass and total number of trabeculations compared with RT3DTTE.[21] Noncompaction images by standard 2D imaging and RT3D imaging, with and without contrast, are shown in **Figures 16-20** to **16-24** (**Videos 16-11** to **16-20**). The combination of 3D imaging and contrast enhancement helped determine the length of the noncompaction; that is, the length of the sinusoids, a key point in differentiating noncompaction from more commonly encountered marked trabeculations. The ratio of the thickness of the myocardium to the thickness of the trabeculations must be less than 0.5 to be consistent with noncompaction.[22] The number of sinusoids has been cited by some investigators as also being important.

Thrombi

Atrial thrombi commonly are encountered; the main challenge they present is differentiation from other intracardiac masses, such as myxomas. RT3DE frequently can pinpoint attachment points; thrombi are rarely attached to the

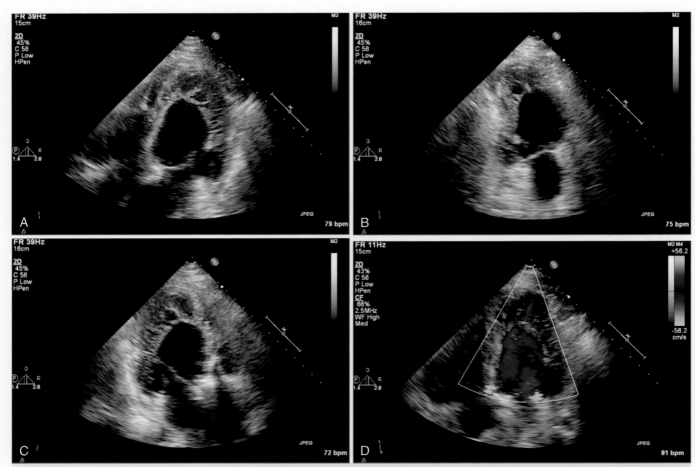

Figure 16-20 Two-dimensional images of left ventricular noncompaction. **A,** Apical four-chamber view. **B,** Apical two-chamber view. **C,** Apical long-axis view. **D,** Color Doppler emphasizes the individual apical sinusoids (see Videos 16-11 to 16-14).

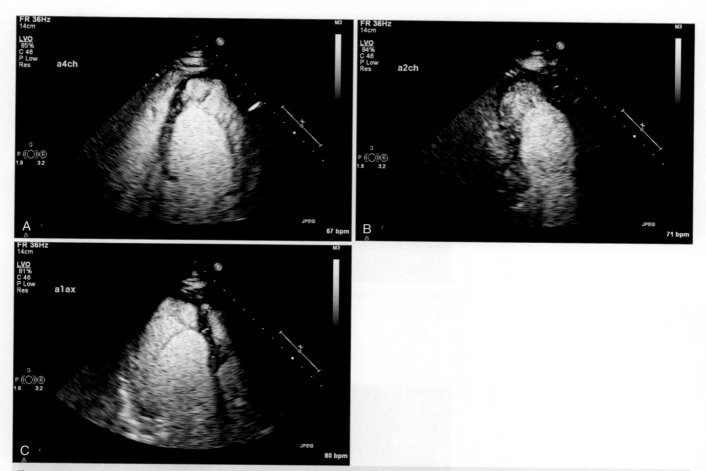

Figure 16-21   Left ventricular noncompaction with contrast. **A,** Apical four-chamber view. **B,** Apical two-chamber view. **C,** Apical long-axis view. As with two-dimensional (2D) color, the 2D contrast accentuates the apical sinusoids. The length of the sinusoids compared with the length of the endocardium can easily be estimated (see Videos 16-15 to 16-17).

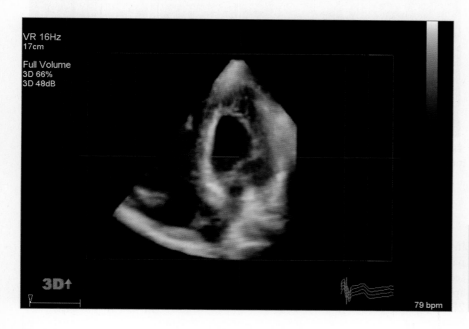

Figure 16-22   Three-dimensional transthoracic echocardiography of a patient with noncompaction showing the prominent area of trabeculation in the apex compared with noncompaction (see Video 16-18).

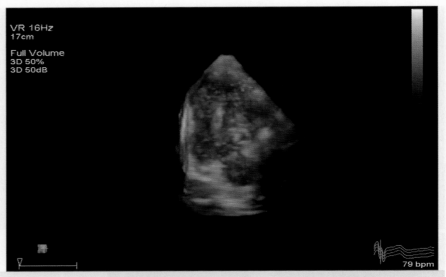

Figure 16-23   Noncompaction of the left ventricle in three dimensional echocardiography (see Video 16-19).

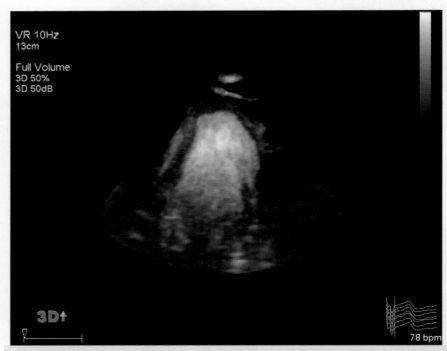

Figure 16-24   Three-dimensional acquisition with contrast from a patient with noncompaction of the left ventricle (see Video 16-20).

interatrial septum, whereas atrial myxomas frequently are. In addition, 3DE, particularly RT3DTEE, occasionally identifies left atrial appendage thrombi not seen by 2DTEE. An even greater benefit to RT3DTEE with regard to left atrial appendage thrombi is its ability to exclude thrombi that are "suspected" by 2DTEE. The advantage RT3DTEE provides left atrial appendage analysis lies in

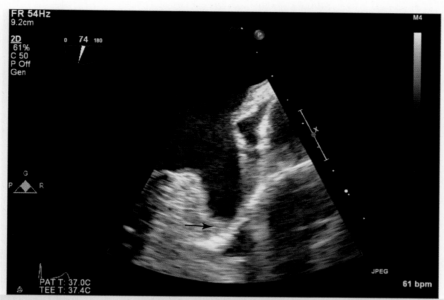

Figure 16-25 Suspected thrombus by two-dimensional transesophageal echocardiography (*arrow*). In what turned out to be left atrial appendage trabeculations (see Figure 16-26), in this view the findings in the left atrial appendage could easily be diagnosed as thrombus (see Video 16-21).

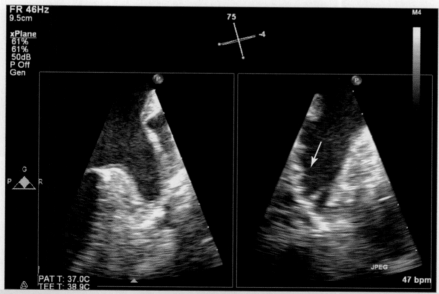

Figure 16-26 Using the three-dimensional transesophageal echocardiography transducer in the X-plane mode allows simultaneous orthogonal views of the left atrial appendage. The first view has the appearance of a thrombus in the 90-degree orthogonal plane view, but it actually is a trabeculation. *Arrow* points to multiple left atrial appendage trabeculations (see Video 16-22).

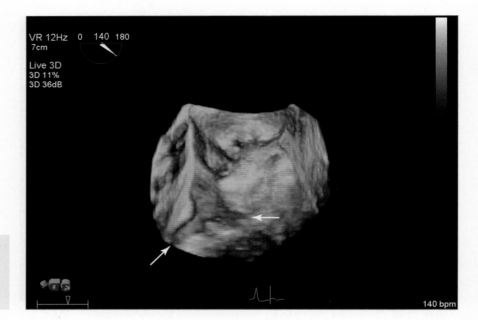

Figure 16-27 A bifid left atrial appendage viewed by real-time transesophageal three-dimensional echocardiography. *Arrows* show the two lobes (see Video 16-23).

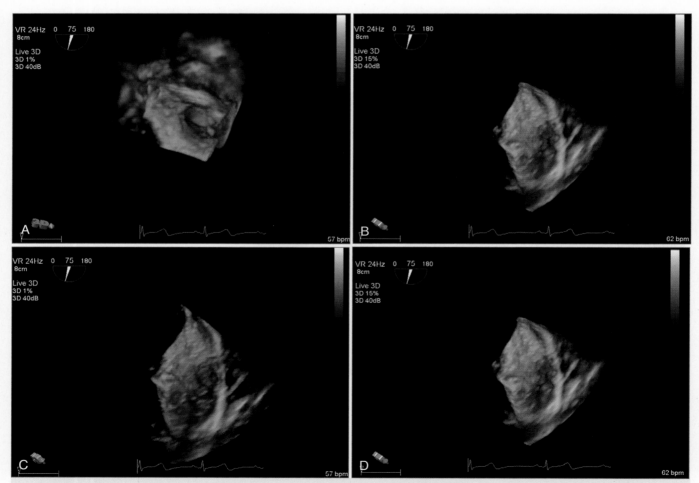

Figure 16-28 Left atrial appendage with suggested thrombus imaged by echocardiography. **B** to **D,** Multiple views showing trabeculations within the left atrial appendage but no thrombus (see Videos 16-24 to 16-26).

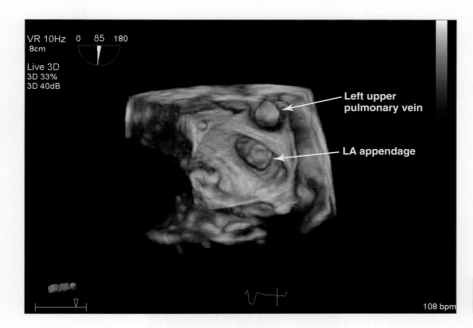

VR 10Hz   0   85   180
8cm

Live 3D
3D 33%
3D 40dB

Left upper
pulmonary vein

LA appendage

108 bpm

Figure 16-29   Example of left atrial (*LA*) appendage cropping.

its ability to differentiate the normal trabeculations of the "rough" area of the appendage from thrombi. This is accomplished by the combination of X-plane 2D imaging, which allows simultaneous orthogonal views of multiple 2D planes, as well as real-time 3D imaging (**Figures 16-25** to **16-28**; **Videos 16-21** to **16-26**) The advantages of the RT3DTEE imaging are the ability to see the opening of the appendage en face and the ability to crop the appendage from the opening into the left atrium all the way to the apex (**Figure 16-29**). The adjacent structure, the left upper pulmonary vein, is a useful landmark for probe orientation.

Thrombi within the left ventricle have been imaged and described by 3DTTE.[23] The 3D approach allowed the thrombus to be easily viewed from the lateral projection, helped identify the site of attachment, and, by cropping the 3D images, identified the degree and extent of lysis within the thrombus (large echo void within the mass consistent with thrombus lysis). The identification of lysis within the thrombi suggests efficacy of the anticoagulation regimen. The identification of left ventricular thrombus lysis was described by Sinha and associates[23] in a patient with postpartum cardiomyopathy. Thrombus was observed by 2DTTE, but only RT3DTTE showed large echolucent areas consistent with lysis within the thrombi (**Figures 16-30** and **16-31**).

In a study by Anwar and colleagues,[24] RT3DE was found to be superior to 2DE for the assessment of thrombus mobility, differentiation between thrombus and myocardium, and delineation of changes in thrombi structure and volume. The sensitivity of RT3DE in finding thrombi was greater than 90%, and the specificity was greater than 85%. Moreover, RT3DE allowed better visualization of left atrial appendage thrombi (78% vs. 33% by 2DE). In another case study, a thrombus was visualized in the right ventricle by 3DE but not by 2DE (**Figure 16-32**).[25] Three thrombi in the apex in a patient with cardiomyopathy are well visualized in a case described by Lo et al (**Figure 16-33**).[26] Additional examples of apical thrombi are shown in **Figures 16-34** and **16-36** (**Videos 16-27** to **16-30**).

Text continued on page 324

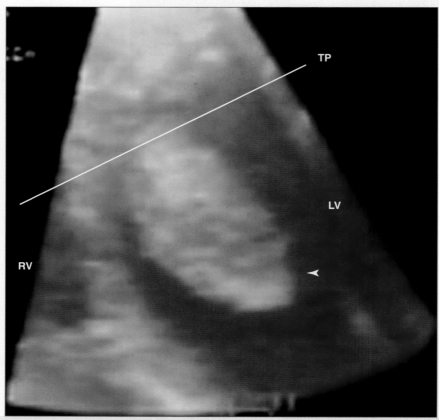

Figure 16-30   Thrombi with echolucent areas consistent with lysis. *LV,* left ventricle; *RV,* right ventricle; *TP,* transverse plane. (From Sinha A, Nanda NC, Khanna D, et al: Morphological assessment of left ventricular thrombus by live three-dimensional transthoracic echocardiography. *Echocardiography* 21:649–655, 2004.)

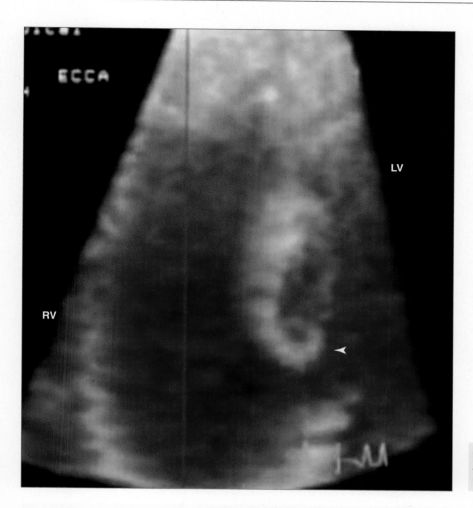

Figure 16-31 Thrombi with echolucent areas consistent with lysis (*arrowhead*). *LV,* left ventricle; *RV,* right ventricle.

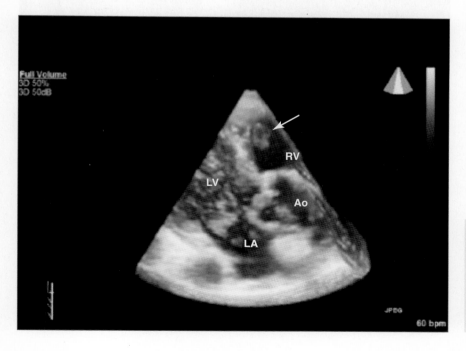

Figure 16-32 Right ventricular thrombus not visualized by two-dimensional echocardiography. Ao, aorta; LA, left atrium; LV, left ventricle; RV, right ventricle. (From Wertman BM, Goland S, Davidson RM, Siegel RJ: Right atrial and ventricular masses of unknown origin. *J Am Soc Echocardiogr* 21:776, 2008.)

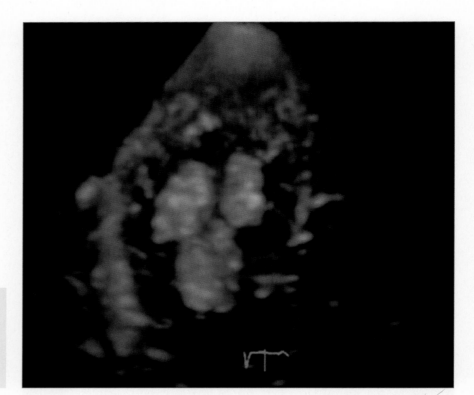

Figure 16-33 Thrombi in cardiomyopathy. (From Lo CI, Chang SH, Hung CL: Demonstration of left ventricular thrombi with real-time 3-dimensional echocardiography in a patient with cardiomyopathy. *J Am Soc Echocardiogr* 20:e9–e13, 2007.)

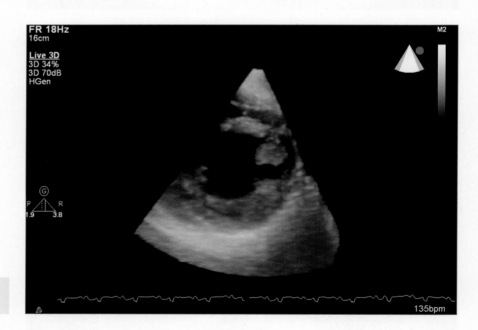

Figure 16-34 Thrombi and attachment point.

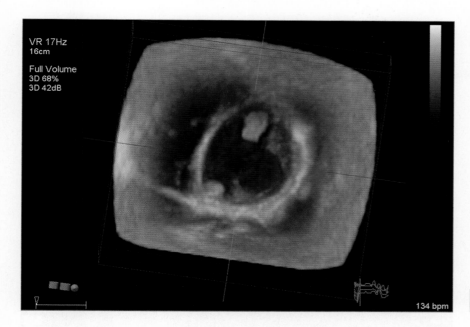

Figure 16-35   Two thrombi.

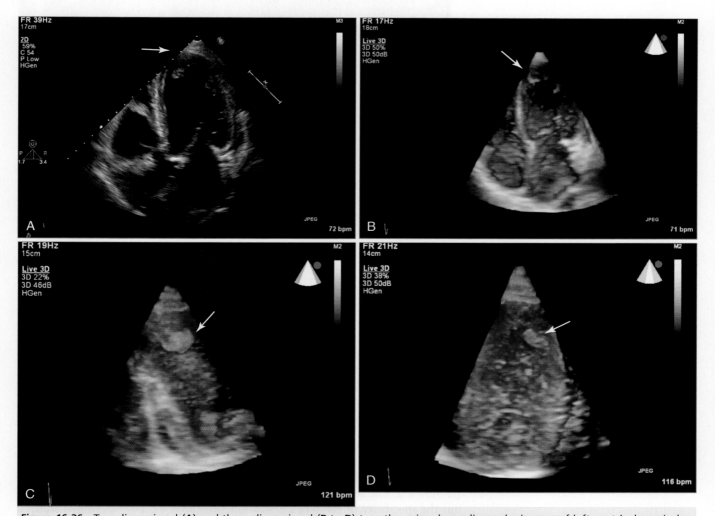

Figure 16-36   Two-dimensional (**A**) and three-dimensional (**B** to **D**) transthoracic echocardiography images of left ventricular apical thrombus (*arrows*) (see Videos 16-27 to 16-30).

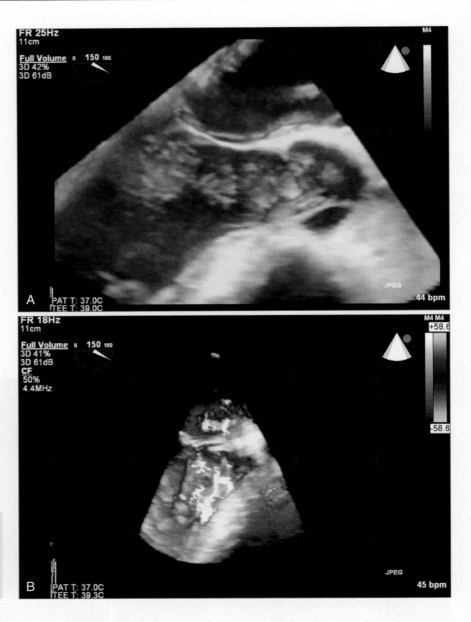

Figure 16-37 **A,** Three-dimensional transesophageal echocardiography image of vegetation on the right coronary cusp of the aortic valve. **B,** The vegetation is a discrete sessile, papillary-appearing mass (see Videos 16-31 and 16-32).

Vegetations

Next to evaluation of left ventricular systolic function, the evaluation of vegetations resulting from infectious endocarditis is arguably the most useful application of 3DE. A series of patients with aortic valve vegetations is shown as well as a case with a hole, or "rent," in the aortic valve (**Figures 16-37** to **16-43**; **Videos 16-31** to **16-38**). The size and extent of valvular vegetations have consistently measured larger by all methods of RT3DE compared with 2DE. In addition to the size, RT3DE helps visualize intricacies of the shape and mobility of vegetations. Accurate vegetation size assessment is clinically relevant because surgical indications can change depending on vegetation size alone. RT3DTEE has been particularly useful for the characterization of complications of endocarditis, such as abscess cavity formation and valve destruction. Our experience supports the detection of abscess with RT3DTEE. A study by Liu and associates,[27] which enrolled 46 patients with endocarditis, compared 2DTTE with RT3DTTE. The sensitivity for detection of endocarditis was very similar (92%), but the specificity of RT3DTTE was superior (88% vs. 100%). In this study, a mobile "nodule" visualized in RT3DE was found to be the most accurate finding

Text continued on page 329

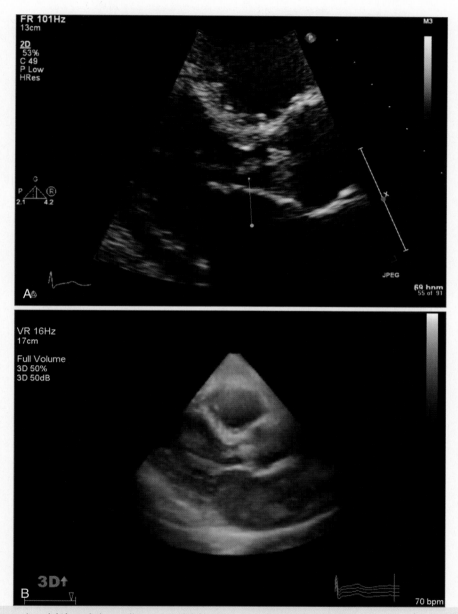

Figure 16-38   Two-dimensional (**A**) and three-dimensional (**B**) transesophageal echocardiography images of a vegetation seen on the ventricular side of the aortic valve. The size, particularly the length, is more easily appreciated by three-dimensional imaging, as is the relationship to the left ventricular outflow tract and the wall of the left ventricle.

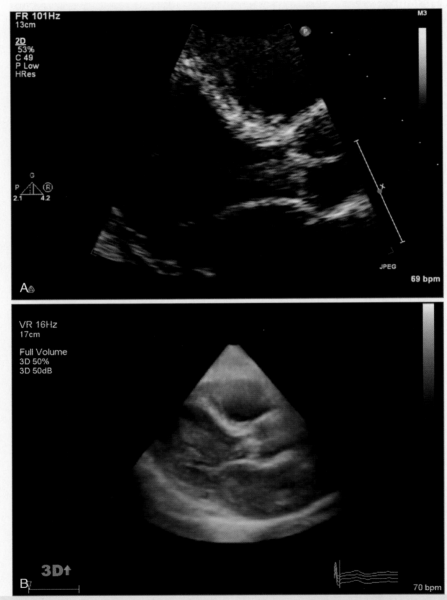

Figure 16-39 Aortic valve vegetation imaged by two-dimensional (**A**) and three-dimensional (**B**) echocardiography (see Videos 16-33 and 16-34).

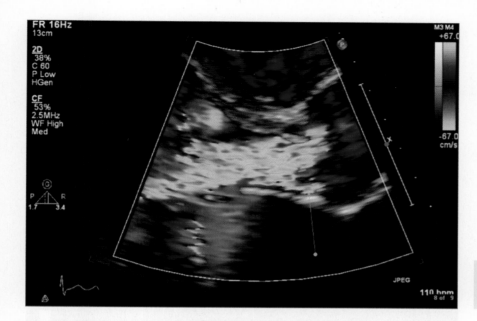

Figure 16-40   Severe aortic valve regurgitation from endocarditis and associated destruction of the valve.

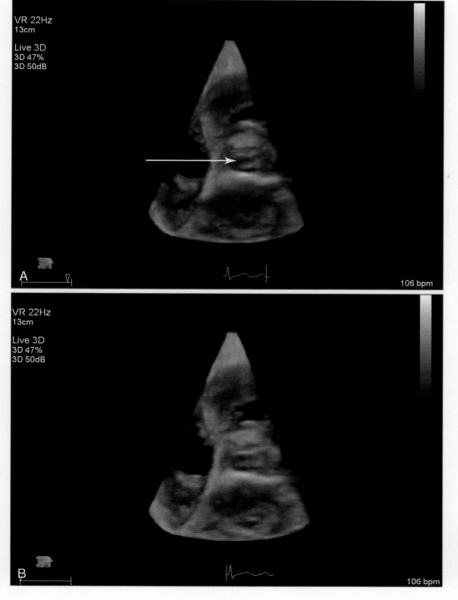

Figure 16-41   **A** and **B,** Patient with aortic valve vegetation showing a rent in the noncoronary cusp, resulting in regurgitation (see Video 16-35).

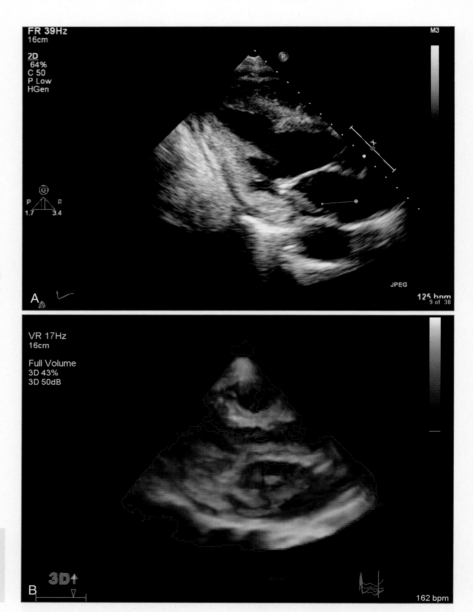

Figure 16-42 Mitral valve vegetation seen by two-dimensional (**A**) and three-dimensional (**B**) transthoracic echocardiography (see Videos 16-36 and 16-37).

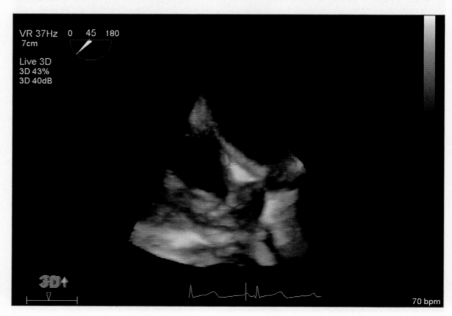

Figure 16-43 Pacemaker vegetation (see Video 16-38).

for diagnosis of infective endocarditis. A smaller study (13 patients) compared 2DTEE to RT3DTEE and found incremental value in RT3DTEE in terms of more accurate sizing of vegetations, the ability to measure volumes, the ability to discover echolucencies within myocardial masses, and improved detection of abscess cavity.[28] The main difference was the ability to visualize the valve leaflets en face and determine the number of mitral valve scallops as well as chordae tendinae involved in the process. The en face visualization also allowed the determination of leaflet perforation as well as measurement of the area of the valve leaflet affected by the endocarditic process.

Although cardiac MRI has shown promise for evaluation of endocarditis, this modality often is not feasible for patients with prosthetic valves, particularly for those with devices in place. At the same time, visualization is sometimes limited in the case of 2DE. RT3DE, particularly RT3DTEE, has therefore become an ideal imaging modality for ruling out prosthetic valve vegetations and device-related vegetations, especially for the mitral valve. It also provides a more precise relationship between the anatomic or prosthetic structures, which can aid in surgical decisions. Since RT3DE became clinically available, case series have been reported of patients with prosthetic valve endocarditis in which RT3DE was able to detect additional smaller vegetations, motion of the sewing rings suggestive of dehiscence, and paravalvular leaks of the prosthetic valves. In addition, at the time of surgical intervention, there was a high correlation between RT3DE and surgical findings.

Masses Associated with Devices

Pacemaker and implantable cardioverter defibrillator (ICD) infections are increasing at an alarming rate and, when present, frequently present a management challenge.[29,30] Paley and colleagues[31] described an infectious vegetation associated with a defibrillator wire. It could not be discerned by 2DTEE whether the mass was attached to the wire. However, with RT3DTEE, it was very clear that the vegetation was attached to the defibrillator wire. Others have described similar evaluation of pacemaker-related vegetations by RT3DTTE.[32] In a case report by Naqvi and associates[33] that included two patients, RT3DE was particularly helpful in differentiating vegetations arising from ICD leads and those arising from the valve itself. In one of the patients with tricuspid annuloplasty ring, it was unclear by 2DE if the vegetation was arising from the tricuspid annuloplasty ring or from the ICD lead, but RT3DE was able to demonstrate that the vegetation was only attaching to the ICD lead. On the basis of this information, the patient only underwent ICD wire removal, after which repeat imaging revealed no residual vegetations. Figures 16-42 and 16-43 (see Videos 16-36 to 16-38) show two examples of masses, in this case vegetations, associated with pacemaker wires. In the first case, the vegetation is attached to the pacemaker wire. In the second case, the vegetation is completely separate from the pacemaker wire; RT3DTEE was instrumental in making that distinction.

Normal Variants

Classic normal variants that frequently arise on 2DE include structures such as a Chiari network, a prominent eustachian valve, Lambl's excrescence, the ligament of Marshall (also known as the "warfarin ridge," the tissue separating the left atrial appendage from the left upper pulmonary vein), and false chords or tendons with either the right or left ventricle. RT3DTTE and RT3DTEE have helped visualize all these normal variants better than traditional 2DTTE and 2DTEE. An example is the false tendon frequently seen in the left ventricle. **Figure 16-44 (Video 16-39)** illustrates a 3D image of a false tendon as well as a case of a prominent and mobile chorda tendinae. Although the variant is clear by either modality, the 3D image allows visualization of the depth of the tendon and its relationship to the back wall of the ventricle. Imaging a prominent crista terminalis and eustachian ridge of the right atrium with RT3DTTE has been

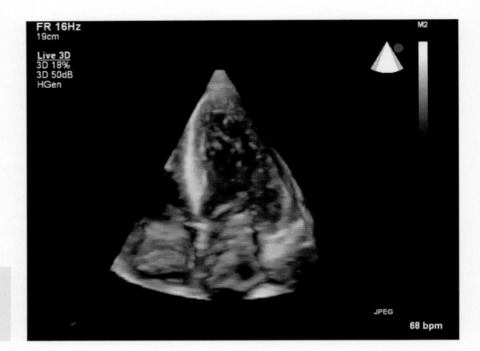

Figure 16-44 Live three-dimensional transesophageal echocardiography of the left ventricle showing marked trabeculations and false tendon (see Video 16-39).

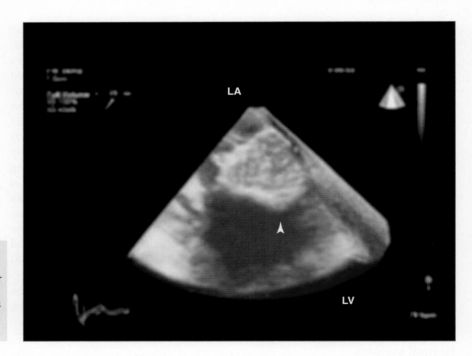

Figure 16-45 Mitral annular calcification (*arrowhead*). *LA,* left atrium; *LV,* left ventricle. (From Assudanni J, Singh B, Samar A, et al: Live/real time three-dimensional transesophageal echocardiographic findings in caseous mitral annular calcification. *Echocardiography* 27:1147–1150, 2010.)

described; the authors advocated imaging with the ventricle foreshortened by angling the transducer posteriorly in the apical four-chamber view.[34]

Calcification of the mitral valve, the aortic valve, or both is common in older patients. Differentiating between calcification and tumor or vegetation occasionally can be challenging. RT3DE has been used to aid in this differentiation and thus avoid unnecessary surgical procedures. A case of caseous mitral annular calcification was described by Assudani and colleagues.[35] RT3DE demonstrated characteristics similar to those of the pathologic specimen that was surgically excised (**Figure 16-45**). These characteristics included echogenic bandlike areas surrounded by a well-defined, highly echogenic border. **Figure 16-46** (**Videos 16-40** and **16-41**) shows an example of mitral annular calcification imaged by

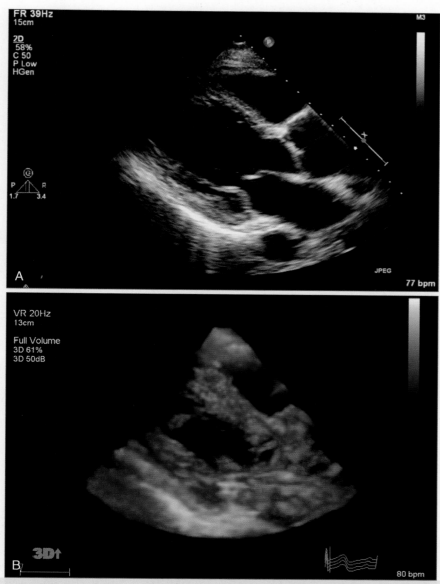

Figure 16-46 Two-dimensional (**A**) and three-dimensional (**B**) transesophageal echocardiography images showing a mitral valve mass that is mostly annular calcification (see Videos 16-40 and 16-41).

2DE and RT3DTTE. Once again, the 3D image provides depth and improves the perspective of the size of the mass. **Figure 16-47** (**Video 16-42**) shows an example of cropping through the 3D dataset. In this case, slight azimuthal movement into the dataset, moving toward the back wall of the left atrium, shows that the mass is no longer seen; hence the thickness of the mitral annular calcification is appreciated.

CASE 1

A 55-year-old woman presented to the emergency department with dizziness and near-syncope. Electrocardiography performed immediately revealed sinus rhythm with complete heart block. A temporary transvenous pacer was placed. The patient had no known history of heart disease. TTE revealed a mass in the left atrium. TEE revealed that the mass was much more extensive and infiltrated both the interatrial and interventricular septa and was present in both atria and

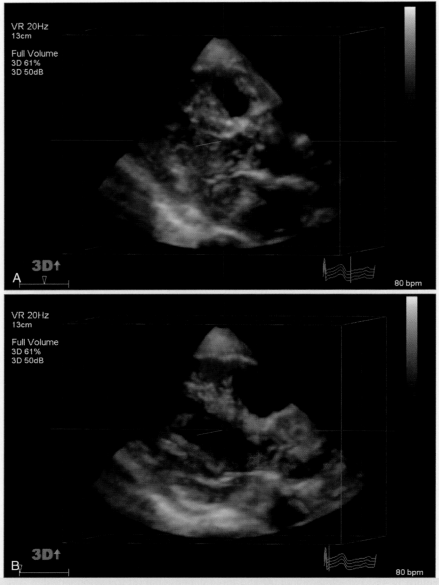

Figure 16-47   A, Cropping of a mitral valve mass. **B,** After cropping further away from the mitral valve, the mass is no longer seen (see Video 16-42).

in the left ventricular outflow tract. Initial presumed diagnosis was a cardiac tumor (**Figures 16-48** to **16-52; Videos 16-43** to **16-46**). It was believed that surgery would be used for diagnosis only and that removal or debulking would not be possible. A permanent DDD pacemaker was placed. After pacemaker placement, a percutaneous biopsy revealed that the tissue was granulomatous and an inflammatory mass, not a tumor. The patient had a history of exposure to tuberculosis and had additional immunologic evidence based on interferon gamma release assay. However, chest radiograph and CT of the chest were not suggestive of pulmonary tuberculosis. Because of the strong suspicion that the mass could be a tuberculoma, the patient was treated for approximately 1 month with four tuberculosis drugs. The patient could not tolerate this treatment, however, and it was stopped. Anti-myeloperoxidase titers, initially positive at 2.0, increased to 7.5. In addition, antineutrophilic cytoplasmic antibody test results,

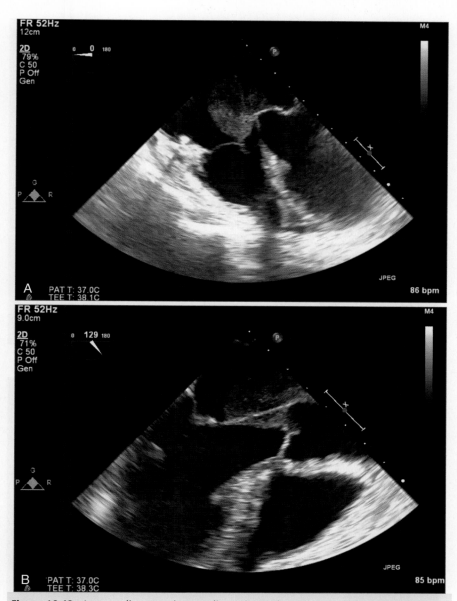

Figure 16-48   Intracardiac mass in two dimensions. The mass spans the interatrial septum and the interventricular septum and invades the anterior leaflet of the mitral valve and the left ventricular outflow tract (see Videos 16-43 and 16-44).

initially negative, became positive at 1:64. Hence the diagnosis of Wegner's granulomatosis was serologically confirmed.

CASE 2

A 45-year-old woman was admitted with an acute left middle cerebral artery cerebrovascular accident. The patient had a history of rheumatic heart disease with mitral valve replacement. She had stopped taking warfarin. An initial 2DTEE showed a thrombus in the left atrial appendage as well as a mass, likely a thrombus, associated with the posterior leaflet of the prosthetic mitral valve (**Figure 16-53; Videos 16-47 and 16-48**). RT3DTEE allowed visualization of the entire valve en face. In addition, RT3DTEE enhanced visualization of the thrombus associated with the mitral valve and, more importantly, showed that it was more than twice as large as was appreciated by 2DTEE.

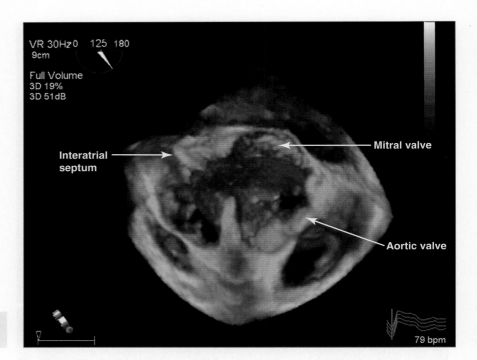

Figure 16-49 An intracardiac mass in three dimensions (see Video 16-45).

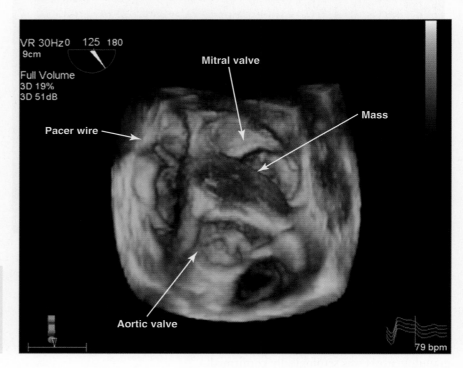

Figure 16-50 An intracardiac mass. In this view, the mitral valve is to the right, the tricuspid valve to the left, and the aortic valve at the bottom of the image. The pacemaker wire is seen in the right atrium traversing through the tricuspid valve.

CASE 3

A 43-year-old man with a known history of a bicuspid aortic valve presented for follow-up echocardiogram 3 years after his last echocardiogram. At the time of his previous echocardiogram he had only mild aortic regurgitation with upper normal ventricular size. At that time, he had been admitted with methicillin-resistant *Staphylococcus aureus* bacteremia. Despite having no discrete vegetation on his bicuspid aortic valve, he met the Duke criteria for endocarditis and was treated with a prolonged course of vancomycin. Surprisingly, 2DTTE and RT3DTTE images on the current presentation showed severe aortic regurgitation and a mass on the right coronary cusp of the aortic valve. 3DTEE was

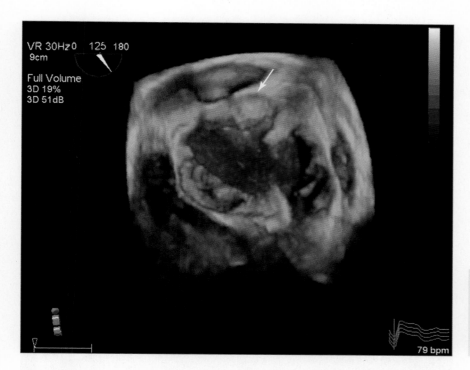

Figure 16-51 Three-dimensional transesophageal echocardiography image of an intracardiac mass. In this view, the heart is shown in the standard surgeon's view, with the aortic valve (*arrow*) at the 11:00 position.

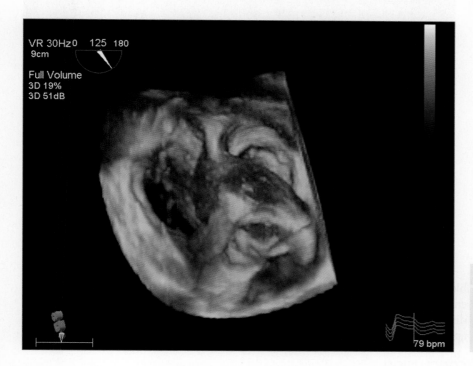

Figure 16-52 The image is tilted slightly from that in Figure 16-51 to show the aortic valve in the optimal en face view. The view of the right atrium is also improved, with the pacemaker wire more prominent (see Video 16-46).

therefore ordered and performed. This confirmed the mass and its presence on the anterior cusp of the bicuspid aortic valve, anatomically where the right coronary cusp should be located. The mass on the right coronary cusp of the valve was consistent either with vegetation or prolapse of the valve leaflet caused by previous endocarditis or chronic degeneration of the valve. With RT3DTEE, the mass was recognized as a more discrete nodule, as opposed to being less clear by 2DTEE and suggestive of an undulating mass consistent with a vegetation (**Figure 16-54; Videos 16-49 to 16-53**). An infectious workup, however, was unrevealing, with no growth from blood cultures, no fever, and no elevated white

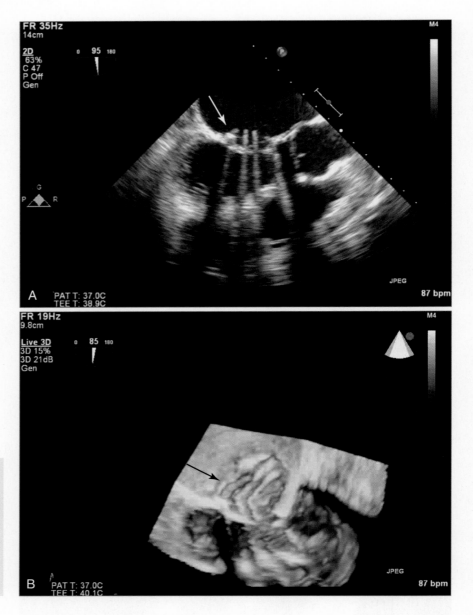

Figure 16-53 Two-dimensional (**A**) and three-dimensional (**B**) transesophageal echocardiography (3DTEE) of a left atrial thrombus attached to a bileaflet mechanical prosthetic mitral valve. The 3DTEE view allowed visualization of the entire thrombus, which was almost as long as the width of the valve and much larger than appreciated on two-dimensional TEE (*arrows*) (see Videos 16-47 and 16-48).

blood cell count. It was therefore apparent that the patient did not have recurrent endocarditis. In this case, the RT3DTEE was clear in terms of identifying a discrete, nodular mass that appeared more chronic rather than acute. The mass appeared more diffuse and mobile by 2DTEE.

CONCLUSION

RT3DE, whether performed as a transthoracic or transesophageal modality, provides previously unprecedented views of intracardiac masses. The ability to view masses in RT3DE eliminates many, if not all, problems that previously plagued earlier modalities, such as gated techniques. The quantification of size, particularly volume, is more easily obtained with RT3DE via direct measurement as opposed to extrapolation from 2DE data. Finally, the appreciation of the relationship of structures adjacent to the intracardiac mass with RT3DE is unparalleled. Future expectations include more rapid and easily obtained volume measurements, expedited image processing, and simultaneous acquisition of 2D and 3D images for real-time, side-by-side comparison.

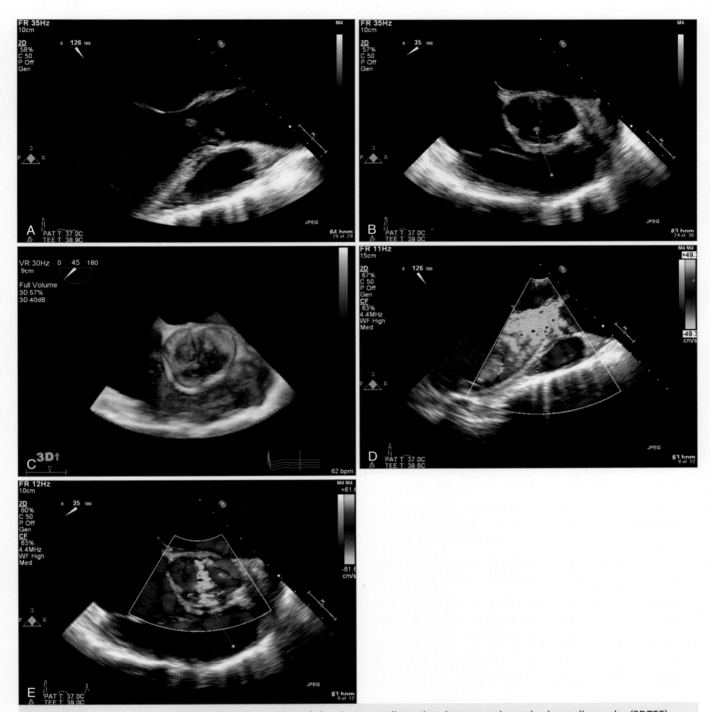

Figure 16-54 Images of a bicuspid aortic valves with nodules. **A,** A two-dimensional transesophageal echocardiography (2DTEE) longitudinal view of the aortic valve showing a mass suspicious for a vegetation. **B,** 2DTEE short-axis view of a nodule on the aortic valve, again suspicious for a vegetation. **C,** Three-dimensional TEE short-axis view of a nodule on the aortic valve showing it to be a discrete nodule rather than an undulating mass, as suggested by 2DTEE. **D,** 2DTEE longitudinal view showing aortic regurgitation, apparently severe. **E,** Short-axis color 2DTEE showing aortic regurgitation though a bicuspid aortic valve. Compared with the longitudinal view, aortic regurgitation appears to be not as severe and shows that the longitudinal view captures an orthogonal view of the jet covering the entire left ventricular outflow tract. As is seen in **E,** however, the short-axis view shows that the jet is narrow and not as severe (see Videos 16-49 to 16-53).

References

1. Burke A, Virmani R: Tumors of the heart and other great vessels. In *Atlas of tumor pathology*, Washington, DC, 1996, Armed Forces Institute of Pathology.
2. Best AK, Dobson RL, Ahmad AR: Best cases from the AFIP: Cardiac angiosarcoma. *Radiographics* 23:S141–S145, 2003.
3. Grebenc ML, Rosado de Christenson ML, Burke AP, et al: Primary cardiac and pericardial neoplasms: Radiologic-pathologic correlation. *Radiographics* 20:1073–1103, 2000.
4. Abraham KP, Reddy V, Gattuso P: Neoplasms metastatic to the heart: Review of 3314 consecutive autopsies. *Am J Cardiovasc Pathol* 3:195–198, 1990.
5. Scohy TV, Lecomte PV, McGhie J, et al: Intraoperative real time three-dimensional transesophageal echocardiographic evaluation of right atrial tumor. *Echocardiography* 25:646–649, 2008.
6. Butz T, Scholtz W, Korfer J, et al: Prolapsing left atrial myxoma: Preoperative diagnosis using a multimodal imaging approach with magnetic resonance imaging and real-time three-dimensional echocardiography. *Eur J Echocardiogr* 9:430–432, 2008.
7. Reddy VK, Faulkner M, Bandarupalli N, et al: Incremental value of live/real time three-dimensional transthoracic echocardiography in the assessment of right ventricular masses. *Echocardiography* 26:598–609, 2009.
8. Culp WC, Jr, Ball TR, Armstrong CS, et al: Three-dimensional transesophageal echocardiographic imaging and volumetry of giant left atrial myxomas. *J Cardiothorac Vasc Anesth* 23:66–68, 2009.
9. Mehmood F, Nanda NC, Vengala S, et al: Live three-dimensional transthoracic echocardiographic assessment of left atrial tumors. *Echocardiography* 22:137–143, 2005.
10. Yang HS, Arabia FA, Chaliki HP, et al: Images in cardiovascular medicine. Left atrial fibroma in Gardner syndrome: Real-time 3-dimensional transesophageal echo imaging. *Circulation* 118:e692–e696, 2008.
11. Howard RA, Aldea GS, Shapira OM, et al: Papillary fibroelastoma: Increasing recognition of a surgical disease. *Ann Thorac Surg* 68:1881–1885, 1999.
12. Singh A, Miller AP, Nanda NC, et al: Papillary fibroelastoma of the pulmonary valve: Assessment by live/real time three-dimensional transthoracic echocardiography. *Echocardiography* 23:880–883, 2006.
13. Le Tourneau T, Polge AS, Gautier C, Deklunder G: Three-dimensional echography: cardiovascular applications. *J Radiol* 87:1993–2004, 2006.
14. Suwanjutah T, Singh H, Plaisance BR, et al: Live/real time three-dimensional transthoracic echocardiographic findings in primary left atrial leiomyosarcoma. *Echocardiography* 25:337–339, 2008.
15. Trifunovic D, Vujisic-Tesic B, Vuckovic M, et al: Multimodality imaging in the assessment of cardiac lymphoma presented as new-onset atrial fibrillation. *Echocardiography* 27:332–336, 2010.
16. Nalawadi SS, Siegel RJ, Wolin E, et al: Morphologic features of carcinoid heart disease as assessed by three-dimensional transesophageal echocardiography. *Echocardiography* 27:1098–1105, 2010.
17. Lokhandwala J, Liu Z, Jundi M, et al: Three-dimensional echocardiography of intracardiac masses. *Echocardiography* 21:159–163, 2004.
18. Chong JJ, Richards DA, Chard R, et al: Two-dimensional and three-dimensional transthoracic echocardiography in surgical planning for right atrial metastatic melanoma. *Eur J Echocardiogr* 9:286–288, 2008.
19. Pothineni KR, Nanda NC, Burri MV, et al: Live/real time three-dimensional transthoracic echocardiographic description of chordoma metastatic to the heart. *Echocardiography* 25:440–442, 2008.
20. Nemes A, Caliskan K, Soliman OI, et al: Diagnosis of biventricular non-compaction cardiomyopathy by real-time three-dimensional echocardiography. *Eur J Echocardiogr* 10:356–357, 2009.
21. Rajdev S, Singh A, Nanda NC, et al: Comparison of two- and three-dimensional transthoracic echocardiography in the assessment of trabeculations and trabecular mass in left ventricular non-compaction. *Echocardiography* 24:760–767, 2007.
22. Chin TK, Perloff JK, Williams RG, et al: Isolated noncompaction of left ventricular myocardium. A study of eight cases. *Circulation* 82:507–513, 1990.
23. Sinha A, Nanda NC, Khanna D, et al: Morphological assessment of left ventricular thrombus by live three-dimensional transthoracic echocardiography. *Echocardiography* 21:649–655, 2004.
24. Anwar AM, Nosir YF, Ajam A, Chamsi-Pasha H: Central role of real-time three-dimensional echocardiography in the assessment of intracardiac thrombi. *Int J Cardiovasc Imag* 26:519–526, 2010.
25. Wertman BM, Goland S, Davidson RM, Siegel RJ: Right atrial and ventricular masses of unknown origin. *J Am Soc Echocardiogr* 21:776, 2008. e5–e7.
26. Lo CI, Chang SH, Hung CL: Demonstration of left ventricular thrombi with real-time 3-dimensional echocardiography in a patient with cardiomyopathy. *J Am Soc Echocardiogr* 20:905, 2007. e9–e13.
27. Liu YW, Tsai WC, Lin CC, et al: Usefulness of real-time three-dimensional echocardiography for diagnosis of infective endocarditis. *Scand Cardiovasc J* 43:318–323, 2009.
28. Hansalia S, Biswas M, Dutta R, et al: The value of live/real time three-dimensional transesophageal echocardiography in the assessment of valvular vegetations. *Echocardiography* 26:1264–1273, 2009.
29. Cabell CH, Heidenreich PA, Chu VH, et al: Increasing rates of cardiac device infections among Medicare beneficiaries: 1990–1999. *Am Heart J* 147:582–586, 2004.
30. Voigt A, Shalaby A, Saba S: Continued rise in rates of cardiovascular implantable electronic device infections in the United States: Temporal trends and causative insights. *Pacing Clin Electrophysiol* 33:414–419, 2010.
31. Paley AJ, Kronzon I: A defibrillator wire vegetation: the contribution of 3D real time transesophageal echocardiography. *Echocardiography* 25:1014–1015, 2008.
32. Pothineni KR, Nanda NC, Patel V, Madadi P: Live/real time three-dimensional transthoracic echocardiographic detection of vegetation on a pacemaker/defibrillator lead. *Am J Geriatr Cardiol* 15:62–63, 2006.
33. Naqvi TZ, Rafie R, Ghalichi M: Real-time 3D TEE for the diagnosis of right-sided endocarditis in patients with prosthetic devices. *JACC Cardiovasc Imag* 3:325–327, 2010.
34. McKay T, Thomas L: Prominent crista terminalis and Eustachian ridge in the right atrium: Two dimensional (2D) and three dimensional (3D) imaging. *Eur J Echocardiogr* 8:288–291, 2007.
35. Assudani J, Singh B, Samar A, et al: Live/real time three-dimensional transesophageal echocardiographic findings in caseous mitral annular calcification. *Echocardiography* 27:1147–1150, 2010.

CHAPTER 17

Use of the Cropping Tool to Show Structures of Interest

Alicia A. Bourne, Terese Tognazzi-Evans, Rachel Karl, Denise McRee, Eric J. Sisk, and Edward A. Gill

SUMMARY

This chapter provides several examples of how to crop a real-time three-dimensional (RT3D) image to show a particular structure of interest. Q-lab, a software program developed by Philips Medical Systems, is used in the examples, but other similar software programs are available. One goal of this chapter is to show how to think in three dimensions and how to eliminate unnecessary parts of the 3D dataset to show the structure of interest. The terms "pulling down" and "pushing up" are used to describe how the track ball on the ultrasound machine or a mouse would be moved to rotate the dataset.

In the 3D datasets, the planes are defined as follows:

Red = X plane
Blue = Y plane
Green = Z plane

AORTIC VALVE CROPPING: TRANSESOPHAGEAL IMAGING

Figure 17-1 (Video 17-1) shows the starting point.

Steps

Step 1 (**Figure 17-2**; **Video 17-2**): Obtain the full volume of the aortic valve. The initial approach is to image the aortic valve in the standard short-axis transesophageal echocardiography (TEE) view. This view typically has the rotational angle at 30 degrees. In this case, the rotational angle is at 75 degrees. When the aortic valve is well visualized, a full volume is obtained.

Step 2 (**Figure 17-3**; **Video 17-3**): After obtaining the full volume, pull the dataset down toward the user with the track ball or mouse.

Step 3 (**Figure 17-4**; **Video 17-4**): Maximize and minimize all the cut planes (X, Y, and Z) to the annulus of the aortic valve cusps.

Step 4 (**Figure 17-5**; **Video 17-5**): Activate "Any Plane" by clicking on "Crop Adjust Plane." Position "Any Plane" to the upper right corner of the right coronary cusp annulus and slide the plane adjust bar one third to the left.

Step 5 (**Figure 17-6**; **Video 17-6**): Remove the crop box and "Any Plane" by clicking on the "Crop Adjust Plane" button.

Step 6 (**Figure 17-7**; **Video 17-7**): Optimize the image by clicking on the "B/W" tab and sliding the Gain, Brightness, Compression, and Smoothing bars until the desired appearance is achieved.

Text continued on page 343

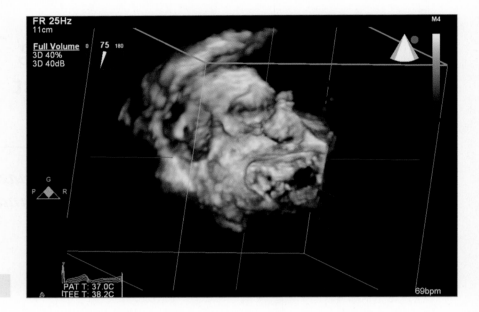

Figure 17-1 Starting point.

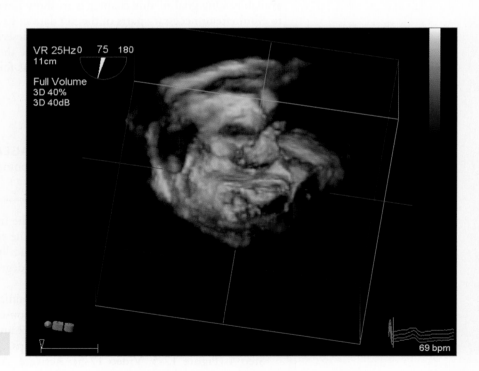

Figure 17-2 Crop box on.

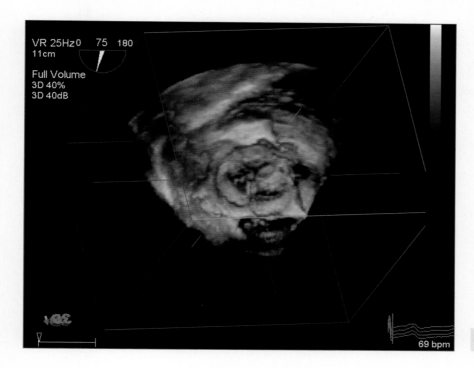

Figure 17-3   Rotating to the aortic valve.

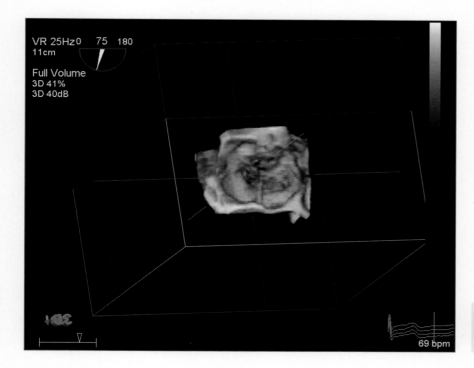

Figure 17-4   XYZ axis. In this case, The Z axis has been brought down approximately halfway from the most superior position.

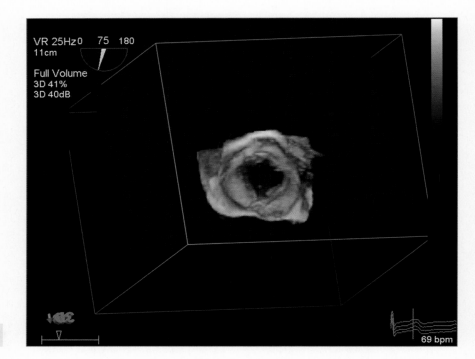

Figure 17-5 Plane adjust 4.

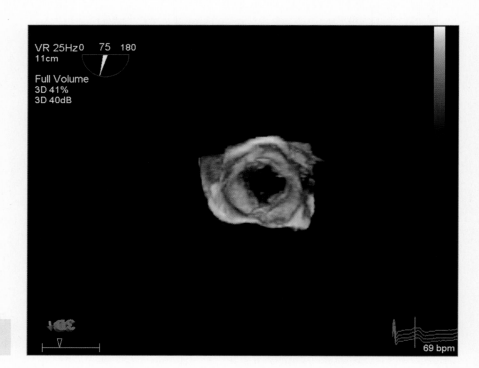

Figure 17-6 Crop box and plane adjust box off.

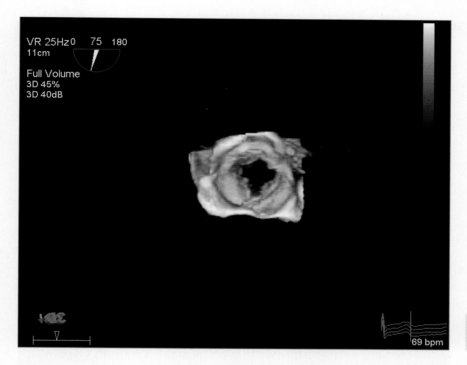

Figure 17-7 Gain and brightness adjustment.

MITRAL VALVE: TRANSTHORACIC IMAGING

Figure 17-8 (Video 17-8) is a setup view showing parasternal long-axis view of the mitral valve and left atrium.

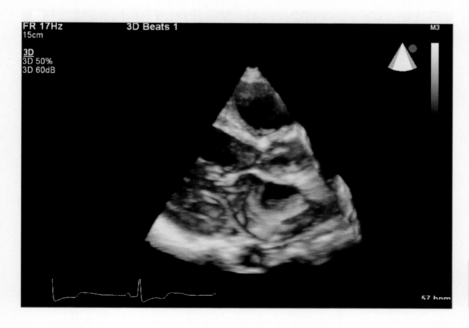

Figure 17-8 Setup view for obtaining full volume of the left ventricle, the left atrium, and the mitral valve.

Steps

Step 1 (**Figure 17-9**; **Video 17-9**): Begin with the parasternal long-axis view and obtain a full volume.

Step 2 (**Figure 17-10**; **Video 17-10**): Rotate the volume rightward to be en face with the X plane.

Step 3 (**Figure 17-11**; **Video 17-11**): Maximize the Z plane to visualize the mitral valve in the short-axis view. That is, when the image initially is called up, it is auto-cropped such that the dataset has the Z plane partially moved in. By maximizing the Z plane, the entire volume is now seen.

Step 4 (**Figure 17-12**; **Video 17-12**): Adjust or minimize the X plane to best see the leaflets.

Step 5 (**Figure 17-13**; **Video 17-13**): Alternatively, turn the volume from 3 completely around to see the mitral valve from the atrial side, pull the volume up slightly, and adjust "X Max" to best see the leaflets.

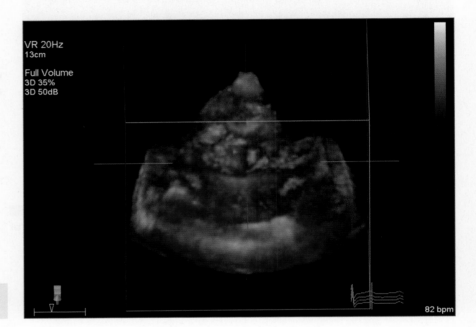

Figure 17-9 Parasternal long-axis view of full volume.

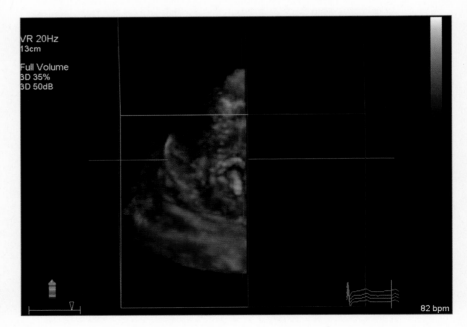

Figure 17-10 Rightward rotation.

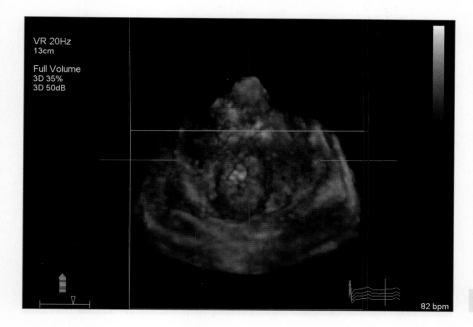

Figure 17-11   Maximizing the Z plane.

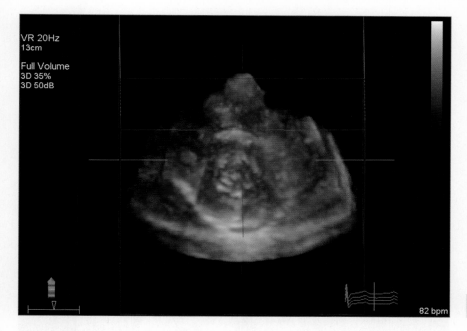

Figure 17-12   Minimizing the X plane.

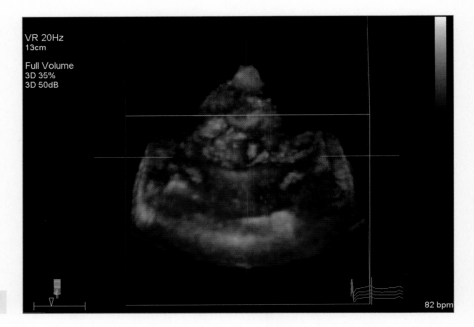

Figure 17-13 Full volume from behind.

Figures 17-14 to 17-16 (Videos 17-14 to 17-16) show the resulting images of the mitral valve on the left atrial and left ventricular sides of the valve.

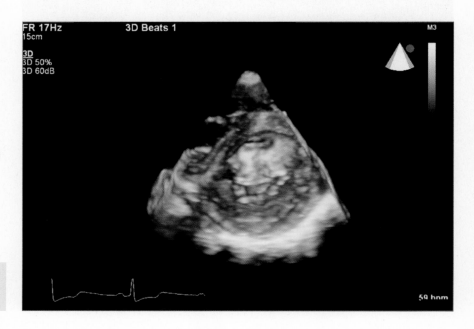

Figure 17-14 Finished product of mitral valve from the left ventricular side, short-axis view.

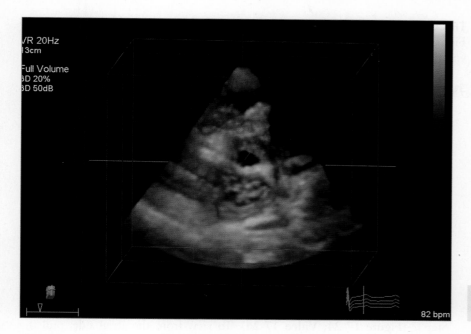

Figure 17-15 Same dataset as in Figure 17-14 viewed from the left ventricular side.

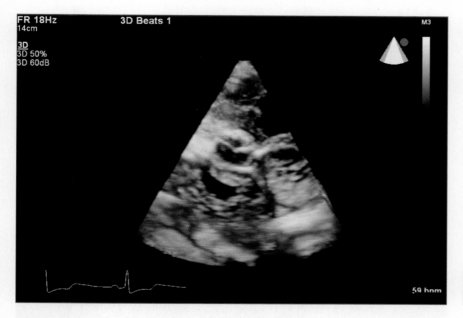

Figure 17-16 Same dataset as Figure 17-15 viewed from the left atrial side.

TRICUSPID VALVE: TRANSTHORACIC IMAGING

Figure 17-17 (**Video 17-17**) shows the starting point—full volume of the right ventricle (RV), the tricuspid valve, and the right atrium.

Steps

Step 1 (**Figure 17-18; Video 17-18**): The image shows the full volume acquired in the parasternal long-axis view. From the full volume that is auto-cropped, maximize the tricuspid valve to full volume from the parasternal long-axis view by maximizing the Z plane.

Step 2 (**Figure 17-19; Video 17-19**): Rotate the full volume rightward to be en face with the X plane.

Step 3 (**Figure 17-20; Video 17-20**): Minimize the X plane to the edge of the tricuspid valve annulus.

Step 4 (**Figure 17-21; Video 17-21**): Minimize the Y plane to one third of the volume just above the leaflet tips.

Step 5 (**Figure 17-22; Video 17-22**): Pull the volume down to show the tricuspid valve and the mitral valve en face from the ventricular side.

Step 6 (**Figure 17-23; Video 17-23**): Remove the crop box by clicking on "Crop Adj Box."

Step 7 (**Figure 17-24; Video 17-24**): To view from the atrial side, pull the volume up to view along the X plane and crop the max back along the X plane to show the tricuspid valve, the mitral valve, and the aortic valve. (Note that the tricuspid valve is on the left side of the volume.)

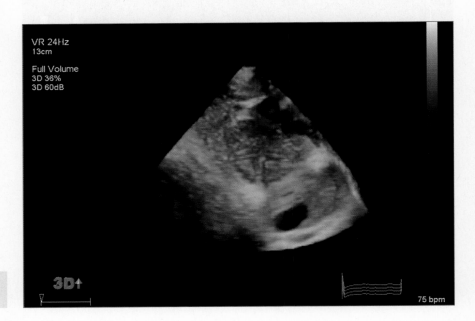

Figure 17-17 Live full-volume starting point.

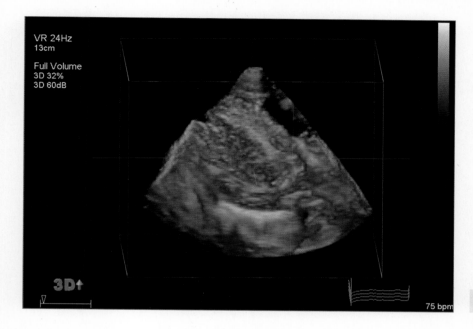

Figure 17-18   Maximizing the Z plane.

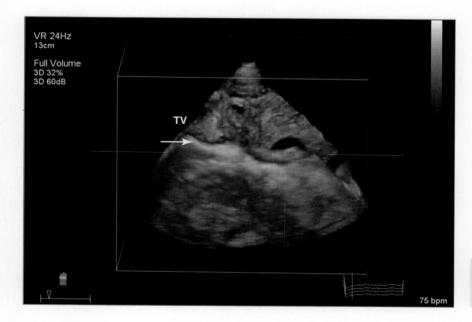

Figure 17-19   Rotating the full volume rightward to be en face with the X plane. *TV,* tricuspid valve.

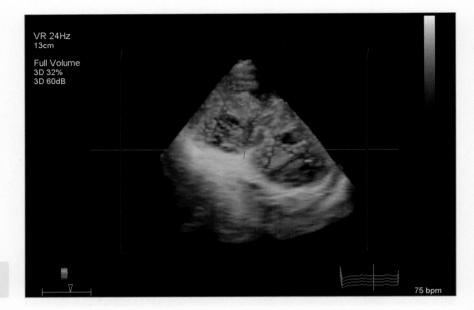

Figure 17-20 Minimizing the X plane to the edge of the tricuspid valve annulus.

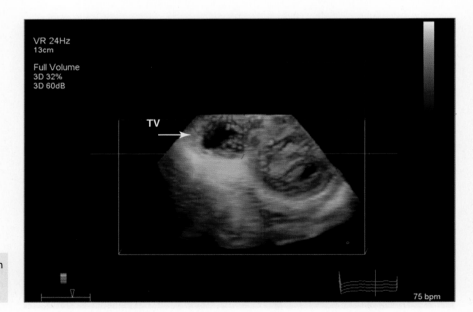

Figure 17-21 Minimizing the Y plane down to one third of the volume (i.e., just above the leaflet tips). *TV,* tricuspid valve.

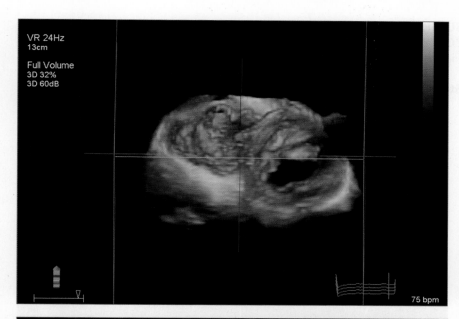

Figure 17-22   Pulling the volume down (track the ball or the mouse down) to show the tricuspid valve and the mitral valve "en face" from the ventricular side.

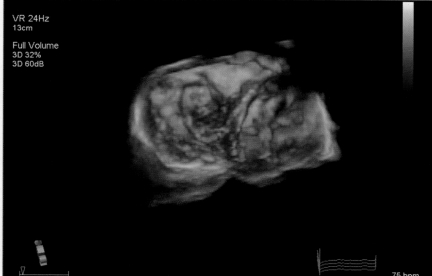

Figure 17-23   Remove the crop box by clicking on "Crop Adjust Box."

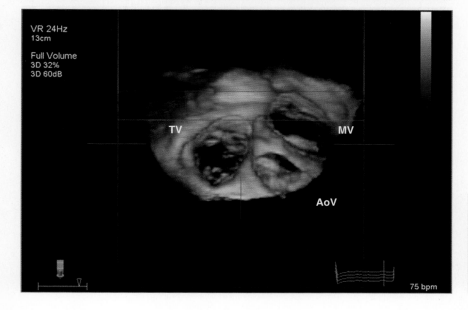

Figure 17-24   To view from the atrial side, pull the volume up to view along the X-plane and crop the max back along the X-plane to show the tricuspid valve (*TV*), mitral valve (*MV*), and aortic valve (*AoV*). Note that the TV is on the left side of the volume.

SUPERIOR VENA CAVA: TRANSESOPHAGEAL THREE-DIMENSIONAL ZOOM VIEW OF THE INTERATRIAL SEPTUM

Figure 17-25 (Video 17-25) shows the starting point.

Steps

Step 1 (**Figure 17-26**; **Video 17-26**): Rotate the volume upward to view the Y plane en face.

Step 2 (**Figure 17-27**; **Video 17-27**): Rotate the volume counterclockwise 90 degrees so the X plane is vertical.

Step 3 (**Figure 17-28**; **Video 17-28**): Crop back from Y max to view the superior vena cava (SVC) (approximately halfway back), the lumen of the inferior vena cava (IVC), and the fossa ovalis.

Step 4 (**Figure 17-29**; **Video 17-29**): Adjust the gains for the desired appearance of vessels.

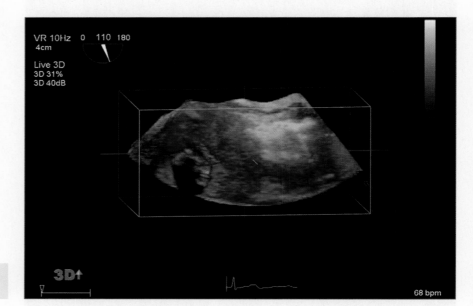

Figure 17-25 Superior vena cava starting point.

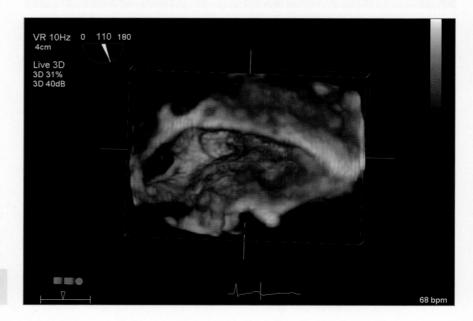

Figure 17-26 Rotating the volume upward to view the Y plane en face.

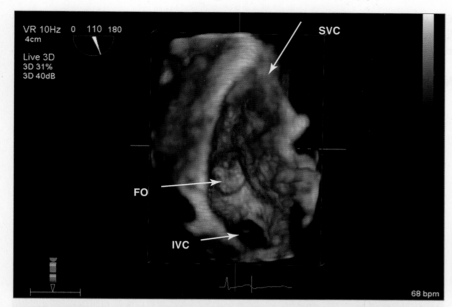

Figure 17-27 Rotating the volume counterclockwise 90 degrees so that the X plane is vertical. *FO,* fossa ovalis; *IVC,* inferior vena cava; *SVC,* superior vena cava.

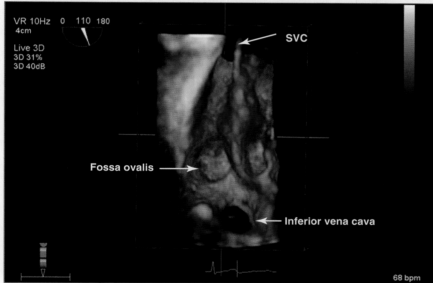

Figure 17-28 Cropping back from Y max to view the superior vena cava (*SVC;* approximately halfway back), the lumen of the inferior vena cava, and the fossa ovalis.

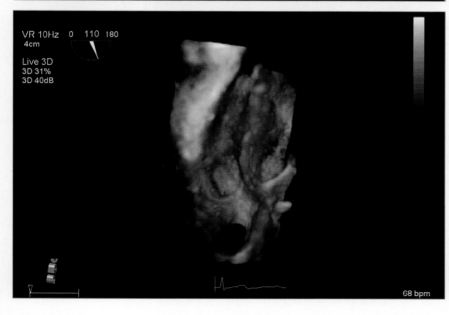

Figure 17-29 Adjust gain for the desired appearance of vessels.

ATRIAL SEPTAL DEFECT CROPPING

Figure 17-30 (**Video 17-30**) shows a 2DTEE image with color flow through the atrial septal defect (ASD) before 3D cropping.

Version 1

Step 1: **Figure 17-31** (**Video 17-31**) shows the start position in original live 3D capture.

Step 2 (**Figures 17-32** and **17-33**; **Videos 17-32** and **17-33**): From the live 3D image, push the volume up to view the right atrial side of the septum. Pull the volume down to visualize the left atrial side of the septum. Maximize and minimize the Y plane to optimize the image. Note the Chiari network.

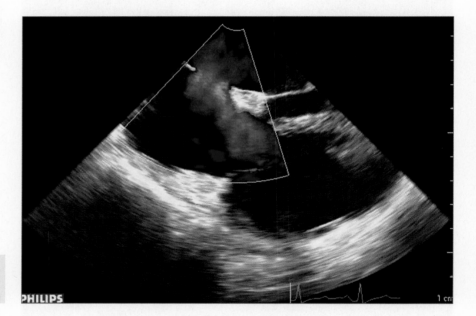

Figure 17-30 Two-dimensional transesophageal echocardiography image of the atrial septal defect.

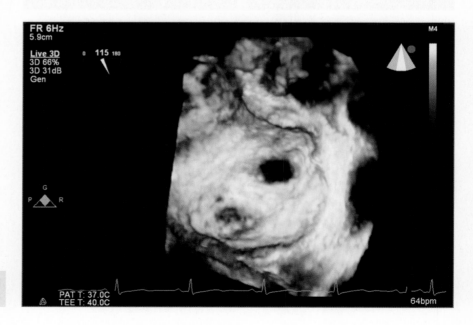

Figure 17-31 Start position: original live, three-dimensional capture.

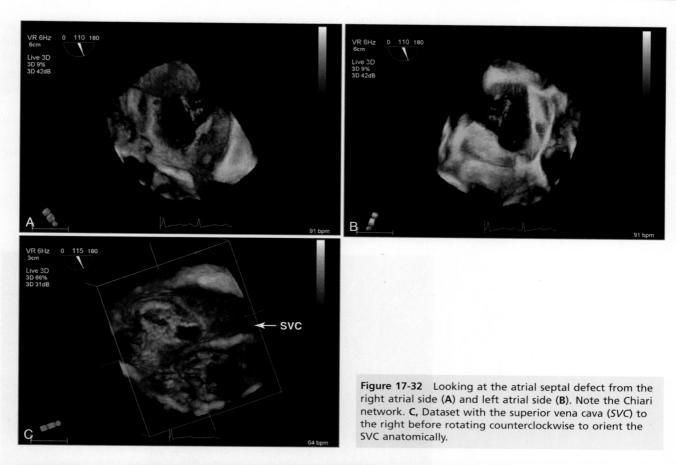

Figure 17-32   Looking at the atrial septal defect from the right atrial side (**A**) and left atrial side (**B**). Note the Chiari network. **C,** Dataset with the superior vena cava (*SVC*) to the right before rotating counterclockwise to orient the SVC anatomically.

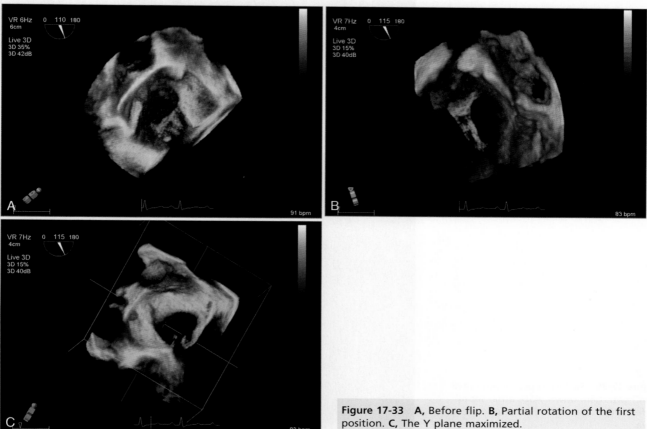

Figure 17-33   **A,** Before flip. **B,** Partial rotation of the first position. **C,** The Y plane maximized.

Step 3 (**Figure 17-34**; **Video 17-34**): Rotate counterclockwise 30 degrees or until the SVC and IVC are aligned vertically, with the SVC superior and the IVC inferior. This particular view is ideal for catheter deployment of closure devices. This shows the ASE and the aneurysmal or outpouching of the fossa ovalis of the septum. It also shows the anatomic correlation between the fossa ovalis and the typical secundum ASD.

Step 4 (**Figure 17-35**; **Video 17-35**): This shows the surface SVC, with Gain down.

Step 5 (**Figure 17-36**; **Video 17-36**): A grid overlay is used to show the size of the defect.

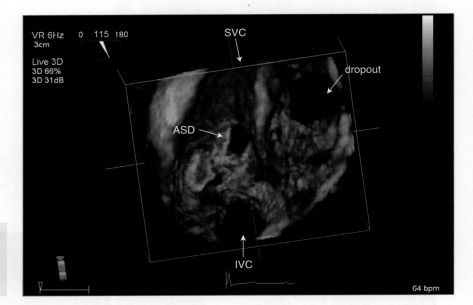

Figure 17-34 Rotating counterclockwise 30 degrees or until the superior vena cava (*SVC*) and inferior vena cava (*IVC*) are aligned vertically with the SVC superior and the IVC inferior. *ASD*, atrial septal defect.

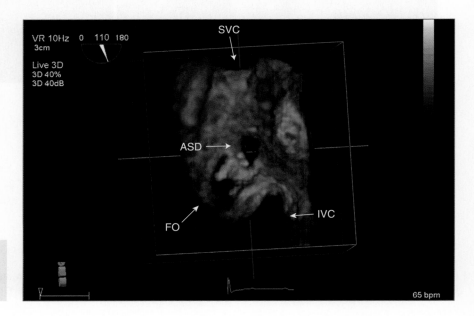

Figure 17-35 Surface superior vena cava (*SVC*) with gain down. *ASD*, atrial septal defect; *FO*, fossa ovalis; *IVC*, inferior vena cava.

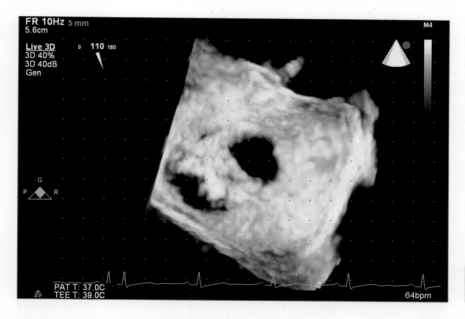

FR 10Hz 5 mm
5.6cm

M4

Live 3D   0 110 180
3D 40%
3D 40dB
Gen

G
P   R

PAT T: 37.0C
TEE T: 39.0C

64bpm

Figure 17-36   Grid overlay to show the size of the defect.

Version 2

Figures 17-37 and **17-38** (**Video 17-37**) show 3DTEE baseline images of the ASD before any cropping.

Step 1 (**Figure 17-39**; **Video 17-38**): Rotate 90 degrees counterclockwise in the same plane (around the Y plane).

Step 2: **Figure 17-40** (**Video 17-38**) shows the result of rotation.

Step 3: **Figure 17-41** (**Video 17-39**) shows the crop box turned on.

Step 4 (**Figure 17-42**; **Video 17-40**): Begin clockwise rotation around the X axis, in this case halfway from the left atrial side to the right atrial side.

Step 5 (**Figure 17-43**; **Video 17-41**): Complete the rotation from the left atrial side to the right atrial side. Now view the right atrial side.

Step 6 (**Figure 17-44**; **Video 17-42**): The crop box has been turned off.

Step 7 (**Figure 17-45**; **Video 17-43**): Adjust the image slightly. Gain initially is at 40, Brightness at 40, 3D Compress at 40, and 3D Smoothing at 5. In this case, Gain has been turned down, Brightness up, Compress down, and Smoothing up. Final numbers are Gain at 26, Brightness at 46, 3D Compress at 19, and 3D Smoothing at 8.

Step 8: **Figure 17-46** is an additional image of the ASD, with grid overlay showing the diameter as roughly 10 × 10 mm.

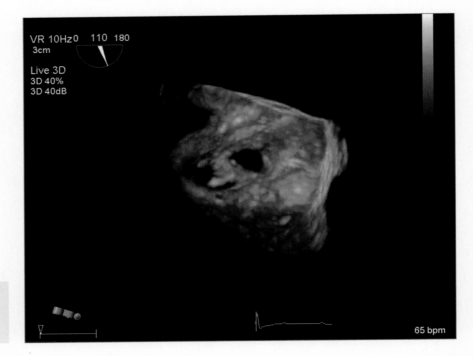

Figure 17-38   Three-dimensional transesophageal echocardiographybaseline images of the atrial septal defect before any cropping.

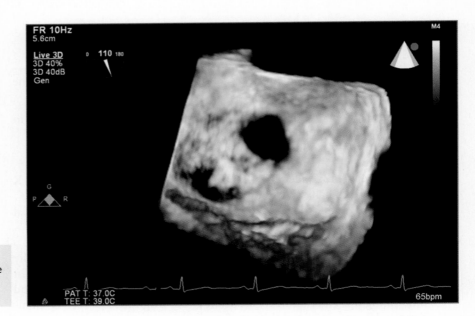

Figure 17-37   Three-dimensional transesophageal echocardiography baseline images of the atrial septal defect before any cropping.

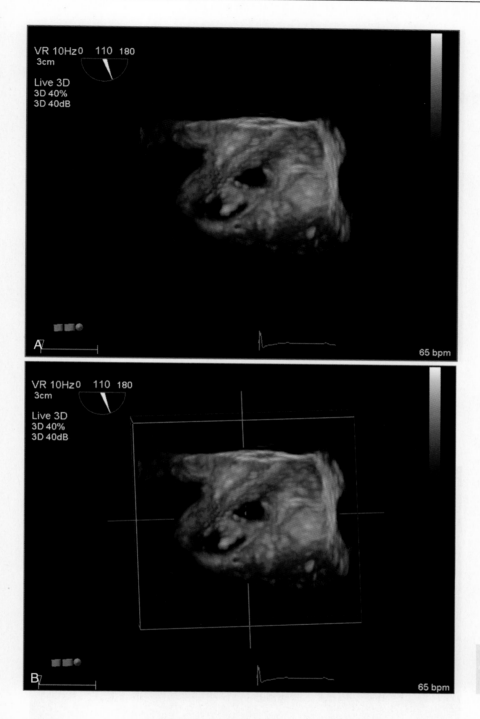

Figure 17-39 Starting counterclockwise rotation, shown without (**A**) and with (**B**) the crop box.

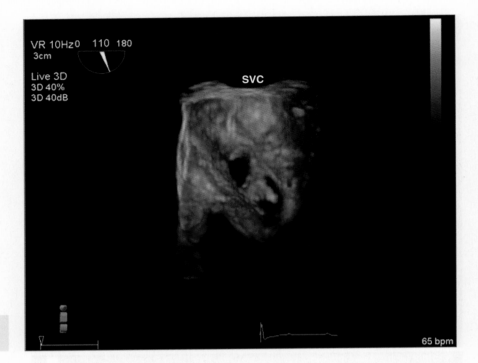

Figure 17-40 Result of counterclockwise rotation. *SVC,* superior vena cava.

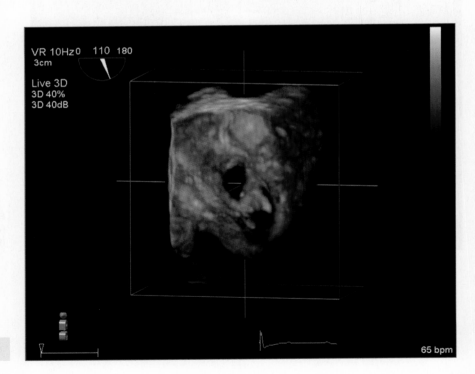

Figure 17-41 Crop box on.

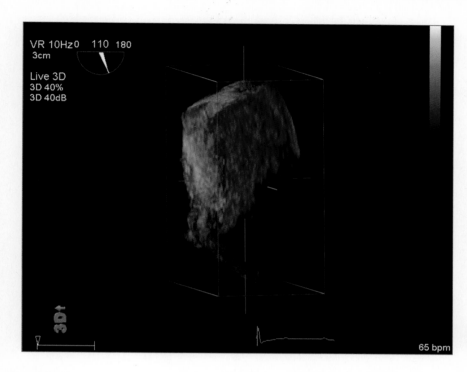

Figure 17-42 Beginning rotation around the X axis.

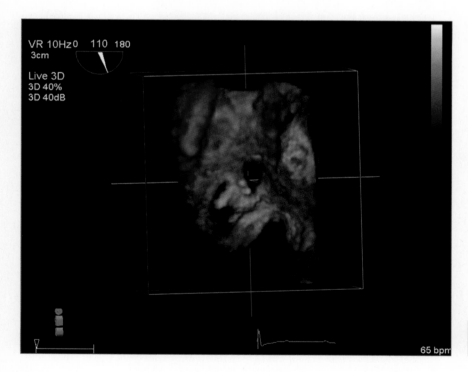

Figure 17-43 Complete rotation around the X plane.

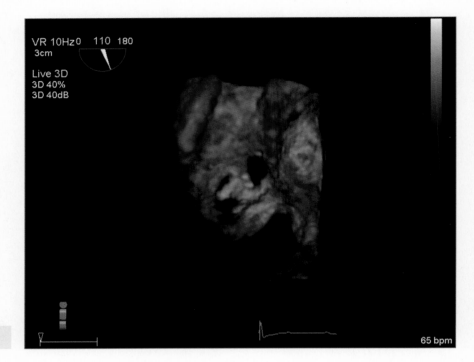

Figure 17-44 Crop box turned off.

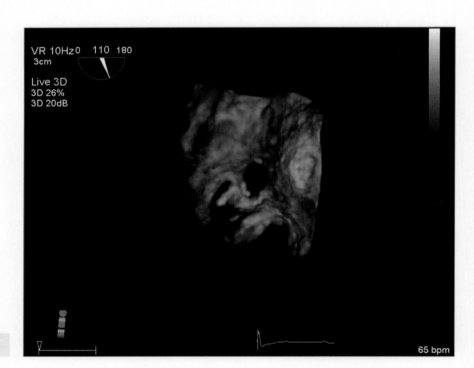

Figure 17-45 Slight adjustment of image.

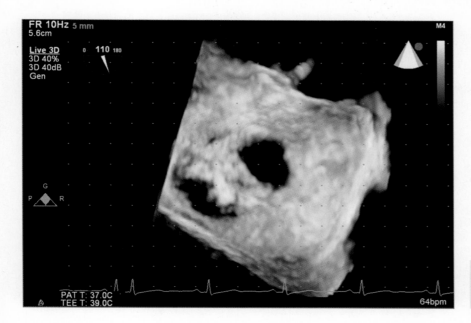

Figure 17-46 The atrial septal defect with grid overlay showing the diameter as roughly 10 × 10 mm.

RIGHT VENTRICULAR PACEMAKER: CROPPING TO SHOW THE PACEMAKER

Steps

Note the 2D image of the right ventricular pacemaker lead (**Figure 17-47**; **Video 17-44**).

Step 1 (**Figure 17-48**; **Video 17-45**): Begin with the parasternal long-axis view and obtain a full volume.

Step 2 (**Figure 17-49**; **Video 17-46**): Rotate the entire volume set to show the pacemaker. In this case, the dataset is rotated around the Y axis; counterclockwise rotation allows visualization of the pacemaker.

Step 3 (**Figure 17-50**; **Video 17-47**): The free plane, sometimes referred to as "any plane," is positioned to cut diagonally into the dataset. An attempt is made to position the free plane at a diagonal angle such that when cutting into the dataset, the cut plane moves toward the pacemaker and removes "tissue" running parallel to the pacer.

Step 4 (**Figure 17-51**; **Video 17-48**): The free plane is locked into a fixed angle and advanced into the dataset toward the pacemaker. As can be seen in the image, the pacemaker is becoming more visible. Note that the tip of the pacemaker does not seem to reach the apex of the right ventricle.

Step 5 (**Figure 17-52**; **Video 17-49**): The free plane has been locked in position after moving into an optimal position. After locking the free plane so that it cannot advance further, the entire crop box can be rotated to see what degree of rotation allows optimal visualization of the pacemaker.

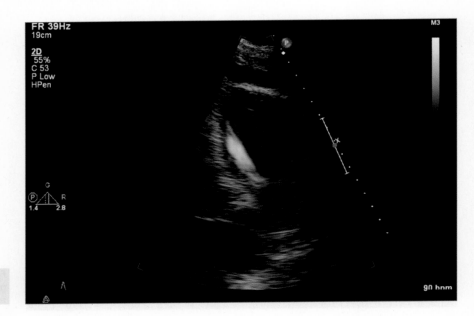

Figure 17-47   Two-dimensional image of the right ventricular pacemaker lead.

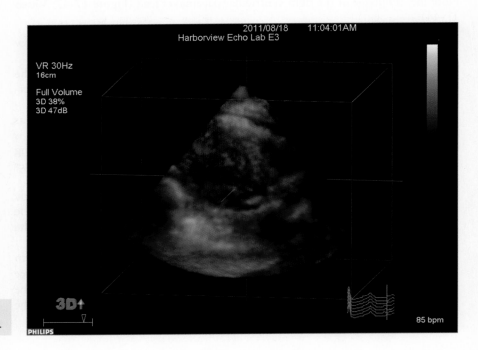

Figure 17-48   Beginning with parasternal long-axis view and obtaining a full volume.

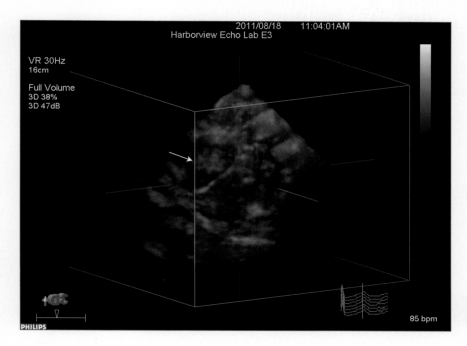

Figure 17-49   Rotating the entire volume set to show the pacemaker (*arrow*).

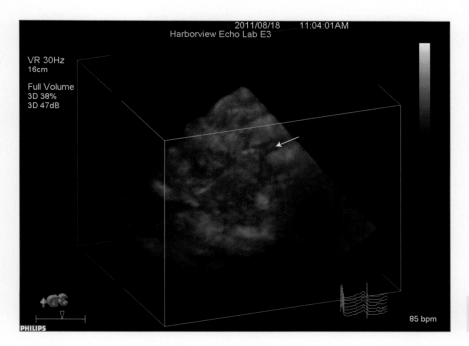

Figure 17-50   Free plane positioned. *Arrow,* pacemaker.

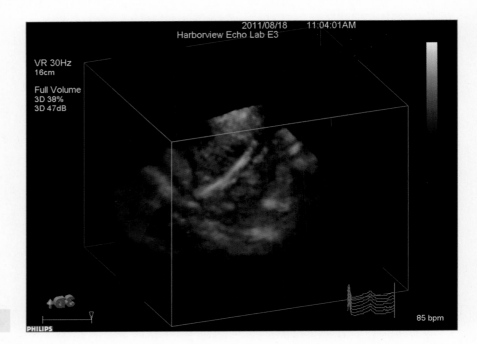

Figure 17-51 Free plane advanced.

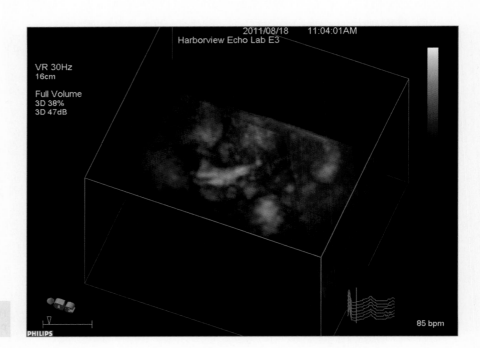

Figure 17-52 Free plane locked and volume rotated.

Index

Page numbers followed by "f" indicate figures, and "t" indicate tables.